CRANIAL SUTURES

CRANIAL SUTURES

Analysis, Morphology &
Manipulative Strategies

MARC G. PICK, D.C., D.I.C.S.

ILLUSTRATIONS
Elisa Graham

PHOTOGRAPHS
Marc G. Pick, D.C., D.I.C.S.

Library of Congress Catalog Card Number: 98-74358
International Standard Book Number: 0-939616-29-7
Printed in the United States of America

2 4 6 8 10 9 7 5 3 1

Book design by Gary Niemeier

DEDICATION

This text is dedicated to the memory of my beloved
mother Beatrice Pick, who taught me patience with
unconditional love; my loving father David Pick, for
his never ending guidance and supportive wisdom;
and my brother Dr. Dennis Pick, who is responsible
for guiding me to Chiropractic and my life's work.

Acknowledgments

I would like to thank Dr. Carl S. Cleveland III for his support in permitting me unlimited access to the dissection lab at Cleveland Chiropractic College in Los Angeles. Without his support and generosity my dissection investigations would have been impossible to perform.

I would also like to give thanks to Elisa Graham for her outstanding illustrations. Her ability to capture the true dimensions of the anatomical form undeniably gives the reader a comprehensible insight into the text's contents.

To my loving wife, Dr. Josephine Pick, I want to give a very special acknowledgment for her unwavering patience and support, which made the endless hours of rewrites endurable.

TABLE OF CONTENTS

PREFACE

Years ago I became acquainted with the cranial studies of Doctors Sutherland and DeJarnette. Since that time, I've found myself frequently confronted with patients that didn't quite fit the classic textbook formulas. I found that I was left with a large void in my attempts to help the individuals seeking my professional care. I began my quest for knowledge with the sutural system of the skull. Being easily accessed and connecting the cranial structures together, it seemed to be the logical place to begin my investigation. Much to my surprise, I quickly realized the abyss surrounding the knowledge of the sutural articular surfaces. I launched my investigation by acquiring as many disarticulated skulls as I could get my hands on. Initially my methods of study were simple and direct. I would sit for hours and alternate between rearticulating and disarticulating the various skulls in my possession. Although I noticed the individual characteristic variations between skulls and their articular surfaces, they all seemed to possess some standard rudimentary morphological attributes that consistently persisted from skull to skull. As time progressed, my investigations became more complex, and I began to notice the intricate interlocking beveled systems of the sutures. I soon realized how contact positioning synthesized with precise directional manipulations made a substantial difference in whether I was sabotaging or successfully influencing the suture's articular junction.

This book was composed for those who find themselves in a similar dilemma and wish to free themselves from the rigid classic textbook bonds for a more creative technique strategy. This text is not meant to replace other techniques, nor is it a technique manual designed to address specific symptoms or diseases. The reader will not find references to conditions or health care tactics. These manipulative approaches can be found in the various technique manuscripts already in existence. Rather, the purpose of this text is to serve as a guide in developing the practitioner's palpatory skills and to impart a deeper understanding of how the sutures articulate morphologically.

Hence, it is my aspiration that the information provided here will endow the practitioner with a comprehensive understanding of the principles involved in influencing the sutures, and will, in the end, emancipate the practitioner to address the individual case needs as they arise.

MARC G. PICK, D.C., D.I.C.S.

Overview and Terminology

The human skull is made up of twenty-two individual bones that are separated from each other by articular seams known as sutures. For years anatomists believed that sutures functioned as primary growth regions of the skull and only served to hold the skull together.[1-3] However, recent studies suggest another important function for sutures: they permit independent cranial bone motion throughout the skull. Pritchard et al. found that within sutural articular seams there are four tissue layers surrounding a fifth central vascular layer, and suggested that these structures form a strong bond between adjacent bones that allow for slight articular motion.[4] In 1971, Baker reported that maxillary arch expansion affected movement of the cranial bones along their sutures.[5] Other studies also found evidence of motion within the sutures of the human skull.[6-13]

Because the skull is essentially a closed structural unit, access to the internal structures via the sutural articular unions would seem to be an obvious mode of entry, for example, the internal meninges infiltrate through the sutural articular seams to become the external periosteum of the cranial vault. With this relationship in mind, it becomes apparent that manipulation of the external cranial structures can alter the structure around and within the brain.[14]

When viewed topographically, the articulations that constitute the sutural seams are often deceiving to the eye. Frequently, what appears to be a simple or direct articular junction may in fact be a complex integration of overlapping beveled surfaces inundated with sockets, ridges, and interlocking subcranial undercuts. Unfortunately, the success of a therapeutic manipulation can be inhibited, or perhaps ultimately negated, by an articulation's concealed characteristics if they are unknown to the practitioner. Consequently, to provide the reader with a more complete view of the suture's morphology, each suture has been sliced along various planes to insure its optimum interarticular exposure (Fig. I-1). Along with this knowledge, it is hoped that the reader will obtain the essential understanding required for successful manipulation.

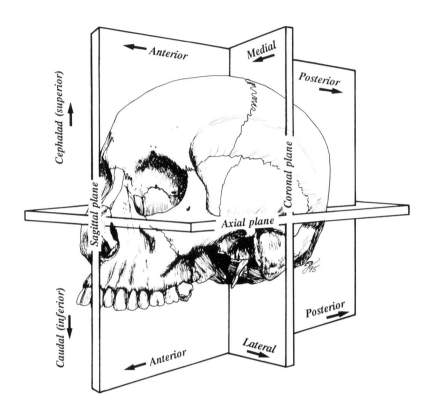

Fig. I-1 Directional planes

The text is divided into three parts: (1) palpation, (2) morphology and osseous manipulative strategies, and (3) soft tissue manipulative strategies. In addition, within the chapters, discussion of the sutures themselves is subdivided as follows:

• *Accessible versus inaccessible.* This division has been created primarily for the text's first two sections.

• *Vault versus face.* The vault includes sutures having a direct association with the dural meningeal tissue, and the face includes those sutures indirectly associated with the dura through the face and its associated periosteum.

Part One, Sutural Palpatory Techniques, is designed to enhance the practitioner's investigative skills in identifying the accessible sutures' topographic locations, configurations, articular aberrations, and degree of mobility. In order to achieve a comprehensive analysis, this section is further subdivided into (1) static, (2) active kinetic, and (3) passive kinetic palpatory procedures.

1. *Static palpation* is used to identify a suture's topographical location, symmetry, and structural aberrations.
2. *Active kinetic palpation* employs the patient's participation to investigate possible deviations of sutural mobility caused by physiological aberrations.
3. *Passive kinetic palpation* is used to identify aberrant structural mobility while the patient remains passive.

Depending on the practitioner's investigative protocol, each procedure may be applied independently or synchronized into static, active, and passive applications as each suture is sequentially addressed.

Unfortunately, sutural aberrations are very prominent throughout the human population and often require a variety of creative approaches when treating cranial lesions. For this reason, a complete sutural analysis is suggested prior to initiating a cranial manipulative series. The sutural analysis should forewarn the practitioner against possible manipulative rejections and establish a reference baseline for future evaluations. Once the initial reference has been established and aberrations recorded, the practitioner may choose to monitor the focal points of aberrations during the course of treatments.

To assure against the development of new aberrations that may occur from manipulation or the environment, a complete reexamination is recommended at six-week intervals. This recommendation is based upon the observation of Meikle et al. that sutures show a significant increase in protein accumulation within six hours of initial stress activation.[15] Consequently, the probability that new palpable aberrations could occur within a few weeks is very feasible and would support the recommended reexamination time table.

Part Two, Sutural Morphology and Osseous Manipulative Strategies, describes the inherent characteristics of each suture and the hidden structural configurations that often inhibit manipulative effects. Each suture's morphological description is followed by a depiction of its encouraged mobility and strategic manipulative procedure. The accompanying strategies optimize articular disengagement and reengagement, and are described to serve as an adjunct to enhance the practitioner's manipulative skills.

Part Three, Soft Tissue Manipulative Strategies, introduces the practitioner to the ancient Chinese manipulative technique of *tuina*. Each hand maneuver is listed under its Chinese name, and the English equivalent follows in parentheses. As is often encountered with abnormal structural changes, aberrant tissue formations often develop to aid in the body's accommodation for survival. Unfortunately, these structural changes often alter the supporting structures and may adversely affect the practitioner's manipulative maneuvers. The purpose of this section is to give the practitioner a variety of maneuvers that can treat the various aberrations and thus enhance the practitioner's armory of tactical manipulative maneuvers to best serve the individual needs of the patient.

Cranial manipulative techniques are not discussed in any detail in this text since there are numerous technical books written on this subject.[16-22]

However, as any type of cranial manipulation must deal with the skull, it is my hope that this text will serve to augment the effectiveness of the various techniques by increasing the practitioner's comprehensive understanding of sutures and their interarticular associations.

Hand Postures and Exercise

Many hand postures have been used within the field of cranial manipulation. Although the various hand postures appear to differ greatly, there seems to be a typical blend of four basic postural positions that consistently manifest in almost all cranial procedures (Fig. I-2).

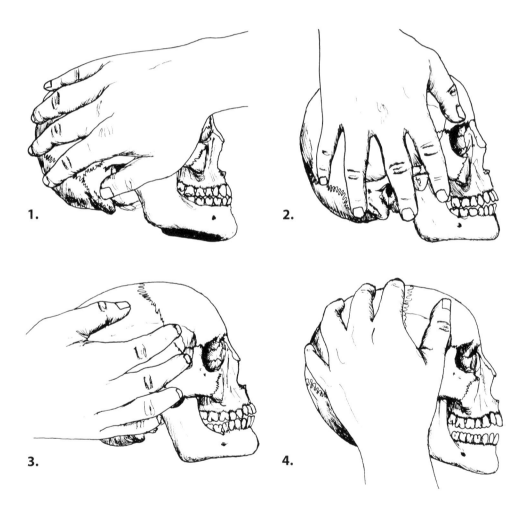

Fig. I-2 Four basic hand postures in cranial manipulation

  1. Radial side is positioned toward the *caudal* aspect of the patient's skull
  2. Fingers are directed *caudal*
  3. Radial side is positioned towards the *cephalad* aspect of the patient's skull
  4. Fingers are directed *cephalad*

The following hand postures are used in the *Focal Point Cranial Protocol System*. Their use will aid the reader in comprehending the procedures described in the palpatory section of this text.

This exercise is meant to familiarize the reader with the different hand postures. The following illustrations (Fig. I-3) are missing their recording codes. Place the correct postural code in the box provided in the illustration.

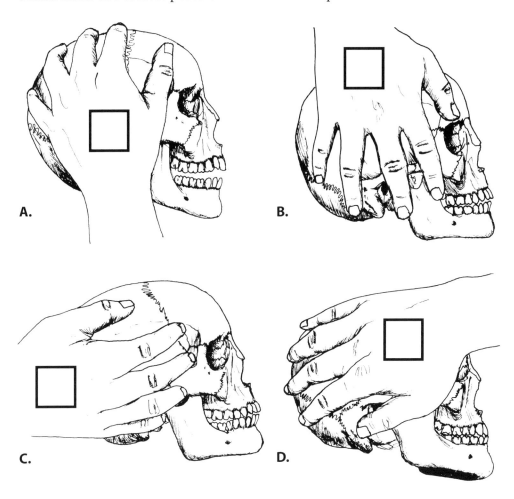

Fig. I-3 Exercise for four basic hand postures.
The missing recording codes are: A: 4, B: 2, C: 3, and D: 1.

Pressure Application Techniques

Degrees of Pressure

Individual constitutions vary, and the practitioner must consider these variations before applying manipulative pressure. The individual variations in patient vitality and structural makeup is so diverse that the use of units for measuring pressure, for example, pounds per square inch or grams per centimeter, is virtually impractical and may prove to be more harmful than beneficial. Because of these differences, the *focal point* method of pressure application has been implemented throughout this text in order to break through the barriers of individual differences and take advantage of the commonality present in all living beings.

Everyone, young or old, heavy or thin, and strong or weak, has three basic pressure levels in common: a surface level, a rejection level, and a working level. Although the manipulative approach and amount of pressure may vary at each level depending upon the individual, relatively speaking the levels are the same from person to person.

SURFACE LEVEL

The surface level is the gentlest level of pressure that the practitioner can apply to the subject and constitutes the initial contact with the subject's topographical surface.

REJECTION LEVEL

The rejection level is reached when there is maximal tissue resistance or pain. As reflected in its name, this level elicits the greatest resistance to the practitioner's access or the greatest level of pain, and represents the maximum point of metabolic endurance by the subject. Since some subjects may report pain well before tissue resistance is encountered, the presence of pain supersedes tissue resistance and can be used to delineate the rejection level.

Although the application of force beyond the rejection level is strongly discouraged, applying pressure into the rejection level may often serve to disperse axonal cytoplasmic congestion or various adhesive formations. For this reason, the rejection level is further subdivided into three sublevels.

1. *Rejection level one* is the beginning stage of the body's rejection of the manipulation and the point where major tissue resistance or discomfort is first initiated.

2. *Rejection level two* is considered midpoint between rejection level one and the intolerable level three. This level is rarely utilized in cranial therapy. However, it may be the pressure of choice when attempting to activate a Golgi-tendon response for certain muscular-system conditions.[23]

3. *Rejection level three* is the final rejection level. The pressure at this level is beyond the tolerance of the subject and has *no* therapeutic value whatsoever.

WORKING LEVEL

The working level is located half-way between the surface and rejection levels, and is the level at which most manipulative procedures begin. Within this level the practitioner can feel pliable counter-resistance to the applied force. The contact feels noninvasive, can be used to initiate an aggressive stage of manipulation, and is usually well within the comfort zone of the subjects. Here the practitioner will find maximum control over the intracranial structures, whether by applying increased pressure to direct away from the area or by releasing pressure to draw toward the contact area.

CODES

The amount of pressure applied within a particular cranial maneuver can be codified. Table I-1 identifies several codes and supplies definitions and brief examples. The table contains only a few examples of pressure codes and is not meant to limit the number of codes that can be assigned. The combinations are limited only by the proficiency of the practitioner and the sensitivity level of the patient.

Table I-1 Pressure codes, with examples

Codes	Definitions and Purpose
S	Pressure is applied at the surface level to calm or mollify the contact region.
S¼W	From the surface level, pressure is applied one-fourth of the distance toward the working level. This degree of pressure is used simultaneously to gently warm and calm the manipulated area.
S/W	Pressure is applied midway between the surface and working levels.
W	Pressure is applied at the working level to stabilize against intruding forces.
W⅓R	Pressure is used to mildly dislodge or disperse aberrant tissue.
W/R	Pressure is applied midway between the working and rejection levels. This degree of pressure is often utilized to strongly alter a structure's physical position.
W⅞R	From the working level, pressure is applied seven-eighths of the distance toward the rejection level. This increased aggressive force is often used to disperse chronic adhesive formations.
R	Pressure is applied at the rejection level. This degree of pressure is considered very aggressive therapy, but it is often utilized to disperse adhesive formations or fluid congestion. →

R¹   Pressure is applied at rejection level one, which is at the surface
            of the rejection level. This level of manipulation may be used on
            patients with deficiencies at the cellular level, but must be
            administered slowly.

R²   This level of force is considered aggressive and is applied at
            rejection level two. It is not recommended for cranial
            manipulations.

R³   Pressure at this level is beyond the tolerance of the subject and
            has no therapeutic value whatsoever. It can cause iatrogenic
            injuries.

R/W   The applied pressure is initiated at the rejection level and is
            released midway back toward the working level. This manipu-
            lation is often used to draw fluids from deep within the brain
            structure toward an area of fluid deficiency.

R⅓W   The applied pressure is initiated at the rejection level and is
            released one-third of the way back toward the working level.
            This manipulation is used to draw blood and cerebrospinal fluid
            toward an area of deficiency.

W/S   The applied pressure is initiated at the working level and is gently
            released midway toward the surface level. This gentle release is
            often used to unwind the dura and release tension from its strut
            formations.

W⅔S   The applied pressure is initiated at the working level and is gently
            released at two-thirds of the distance toward the surface level.
            Like the preceding release, this is used to remove stress from the
            meningeal strut system.

Pressure Application Exercise

To perform this exercise, the reader is required to purchase a standard size
watermelon. Using a knife, cut off a third of the melon from its longitudinal
axis (Fig. I-4A) and scoop out the internal melon, leaving only the outer shell
(Fig. I-4B). (No, this is not a recipe for watermelon surprise!)

Utilizing a bilateral, full-hand contact around the lateral surface area of
the melon shell, concentrate on molding the hands to create a tight contact
with the melon. When the initial contact is made without the application of
pressure, the practitioner is implementing *surface level* force to the melon.
This initial contact should be applied gently with the practitioner's hands in a
soft state of relaxation.

Fig. I-4A Removal of a third of the melon cut perpendicular from its longitudinal axis

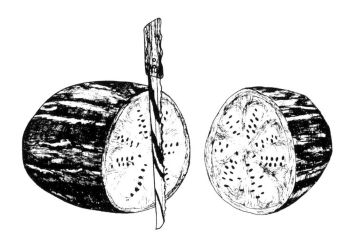

Fig. I-4B Removal of the watermelon's internal fruit

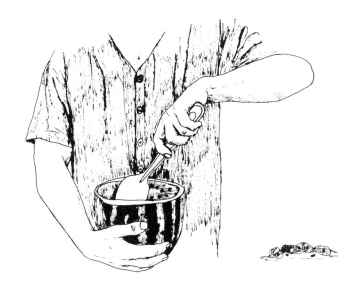

The next phase of this exercise is designed to locate the melon's rejection level. Gently apply even pressure into the melon's shell. As the increased pressure compresses into the shell substance, the practitioner should feel the melon's surface harden to the invasive force. As the melon's surface increases in resistant tension, the musculature of the practitioner's hands should stiffen to mirror the resistant tension perceived from the melon. To truly distinguish the melon's rejection level, you must take special care to keep the intermuscular tension within the hands slightly softer than the tension of the melon's resistant surface. *Rejection level one* is the point at which the melon refuses to give any further and consequently hardens to maximize its resistance. Further compression will create structural deformity to the shell, and this level is termed *rejection level two*. If the practitioner continues to increase the compression, the melon's shell will implode or collapse and this is termed the melon's *rejection level three*. It is worthwhile experimenting to attempt to crush beyond rejection level three, but not until the end of this exercise.

Once rejection level one has been reached, the practitioner should leisurely soften the hands' muscular tension and allow the melon's shell to expand, pushing the hands back toward the surface level. *Repeat this procedure several times until the two levels are easy to perceive.* Now that the surface and rejection levels are tactilely defined, locate the rejection level and again relax the hands to permit the melon's expanding shell to push the hands toward the surface level. However, instead of releasing all the way back to the surface level, only release to a point midway to the surface. This is the *working level* and is the level at which cranial manipulation begins.

Although the watermelon exercise is very effective in developing the practitioner's skills in identifying the various levels, the exercise should also be performed on a whole grapefruit without removing the inner fruit.

References

1. Gray H, Gross CM, eds. *Anatomy of the Human Body,* 29th (American) edition. Philadelphia: Lea & Febiger, 1973:296.

2. Romanes GJ, ed. *Cunningham's Textbook of Anatomy,* 11th edition. London: Oxford University Press, 1972:207.

3. Warwick R, Williams PL, eds. *Gray's Anatomy of the Human Body,* 35th (British) edition. Philadelphia: W.B. Saunders, 1973:389.

4. Pritchard JJ, Scott JH, Girgis FG. The structure and development of cranial facial sutures. *J Anat* 1956;90:73–85.

5. Baker EG. Alteration in width of maxillary arch and its relation to sutural movement of cranial bones. *J Am Osteopathic Assoc* 1971;70:559–564.

6. Retzlaff EW, Michael DK. Cranial bone mobility. *J Am Osteopathic Assoc* 1975;74:869–73.

7. Kostopoulos DC, Keramidas G. Changes in elongation of falx cerebri during craniosacral therapy techniques applied on the skull of an embalmed cadaver. *J Cranialmandibular Practice* 1992;10:9–12.

8. Wood J. Dynamic response of human cranial bones. *J Biomechanics* 1971;4:1–12.

9. Pavlin D, Vukicevic D. Mechanical reactions of facial skeleton to maxillary expansion determined by laser holography. *Am J Orthod.* 1984; 85(6):498–507.

10. Dermant LR, Beerden L. The effects of class ii elastic force on a dry skull measured by holographic interferometry. *Am J Orthod* 1981;79(3): 296–304.

11. Kragt C. Measurement of bone displacement in a macerated human skull induced by orthodontic force, a holographic study. *J Biomechanics* 1979;12:905–910.

12. Moss ML. Extrinsic determination of sutural area morphology in the rat calvaria. *Acta Anat* 1961;44:263–272.

13. McElhaney J, Fogle J, Melvin J, Haynes R, Roberts V, Alem N. Mechanical properties of cranial bones. *J Biomechanics* 1970;3:495–511.

14. Pick MG. A preliminary single case magnetic resonance imaging investigation into maxillary frontal parietal manipulation and its short-term effect upon the intercranial structures of an adult human brain. *J Manipulative Physiological Therapeutics* 1994;17(3):168–173.

15. Meikle MC, Sellers A, Reynolds JJ. Effects of tensile mechanical stress on the synthesis of metalloproteinases by rabbit coronal sutures in vitro. *Cal Tissue Int* 1980;30:77–82.

16. DeJarnette MB. *Cranial Manual*. Nebraska City, NE: Sacro-Occipital Technique Organization, 1979–1980.

17. Magoun HI. *Osteopathy in the Cranial Field,* 2nd edition. Kirksville, MO: Journal Printing Co., 1966.

18. Upledger JE, Vredevoogd JD. *Craniosacral Therapy*. Chicago: Eastland Press, 1983.

19. Sutherland WG. *The Cranial Bowl*. Mankato, MN: Free Press Company, 1939.

20. Walther DS. *Applied Kinesiology*. Pueblo, CO: Systems D.C., 1976: 132–153.

21. Brookes D. *Lectures on Cranial Osteopathy*. Wellingborough, Northamptonshire: Thorsons Publishers Limited, 1981.

22. Gehin A. *Atlas of Manipulative Techniques for the Cranium and Face*. Seattle: Eastland Press, 1985.

23. DeJarnette MB. *Sacro-Occipital Technic*. Nebraska City, NE: Sacro-Occiptial Technique Organization, 1984:116–42.

Sutural Palpatory Techniques

This part is devoted to the education and improvement of the practitioner's palpatory skills in sutural identification and analysis. It is hoped that this text will help practitioners improve their tactile ability in identifying sutures and discerning abnormalities that might interfere with a suture's normal mobility. To aid in this endeavor, the subject has been divided into four chapters.

Chapter 1 addresses issues in palpatory assessment of *sutural aberrations*. In this chapter the practitioner is introduced to the various anomalies often found within the skull's sutural structure.

Chapter 2 discusses *static sutural palpation* and supplies the reader with normal findings that are frequently misinterpreted as aberrations by inexperienced examiners.

Chapter 3 guides the practitioner through the

protocols for *active kinetic palpation*, in which the patient actively participates in the motion analyses.

Chapter 4 guides the practitioner through the protocols for *passive kinetic palpation*, during which the patient is passive while the examiner conducts the manipulative investigation.

To enhance the organization of the material in Chapters 2 through 4, these chapters have been further divided into two subsections, denoting the sutures by their topographic location. In each chapter the first half is devoted to palpation of the cranial vault sutures while the second half is devoted to palpation of the facial sutures.

Although the average human skull consists of approximately sixty sutural articulations, not all of the sutures are accessible to palpation. Of the twenty-three sutures in the cranial vault, only fifteen are actually accessible, and only seventeen of the thirty-nine facial sutures are considered accessible. Since this portion of the text is concerned primarily with the development of the practitioner's palpatory skills, the following information will address only those sutures that are discernibly accessible. To guide the reader through the most judicious palpatory procedure and to create a unified method for analysis, the sutures have been presented in a specific succession that parallels the order of the palpatory exam.

CHAPTER ONE

Palpatory Assessment of Sutural Aberrations

THE CRANIAL SUTURES articulate along beveled surfaces that appear to allow for independent functional mobility of the cranial bones. Should aberrant formations develop, their presence may interfere with the suture's functional expression and, consequently, may hinder the practitioner's manipulations. This portion of the text will address the various sutural aberrations and describe their palpatory characteristics. However, it should first be noted that some sutures consistently display areas that resemble aberrant displacements but are considered acceptable, benign variations. These displacements have no clinical significance. For example, the overlap of the frontal and parietal bones in the middle third of the coronal suture has characteristic fluctuations. These alternating interdigitations can often be mistaken as aberrant sutural displacement because of their trench-like configuration.

To assist in the identification of these acceptable variations, Chapter 2, Static Sutural Palpation, lists the range of *normal findings* for many of the sutures. When this is present, the palpatory distortions and their topographical locations are delineated. However, should these variations be found in conjunction with pain or deformities, the finding is almost always considered pathological.

To comprehensively address the various abnormalities that are most frequently encountered during palpatory examinations, this section has been divided into the following five major topics:

1. Displacement
2. Deformities
3. Sensory distortions
4. Temperature abnormalities
5. Tensile strength abnormalities

Displacement

Abnormal positioning of a cranial bone along a suture's articulation is called *displacement*. The following four displacements are those that are most often found along sutural articular seams:

1. *Sutural jamming.* This displacement is often perceived as a mountainous peak along the suture's seam. The articular surfaces are jammed together, which creates an intra-articular stress that actively generates bone peak formation (Fig. 1-1).

2. *Sutural spreading.* This distortion is perceived as an open trench and creates the impression that the suture is separated along its articular seam. However, several sutures, for example, those of the coronal, lambdoid, and frontozygomatic, may have areas that are frequently mistaken for this kind of distortion, and the absence of pain or adhesive formations would indicate that the trench-like formations are normal for this articular surface. Rather than being considered examples of sutural spreading, these regions appear to be beveled transitions rather than separations (Fig. 1-2).

3. *Sutural obliteration.* This distortion is identified as an area of bony overgrowth and is usually perceived as a continuous bone over an area where sutural indentation is expected. This deformity is repeatedly found over the sagittal suture (Fig. 1-3).

4. *Sutural overlapping.* Although sutural overlapping is common throughout the cranial sutural system, this distortion is frequently related to an unusual step up or down from one bone to another over a suture's articular seam. This distortion is considered abnormal when (a) the area is perceived to contain a reversal in the natural beveled overlap position of the suture, or (b) the step is blatantly obvious, as in the case of frontal jamming along the region of the coronal bregma (Fig. 1-4).

Deformities

An abnormal formation anchored into or over a suture's articular seam is called *deformity*. The following five deformities are the ones found most often along sutural articular seams:

1. *Fibrous adhesions.* This deformity is often perceived as a wire-like formation traversing a suture's articular seam. These adhesions are frequently composed of avascular collagen tissue that are fibrous in nature (Fig. 1-5).

2. *Bone spurs.* Perceived as a bony bridge crossing a suture's seam, this deformity frequently represents the morphological osteoblastic alteration of a fibrous adhesion into a chronic spur formation (Fig. 1-6).

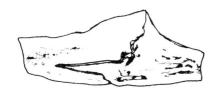

Fig. 1-1. Jamming of a suture's articular margins. The palpable peak is the consequence of stress-precipitated osseous hypertrophic growth along the suture's marginal surface.

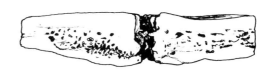

Fig. 1-2. Spreading of a suture's articular margins. The palpable furrow is a consequence of the suture's marginal separation.

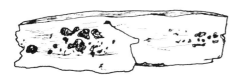

Fig. 1-3. Articular obliteration along a suture's marginal surface. Since this distortion is usually genetic in origin, the surface is usually undefined and lacks palpable hypertrophic growths.

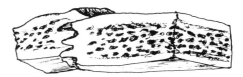

Fig. 1-4. Articular overlapping along a suture's marginal surface. This distortion is generally perceived as a step up or down from one osseous structure to another along a suture's articular margin.

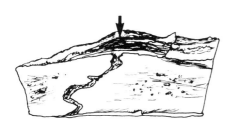

Fig. 1-5. Fibrous adhesion crossing the articular seam of a suture

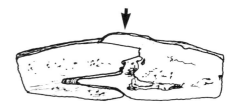

Fig. 1-6. A bony spur traversing a suture's articular seam and partially obliterating the suture

3. *Pliable nodular adhesions.* This deformity is identified as an area of soft or somewhat pliable tissue overlapping the suture's articular seam in a nodular formation. Although the nodule is soft to touch, it is distinctly fibrous in its makeup. Just like with fibrous adhesions, the tissue in pliable nodular adhesions are often composed of avascular collagen tissue. However, unlike fibrous adhesions, pliable nodular adhesions have infiltrated into the periosteum over the skull and possibly into the periosteal layer of the meninges inside the vault. Even though nodular adhesions appear to be more invasive than simple fibrous adhesions, they are nevertheless pliable, suggesting that they are still within an early phase of development (Fig. 1-7).

4. *Solid nodular adhesions.* These adhesions represent a more advanced or chronic nodular adhesive stage. This deformity feels hard or bone-like in nature (Fig. 1-8).

5. *Fluid nodular adhesions.* This deformity feels like an edematous nodule and may consist of a lipoma or cystic formation crossing the suture's articular seam. Moving the nodule from its original position may reveal the depth of the formation's roots. If the nodule is fixed and immovable, chances are it is rooted deep within the suture's articular surface and may even extend into the meningeal layer of the vault (Fig. 1-9).

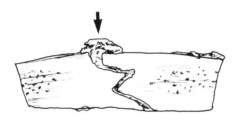

Fig. 1-7. Pliable nodular adhesion, viewed from a transverse sectional cut, rooted within a suture's articular formation

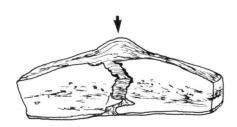

Fig. 1-8. A solid nodular adhesion, viewed from a transverse sectional cut, has infiltrated through a suture and reached the dural meningeal tissue along the inner cranial surface.

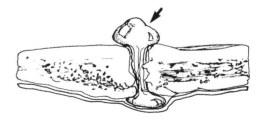

Fig. 1-9. The fluid-filled nodule, viewed from a transverse sectional cut, extends into the vault and is infiltrating the dural region. The nodule is causing the periosteal dura to separate from the cranial bone.

Sensory Distortions

An abnormal sensation in or around a suture's perimeter is called *sensory distortion*. Examiners need to be aware of the following issues when they come across this abnormality:

1. ***Manifested versus latent sensory distortions.*** Manifested sensations are felt even in the absence of external stimuli. Latent sensations are felt when external influences are applied to a region. Latent pain may exist without the presence of manifested pain and may be caused by a diminished capacity of the neuron to reach its action potential. The diminished neuronal action potential may be the result of hyperpolarization of the nerve fiber or neuron. Consequently, latent discomfort can exist in the absence of manifested discomfort when subthreshold stimuli is elevated to threshold level by increased stimulus of the mechanoreceptors through pressure, temperature, or vibration.

2. ***Depth of the sensory distortion.*** The depth of the discomfort is often noted since it can assist the examiner in determining the level of a sutural aberration. Superficial discomfort frequently suggests external conditions, whereas deep discomfort may be caused by an intracranial vascular condition that may require a closer investigation through various scanning modalities.

3. ***Sensory types.*** Some sensory distortions appear as abnormal sensations while others are characterized by a lack of sensation. The following are the most common types of sensory distortions:

- Sharp or stabbing pain. This is usually indicative of an acute condition and may also represent blood stagnation.

- Dull or knotting pain. This kind of pain is frequently attributed to cerebrospinal fluid imbalance or meningeal tension. It may also indicate chronic deficiency around the involved area.

- Explosive pain or pressure. If the sensation is aggravated by touch, the condition is deemed excessive and direct physical contact of the area should be avoided. Explosive pain is usually caused by excessive cranial blood intake and deficient blood outflow. A fine example of this is stenosis of the jugular veins with increased cardiovascular activity.

- Crushing pain. This condition is frequently caused by increased cardiovascular drainage from the vault with diminished blood flow into the head. Arterial spastic conditions are a prime example of this kind of pain.

- Numbness. This condition usually originates from exposure to toxic chemicals, compression, viral infiltration, or vascular insufficiency resulting in sensory axonopathy or neuron destruction. However, it may also be produced by depletion of the ion transfer pump or neuron hyperpolarization.

     If numbness is accompanied by wallerian degeneration, that is, fatty degeneration of a nerve fiber which has been severed from its nutritive sources, the condition may be due to destruction of Nissl bodies in sensory neurons. This causes destruction of the axonal cytoplasmic ectoplasm. However, it may also be produced by a depletion of the neuronal sodium pump or hyperpolarization of the nerve fibers.

Temperature Abnormalities

Temperature abnormalities often reflect conditions of blood excess or deficiency. For example, temperature abnormalities combined with edema in a fluid nodular adhesion may reflect trauma or infection. The following are the four most common types of temperature abnormalities found along sutural seams:

1. *Excessive heat.* This condition is often created by excessive blood accumulation, acute infection, or acute trauma. In the case of trauma or infection, the heat is also accompanied by edema in the surrounding tissue.

2. *Deficiency heat.* This low-grade heat condition is frequently caused by a minor infection or by dehydration of the suture's collagen tissue.

3. *Excessive cold.* This condition is usually generated by blood deficiency. Alternatively, the affected area may also be experiencing a chronic degenerative condition such as the collapse of the bone's trabecular structure, as in advanced cases of osteoporosis or in severe anemia.

4. *Deficiency cold.* This condition is characterized by slightly cooler temperature and usually reflects deficiency of blood caused by scar tissue formation or mild anemia.

Tensile Strength Abnormalities

When it is combined with a finding of displacement, deformity, sensory distortion, or abnormal temperature, a finding of tensile strength abnormality around a suture can alert the practitioner to conditions of excess or deficiency. The following are the two most common distortions found when assessing sutures for tensile strength:

1. *Hardening.* This condition is often associated with chronic adhesive scarring and post-traumatic injuries that are more than two years old.

2. *Softening.* This condition is often associated with deficiency conditions and degenerative diseases of short or long duration.

CHAPTER TWO

Static Sutural Palpation

Theory and Purpose

THE MAJORITY OF practitioners who manipulate the skull inspect sutures while their subjects lie supine on examination tables. Although this position is often acceptable for facial and passive kinetic analyses, it is not encouraged during static and active cranial vault palpation for the following reasons:

1. The sutures that rest adjacent to the examining table's headpiece are often cumbersome to access, thereby making their palpation unnecessarily difficult for the examiner.
2. Gravity could conceivably initiate a compressive strain on the sutures touching the table's headpiece and consequently cause an incessant global articular fixation throughout the cranial vault. Although this contention is only theoretical at this time, the following exercise and facts are presented to substantiate the claim.

When a subject is lying supine, gravity pulls the intracranial contents toward the cranial vault's lowest point. The following exercise is designed to demonstrate this effect as the vault's lowest point is altered and the weight of the intracranial contents moves to accommodate this shift. To implement the exercise, the subject should lie supine with the examiner seated at the head of the table.

1. Cup your hands together and place them under the subject's occipital region.
2. Notice the weight of the subject's head and whether it feels heavier on one side compared to the other.
3. Rotate the subject's head so the face is turned toward the side that feels lighter. This will shift the vault's lowest point into the lighter weight region. Notice the shift in weight as the once lighter region becomes heavier and the once heavier region becomes lighter.
4. Return the subject's head to its original position, and notice how the head's weight distribution once again shifts back to its original stature.
5. With the subject's head in its original position, elevate the head so as to support it with your fingertips. Notice the increased stress and fatigue of your fingers as they attempt to support the head against the constant gravitational pull.

As suggested by the prior exercise, the shift in the vault's weight is due to gravity's effect on the intracranial contents. The plausible outcome from this reaction would be shifts in the internal compression of the posterior meninges. In addition, since the subject's head is resting on the examining table's headpiece, the headpiece's counter-resistant surface produces an increased strain within the posterior sutures, further impeding their natural mobility Ultimately, the acquired intrasutural strain would infiltrate the interlocking beveled systems of the adjacent vault sutures and increase the probability of global sutural fixation. This conclusion appears to be corroborated by the studies discussed below.

In 1956, Pritchard et al. found that the connective tissue passes through the articular seams of the sutures, linking the skull's outer periosteal tissue layer to the periosteal dura inside (Fig. 2-1).[1] This study noted the presence of five distinct tissue layers within a the suture's articular seam, with the middle layer being less dense and very vascular. These findings suggest that a suture's articular seam is somewhat flexible and vulnerable to compression because of the softer middle zone.

In 1972, Herring noted that slippage of one bone upon another would be expected if pressure was applied along a suture's beveled axis.[2] Since the articular beveled axis between the occiput, parietal, and mastoid margins runs in an anterolateral to posteromedial direction, then, in accordance with Herring's finding, the expected axial slippage from the posterior pressure of the headpiece should increase articular compression to the lambdoid and occipitomastoid sutures.

Markens and Oudhof divided the sutures into external and internal portions and noted that (1) the sutures appear to function like hinges, and (2) the greatest displacement was at the external parts, also known as the pars externa.[3] Oudhof further found that the fibers around the pars externa are able to resist forces that would either widen or narrow a suture's articular seam.[4] Consequently, the compression of a skull's external portion and its fibers by the weight of the subject's head could conceivably activate a counter-response that is felt by a suture's articular seam. Other studies found that one to two

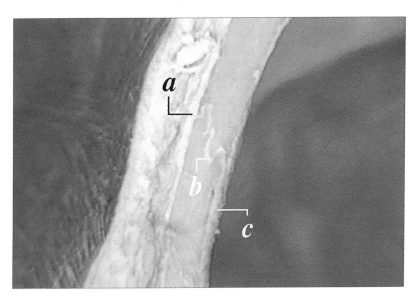

Fig. 2-1 Axial slice through the right coronal suture, delineating the external periosteum as it passes through the suture's articular seam to join with the periosteal layer of the dura inside the cranial vault

a. External periosteum of the skull
b. Periosteum within the suture
c. Dura

pounds of continuous force is all that is required to maintain a measurable separation of the maxillary segments in rhesus monkeys and humans.[5,6]

Based upon these findings, Blum postulated that (1) it would not be unreasonable to assume that even low-level forces might be sufficient to transmit mechanical stresses within adjacent cranial structures, and (2) short-term forces exerted on the cranium can cause associated changes in the intra-sutural tissues with the deposition of Type III collagen.[7] Meiklel found significant protein accumulation within six hours of the initial onset of stress upon a suture, which suggests that mechanical stress can effectively modulate biosynthetic activities.[8] Meiklel et al. extended these observations and found that sutural connective tissue appears to respond to stress with collagen production as well as collagen hydrolysis.[9] From these findings, it appears highly likely that the amount of force generated by the weight of a supine subject's head against a table's headpiece is sufficient to activate an immediate intra-sutural tissue response by the sutures closest to the site of compression.

In 1971, Baker was able to record sutural movements within the cranial vault by widening the maxillary arch, suggesting an integrated functional relationship between sutures.[10] Kostopoulos and Keramidas demonstrated the effects of external manipulation upon the falx cerebri of an embalmed cadaver and were able to measure changes in its elongation.[11] All of the preceding studies support the contentions that (1) all sutures are functionally integrated through dural association and interlocking beveled formations, and (2) compressive stress placed on a suture will likely result in changes throughout the cranium, conceivably interfering with the mobility of distant sutures.

In conclusion, a subject that is resting supine is subject to the influences of gravitational pressure as the weight of the head is compressed against the examining table's headpiece. Consequently, should the occipital region be pressing against the headpiece, the weight of the brain and intracranial fluids will be drawn to the vault's lowest point and exert pressure against the internal wall around the occiput and parietomastoid regions. As the head encounters external resistance from the surface tension of the headpiece, the resulting compressive stress could generate local resistance and fixation in the sutures closest to the area. However, because of the integration of the sutural system as a whole, the functional incapacitation would probably affect other sutures as well and inhibit a practitioner's chances of performing an accurate analysis.

With the subject seated, however, the intracranial material spreads across the entire floor of the cranial vault and thus evenly distributes the intracranial pressure and weight on the those parts of the cranium which embryologically evolved from cartilage. The dural membranes are suspended to eliminate accumulative strain in a particular intracranial region. In addition, the skull is balanced on the occiput's condyle surface, thus eliminating any possible external counter-resistance that could place unforeseen stress on the cranial suture system. For this reason, the approach advocated in this book is to perform static and active vault examinations with the subject seated.

Cranial Vault Palpation

Practitioner-Patient Examining Posture

The patient is seated facing the examiner, who is either seated on a higher stool or standing facing the patient (Fig. 2-2).

Coronal Suture

To enhance the examiner's comparative analysis, both sides of the coronal suture are palpated simultaneously. Palpation is initiated at the patient's bregma (Fig. 2-3A). The bregma can be located by placing the heel of the patient's right hand on the junction of the nasion. With the palm and fingers resting against the frontal squamosal surface and the middle finger on the sagittal midline, the distal phalange of the middle finger will perch on the bregma (Fig. 2-3B).

Utilizing the standard zig-zag or traversing method of palpation, the examiner bilaterally descends along the coronal suture, ending at the junctions of the coronal suture with the right and left greater wings of the sphenoid bone (Fig. 2-3C and D). *Note:* The coronal suture curves in an anterior direction as it descends to the junction with the sphenoid bone (Fig. 2-3E).

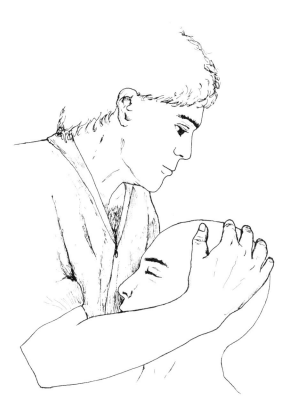

Fig. 2-2 Postural positions of examiner and patient during the sutural palpation procedure of the vault

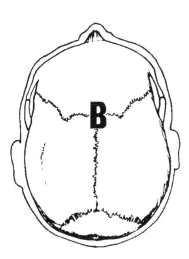

Fig. 2-3A B represents the location of the bregma

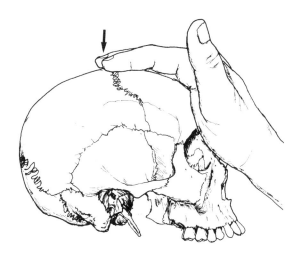

Fig. 2-3B Placement of the patient's right hand when locating the bregma

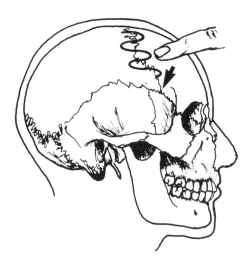

Fig. 2-3C Location of area 2 and palpation in a zig-zag direction along the right coronal suture

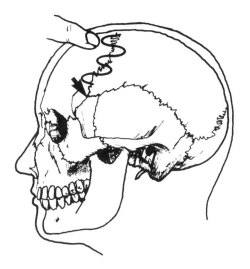

Fig. 2-3D Location of area 10 and palpation in a zig-zag direction along the left coronal suture

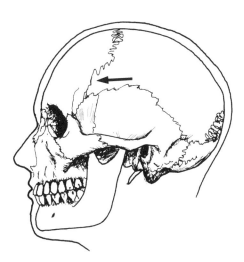

Fig. 2-3E Anterior curve of the coronal suture as it descends from the bregma toward its termination at the superior surface of the sphenoid's greater wing

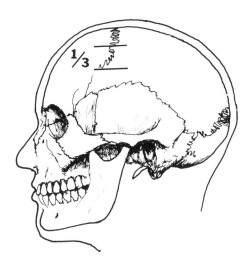

Fig. 2-3F Division of the left coronal suture into three equal regions and the location of the middle region

Normal findings: When the suture is divided into thirds from the bregma to the sphenoid's greater wing, the middle region will feel like an open trench. The examiner has the impression that the suture has spread apart (Fig. 2-3F).

Sphenofrontal Suture

In the previous section, the examiner descended along the coronal suture to terminate at the junctions of the right and left greater wings of the sphenoid bone. From this position, the examiner's palpating fingers need to shift approximately forty-five degrees in an anterocaudal direction. The fingers then begin traversing the sphenofrontal suture in a cephalad-caudal direction (Fig. 2-4A). *Note:* The examiner will find that the frontal bone's lateral surface bulges externally. When attempting to locate the sphenofrontal suture, follow the lower portion of the bulge as it tucks back into the skull. This region will often feel as if it abruptly ends on a flat plate of bone. The plate is the sphenoid's greater wing. Once the plate has been located, the palpating fingers should reascend from the plate onto the frontal bulge. The suture is usually located within 1cm above the plate of the sphenoid bone, on the inferior aspect of the frontal bulge (Fig. 2-4B).

Normal findings: The sphenoid bone overlaps the frontal bone in this region but may feel like a slight upward step in the cephalad direction from the sphenoid bone to the frontal bone's bulging surface (Fig. 2-4B).

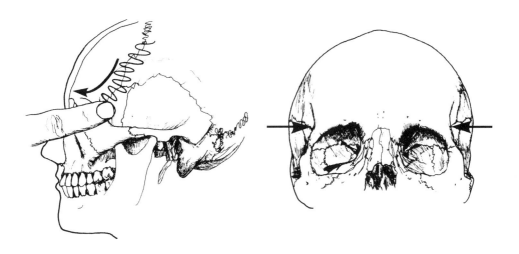

Fig. 2-4A Examiner's altered direction when shifting from the coronal to the sphenofrontal suture

Fig. 2-4B Sphenofrontal suture's location relative to the frontal bone's lateral bulge

Sphenoparietal Suture

The sphenoparietal suture is continuous with the sphenofrontal suture and rests posterior to the coronal suture. To locate the sphenoparietal suture, simply retrace the sphenofrontal suture back to its junction with the coronal suture. When the examining fingers move posterior to the coronal-sphenoid junction, they have commenced palpating the sphenoparietal suture. *Note:* The length of this suture will vary from skull to skull. Based on my own observations of hundreds of skulls, normal sizes vary from those that are undetectable to those that are as much as 12mm in length. The suture's length can be evaluated by noting the distance between the coronal-sphenoid junction and the junction of the sphenoparietal suture with the sphenosquamous suture (Fig. 2-5).

Normal findings: Although the sphenoid bone overlaps the parietal bone along this suture, the suture is often palpated as an upward step in the cephalad direction from the sphenoid's greater wing plate to the parietal bone.

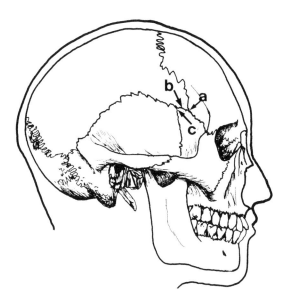

Fig. 2-5 Relative position of the sphenoparietal suture relative to the coronal-sphenoid and sphenosquamous sutures

a. Coronal-sphenoid junction
b. Sphenoparietal suture
c. Junction of the sphenosquamous suture and the sphenoparietal suture

Sphenosquamous Suture

The sphenosquamous suture originates at the posterior aspect of the spheno-parietal suture. The examiner's palpating fingers shift between 90 and 110 degrees to descend in an anterocaudal direction over the sphenosquamous suture. The suture is traversed with a back and forth anteroposterior motion (Fig. 2-6A). *Note:* This suture is usually found anterior to the sideburn hair line and is often located approximately 3.5cm anterior to the center of the external auditory meatus (Fig. 2-6B).

Normal findings: Although the temporal bone overlaps the sphenoid bone in the upper half of this suture and is serrated in its lower half, the suture will usually feel like a firm ridge running in the cephalad to caudal direction. This ridge is often mistaken as sutural jamming.

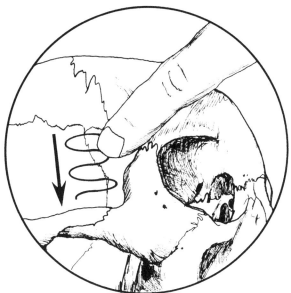

Fig. 2-6A Anteroposterior caudal motion used in palpating the sphenosquamous suture

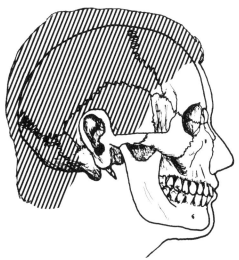

Fig. 2-6B Relative position of the sphenosquamous suture to the anterior sideburn line and the center of the external auditory meatus

Squamoparietal Suture

The squamoparietal suture, also known as the temporoparietal suture, extends in a posterior superior direction from the junction of the sphenoparietal and sphenosquamous sutures. To find the squamoparietal suture, the examiner's fingers should reascend the articular surface of the sphenosquamous suture until they contact the sphenosquamous-sphenoparietal junction. From this point, the examiner's fingers commence palpating the squamoparietal suture. Traversing in a perpendicular direction to the external auditory meatus, the examiner can follow the suture along its arched seam toward the vertex of the auricular helix (Fig. 2-7A and B). *Note:* When the auricle's superior aspect is compressed in a medial direction against the head, the suture is often found descending medially to the vertex of the helix in the direction of the parietomastoid junction (Fig. 2-7B).

Normal findings: This suture has a very tight and thin articulation, which makes its identification very difficult. If the examiner is persistent, a slight upward step from the parietal bone to the temporal squamous bone may be perceived (Fig. 2-7C).

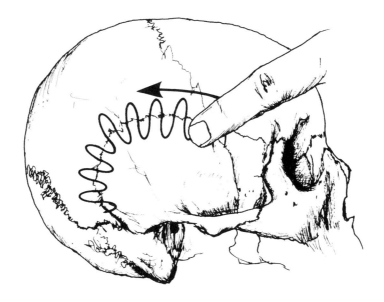

Fig. 2-7A Traversing path used to palpate the squamoparietal suture

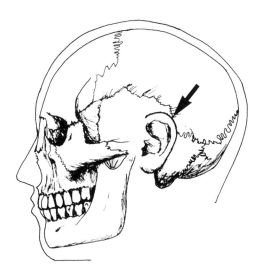

Fig. 2-7B Position of the squamoparietal suture relative to the top of the auricular surface

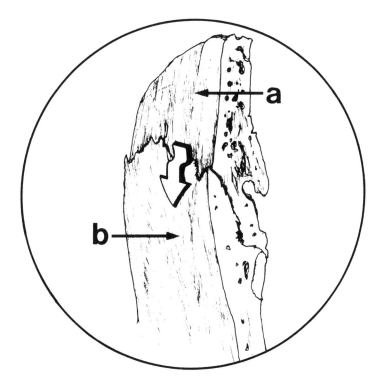

Fig. 2-7C Coronal slice of the squamoparietal suture. The upward step from the parietal surface to the temporal squamous is shown.

a. Parietal bone
b. Temporal squamous bone

Parietomastoid Suture

The parietomastoid suture commences at the termination of the squamoparietal suture and is located in a posterosuperior direction relative to the ear. The junction of the right squamoparietal suture with the right parietomastoid suture is often located around 10 or 11 o'clock relative to the external auditory meatus. The left junction is often located at approximately 1 or 2 o'clock relative to the left external auditory meatus (Fig. 2-8A). The suture ascends in a posterosuperior direction toward the asterion. The asterion is the point on the surface of the skull where the lambdoid, parietomastoid, and occipitomastoid sutures meet and is located at the superior apex of the mastoid process. *Note:* An alternate method for locating this suture is to traverse the superior portion of the mastoid's body from an anterior to posterior direction. The suture will feel like a furrow along the mastoid's anterosuperior border (Fig. 2-8B).

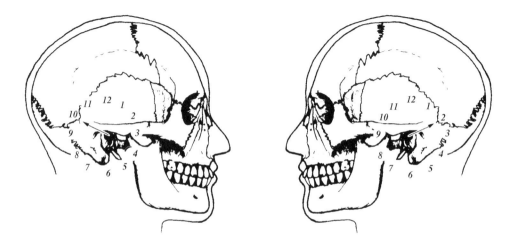

Fig. 2-8A Position of the junction between the parietomastoid and squamoparietal sutures relative to the external auditory meatus

Fig. 2-8B Course used to traverse the parietomastoid suture is highlighted at "a" while the alternate method for locating the parietomastoid suture is highlighted at "b"

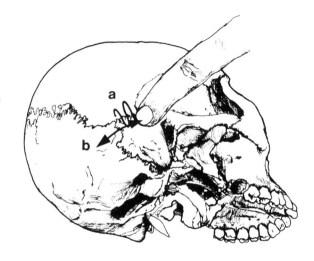

Occipitomastoid Suture

The occipitomastoid suture commences at the junction of the parietomastoid suture with the asterion. Remember that sutures are always palpated in a zigzag method, thus traversing the articulations. From the asterion, the examiner's fingers alter their direction and traverse down along the posterior aspect of the mastoid's process and body (Fig. 2-9A). The suture is located approximately 2mm in a posteromedial direction relative to the mastoid's posterior border (Fig. 2-9B).

Normal findings: The area posterior to the mastoid bone is often felt as a valley with the mastoid bone and the occiput's inferior squamous as the outer edges. The suture is located along the occiput's edge and is often felt as a step into a furrow along the mastoid's posteromedial border. This is often misinterpreted as an open suture by the inexperienced practitioner.

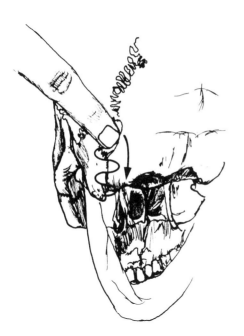

Fig. 2-9A Descending method used to palpate the occipitomastoid suture

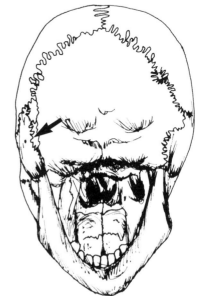

Fig. 2-9B Location of the occipitomastoid suture relative to the posterior mastoid process

Lambdoid Suture

To locate the lambdoid suture, the examiner reascends the occipitomastoid suture, retracing the articulation to the asterion. The lambdoid suture branches posterosuperior from the asterion and terminates at the junction of the opposite lambdoid suture and the posterior aspect of the sagittal suture. Palpation of the lamdoid suture is accomplished by traversing its articular surface in an anteroposterior direction from the asterion to its junction with the sagittal suture at the lambda (Fig. 2-10A).

Note: An alternate method for locating this suture is to cup both hands together with the radial surfaces of the index fingers touching. The cupped hands are placed over the occiput with the palmar surface down. The finger tips are placed on the occiput's squamous plate. The examiner then sweeps the fingers from the occiput's squamous bone to the parietal bones. This sweeping action will usually reveal the lambda and lambdoid sutures (Fig. 2-10B). The lambda is often perceived as an indentation with a right and left posterolateral groove extending from it. The grooves are the superior articular surfaces of the lambdoid sutures.

Normal findings: The lambda often feels like an indentation. However, it may also feel like a small downward step from the occiput onto the parietal bones. The lambdoid suture is often identified as a wide or open suture. This gives the illusion that the suture is spread apart. However, because of the lambdoid suture's serrated articular surface, this feature is considered normal.

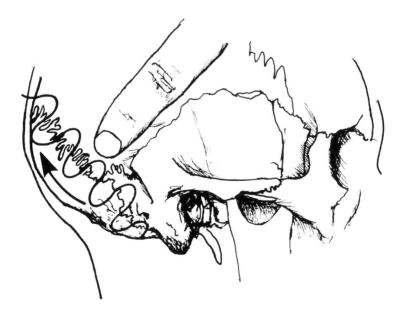

Fig. 2-10A Palpatory route taken by the examiner's fingers when retracing from the occipitomastoid suture to the asterion and along the lambdoid suture to the lambda

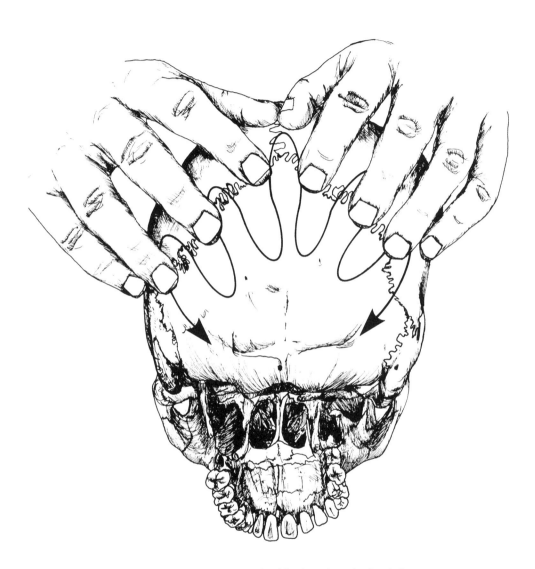

Fig. 2-10B Alternate method for locating the lambda and lambdoid sutures

Sagittal Suture

The sagittal suture is the last of the vault sutures to be palpated. This suture runs in a posterior to anterior direction along the sagittal midline at the top of the vault. Posteriorly, the suture connects to the lambda. Anteriorly, it terminates at the coronal suture, thus creating the bregma (Fig. 2-11A). As the examiner's fingers ascend the right and left lambdoid sutures to meet at the lambda, the index and middle fingers interlace and shift anteriorly to traverse the sagittal suture. This anterior traverse continues until the fingers reach the coronal suture (Fig. 2-11B). *Note:* The sagittal suture is not found on every skull. If this suture is absent, the examiner will feel a hard continuous ridge over the midsagittal crest of the vault in this area.

Normal findings: The posterior third of the suture is often perceived as an open valley or mistaken for being spread apart. This is considered to be normal because the serrated edges in this region of the suture are often larger than those found in the anterior third of the suture.

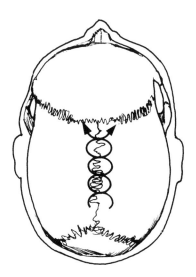

Fig. 2-11A Position of the sagittal suture between the lambda and bregma. The traversing lines indicate the figure-8 motion used in palpating this suture.

Fig. 2-11B Interlaced posture of the examiner's fingers during the palpation of the sagittal suture

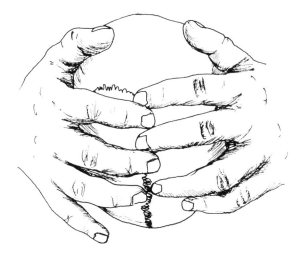

Wormian Bones

Wormian bones are extra bones that are found on many skulls. These are not considered pathogenic by most anatomists. They are simply a product of genetics and seem to function as part of the bones in which they reside. The majority of wormian bones appear along the occipitomastoid and lambdoid sutures. They often appear as extra bones of the occiput. However, these bones may be found anywhere. They usually range in size from 4mm to 6cm but can sometimes be larger (Fig. 2-12). An eight-finger sweep over and around the skull should be performed to digitally determine the presence of extra sutures in regions that usually do not contain them.

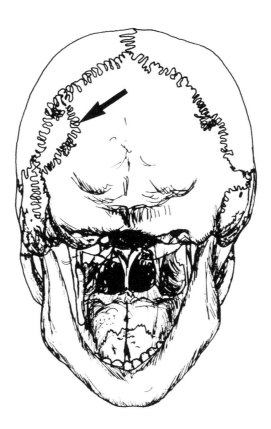

Fig. 2-12 Large wormian bone on the left squamous of the occiput

Metopic Suture

The metopic suture is considered to be an extra suture when found on the adult skull. The suture is usually present on all skulls at birth and remains until the fifth or sixth year of life. According to Berry, the appearance of this suture in adults varies from zero to seven percent, depending on ethnicity.[12] Although it is rare to find this suture in an adult, its presence is not considered pathological.

The suture is found anterior to the coronal suture along the superior mid-sagittal crest of the frontal bone. It is often considered an anterior extension of the sagittal suture (Fig. 2-13). Should this suture exist, the examiner should treat it as an extension of the sagittal suture. Therefore, when palpating the sagittal suture, simply continue anteriorly to the coronal-sagittal junction to detect its existence.

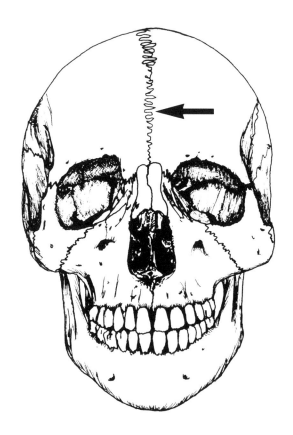

Fig. 2-13 Location of the metopic suture in an adult skull

Facial Palpation

Practitioner-Patient Examining Posture

Unlike the sutures of the vault, the facial sutures lack a direct attachment with the intracranial meninges. The facial sutural system, therefore, is somewhat autonomous with respect to the cranial vault, and its articulations do not need to follow the austere regulations of postural positioning that govern the vault sutures.

The examiner is seated at the patient's head (Fig. 2-14). Palpation commences with the most inferolateral facial suture and moves superomedially. Paired facial sutures are palpated simultaneously to enhance the examiner's comparative analysis.

Recommendation: It has been my observation that the proper selection of a supportive pillow is essential when administering a facial examination. For example, thick pillows elevate the head and lead to cervical flexion. This closes the patient's mouth and impedes the examiner's attempts to contact the maxillary and palatine sutures. Pillows that are too hard can be irritating and lead to an increase in facial muscle tension. Those that are too soft often fail to support the patient's head adequately when positional stability is required. Consequently, the head should be supported by a pillow of moderate tensile strength that does not restrain cranial rhythms. It should uniformly brace the patient's head and neck, regardless of their shape or weight distribution.

I believe the Tempur-Pedic™ pillow meets these criteria and is the best choice for this procedure.[13] Developed by Swedish scientists for NASA's space program, this pillow has thermal sensitivity foam. This gives it a contour-conforming quality that superficially softens to encourage rhythmic motion while maintaining a deep-seated tone for uniform stability of the head and neck.

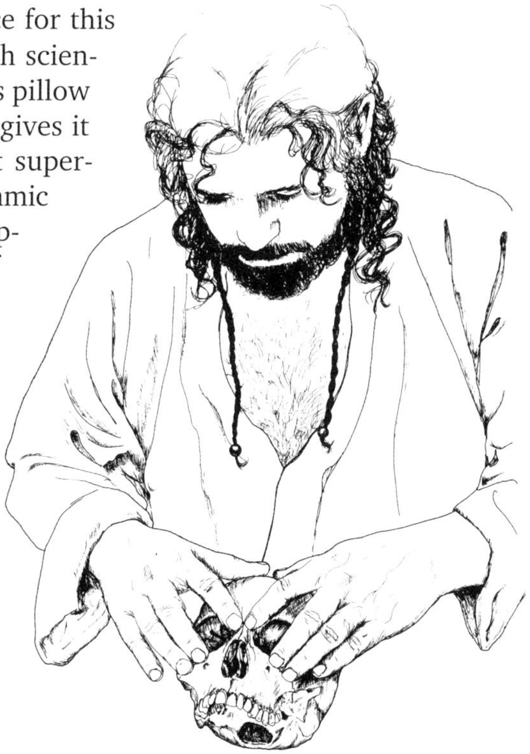

Fig. 2-14 Postural position of the examiner relative to the patient during the sutural palpation procedure of the cranial-facial articulations

Zygomaticotemporal Suture

The zygomaticotemporal suture is located on the zygomatic arch, approximately 1cm posterior from the posterior zygomatic temporal process angle (Fig. 2-15A). The examiner's index or middle finger traverses the suture in an anterior (toward the patient's face) to posterior (toward the patient's mastoids) direction (Fig. 2-15B).

Normal findings: This suture is usually easy to distinguish and frequently presents as an open furrow. To the inexperienced practitioner, this might be mistakenly diagnosed as a separated articular connection. However, in most instances, the opened furrow is considered normal unless accompanied by pain or the presence of a nodular formation.

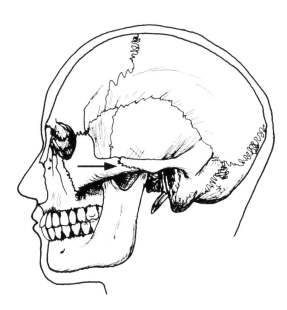

Fig. 2-15A Location of the left zygomaticotemporal suture

Fig. 2-15B Directional method of palpation for the zygomaticotemporal suture

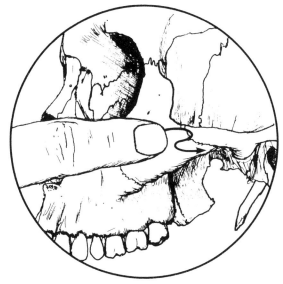

Zygomaticomaxillary Suture

Palpation begins on the inferior osseous rim of the eye socket directly below the pupil (Fig. 2-16A). This is the superior articular region of the zygomaticomaxillary suture. The suture descends laterally as the examiner traverses the suture to its inferior termination point (Fig. 2-16B). The zygomatic bone overlaps the maxilla along its superomedial articular region, and the maxilla overlaps the zygomatic bone along its inferolateral articular region.

Normal findings: The superior articular region of this suture is usually felt as a medial step down from the zygomatic bone onto the maxilla. It is also considered normal to find a slight gap within the step, giving the illusion that the suture is spread apart. On the inferior aspect of this suture the roles reverse and the examiner will usually feel a step up from the zygomatic bone onto the maxilla (Fig. 2-16).

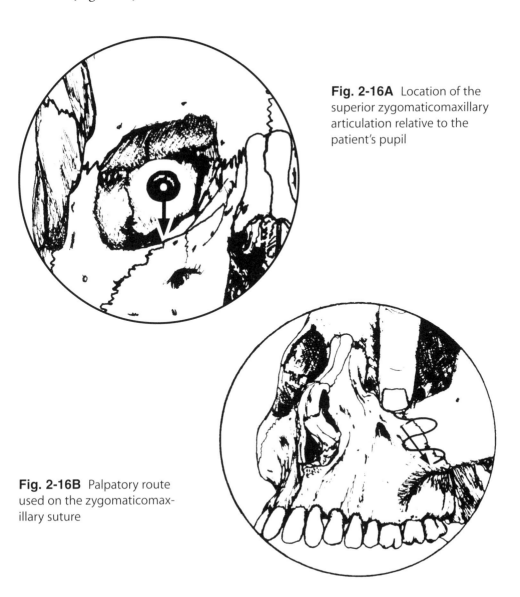

Fig. 2-16A Location of the superior zygomaticomaxillary articulation relative to the patient's pupil

Fig. 2-16B Palpatory route used on the zygomaticomaxillary suture

Intermaxillary Suture

Palpation and visual analysis are frequently used to inspect the intermaxillary suture. The examiner may choose to visually inspect the maxillary incisors near the gum line to acquire information pertaining to this suture (Fig. 2-17A). If the suture has spread apart, the distance between the incisors will be obvious and the hard palate will appear unusually wide. If the suture is jammed, the hard palate will appear steeple shaped and the lower medial edges of the anterior incisors will be compressed, which usually establishes an anterior overlap of two teeth. Should superior to inferior overlapping occur, one gum line will appear lower than the other.

The suture is palpated with the index or middle finger. The use of a finger cot or latex glove is strongly recommended. Initial contact is made posterior to the maxillary incisors along the hard palate's sagittal midline. The examiner maintains contact along the suture while traversing it from side to side until its termination at the soft palate (Fig. 2-17B).

Normal findings: A small hairline ridge is often felt by the examiner. This suture has also been known to feel like a small groove. With the absence of pain or other artifacts, these palpable characteristics are usually considered nonpathological and within acceptable limits.

Variations: A common variant, known as *torus palatinus,* is an overgrowth of bone extending along the region of the intermaxillary suture. While it is considered benign, this hypertrophic extension resembles the growth patterns of sutures placed under tension stress and suggests the possibility of interarticular jamming.

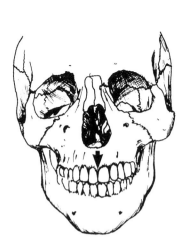

Fig. 2-17A Visual analysis of the maxilla

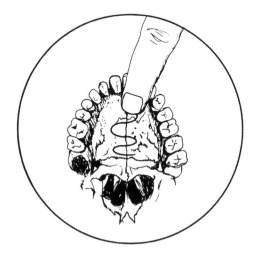

Fig. 2-17B Palpatory route used on the intermaxillary suture

Interpalatine Suture

The interpalatine suture is continuous with the posterior terminal of the inter-maxillary suture and resides along the midsagittal plane (Fig. 2-18A). To locate the suture, simply continue traversing the midsagittal ridge of the intermaxillary suture to its termination at the palatine-maxillary junction. The junction is often felt as a small ridge that crosses the midsagittal region perpendicular to the intermaxillary suture. The interpalatine suture is posterior to this point and the finger continues traversing the articular surface until the soft palate is reached (Fig. 2-18B). Like the intermaxillary suture, the interpalatine suture is palpated with the index or middle finger. The use of a finger cot or latex glove is, again, strongly suggested.

Normal findings: Since the suture is often ridged along its articular surface, it is frequently misinterpreted as being jammed. However, the presence of ridges is normal unless accompanied by pain or discomfort upon compression.

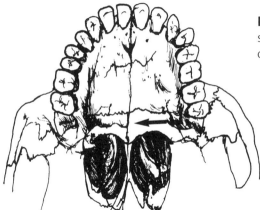

Fig. 2-18A Position of the interpalatine suture relative to the posterior terminal of the intermaxillary suture

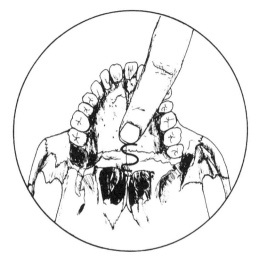

Fig. 2-18B Palpatory route used on the interpalatine suture

Palatomaxillary Suture

The palatomaxillary suture perpendicularly crosses the junction of the inter-maxillary-interpalatine sutures and transverses the hard palate's horizontal plate along one-fifth of its posterior surface area (Fig. 2-19A). To locate the suture, the index finger contacts the internal surface of the maxillary teeth level with the internal gum line. Gliding posteriorly along the inner surface of the teeth, the index finger halts its posterior pilgrimage at the posterior edge of the second molar. This is where the lateral edge of the suture begins. To palpate the suture, simply move the examining finger back and forth antero-posteriorly as it moves horizontally across the upper palate to the opposite second molar's posterior edge (Fig. 2-19B).

Normal findings: Because the maxilla has an inferior articular junction relative to the palatine's horizontal plate, the suture is frequently palpated as a down-ward caudal step from the palatine to the maxilla. However, as the palpating finger approaches the sagittal midline, the suture's articular beveled surfaces reverse and often create a small caudal osseous mound. When it is manifestly painful or painful to external pressure, the mound may be considered abnor-mal. Nevertheless, a nonpainful mound usually indicates a normal variance in the articular junction and is clinically insignificant.

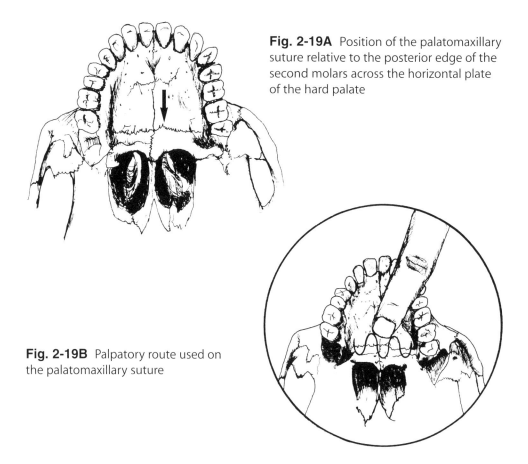

Fig. 2-19A Position of the palatomaxillary suture relative to the posterior edge of the second molars across the horizontal plate of the hard palate

Fig. 2-19B Palpatory route used on the palatomaxillary suture

Frontozygomatic Suture

Located on the outer osseous rim of the eye socket, the frontozygomatic suture is located between 10 and 11 o'clock on the right and between 1 and 2 o'clock on the left (Fig. 2-20A). Palpation commences at the eye socket's outer osseous rim lateral to the commissure ligaments of the eyelids. The examiner then sweeps the lateral osseous eye rim, moving in a cephalad direction (Fig. 2-20B). An indentation in the bone will be felt when the suture is passed over.

Normal findings: Although the zygomatic bone overlaps the frontal portion at this articulation, the suture often feels open. The examiner perceives the illusion of the suture being spread apart.

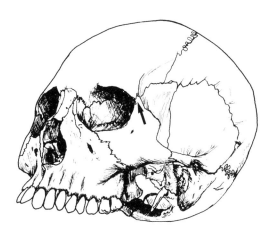

Fig. 2-20A Position of the fronto-zygomatic suture relative to the lateral corner of the eye

Fig. 2-20B Palpatory route used on the frontozygomatic suture

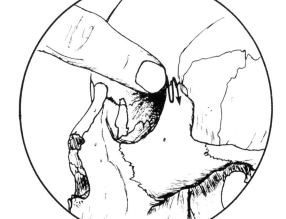

Nasomaxillary Suture

The nasomaxillary suture is located midway between the midsagittal line of the nasal bridge and the medial border of the eye socket. Palpation is initiated at the anterosuperior midsagittal aspect of the nasal bridge. Sweeping laterally over the nasal bone's surface, the examiner's palpating finger will encounter a shallow furrow medial to a ridge. This furrow is the suture, and the ridge is the nasal articular surface of the maxillary-frontal process. After following this procedure to locate the suture, traverse the suture from its origin (inferior to the nasion) to its inferior termination with the nasal cartilage (Fig. 2-21). *Note:* The average suture is 2.5 to 3cm in length.

Normal findings: This suture often feels like a small furrow medial to a slight ridge. Because of the close association of the two structures, examiners often find themselves confused between sutural jamming and spreading. In actuality, this finding is considered normal, and lesions are determined by the presence of pain or nodular formations.

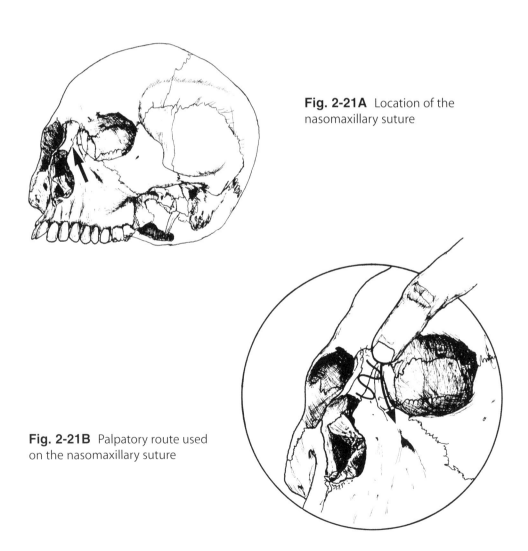

Fig. 2-21A Location of the nasomaxillary suture

Fig. 2-21B Palpatory route used on the nasomaxillary suture

Internasal Suture

The internasal suture is located between the two nasal bones; superiorly the suture intersects the nasion, and caudally it terminates at the rhinion (Fig. 2-22A). Palpation with the index finger commences at the nasion and continues traversing the suture's course until its termination with the nasal cartilage (Fig. 2-22B).

Normal findings: The cephalad fourth of this suture is often overlapped to the left by 3 to 4mm (Fig. 2-22A). This deviation is considered nonpathological and should be considered a normal variance. Palpation often reveals a 1mm flattened surface over the suture.

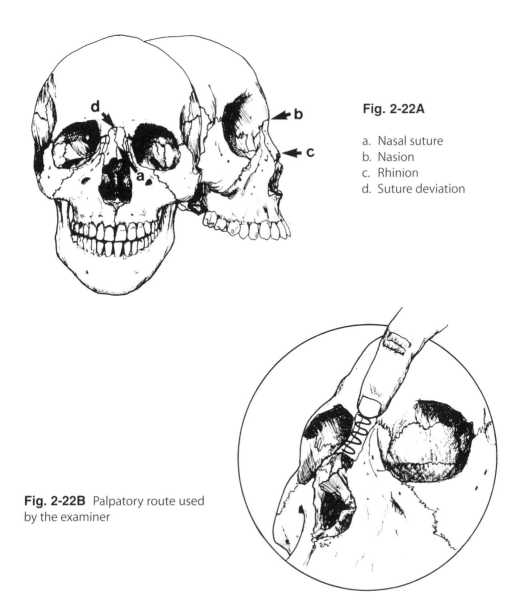

Fig. 2-22A

a. Nasal suture
b. Nasion
c. Rhinion
d. Suture deviation

Fig. 2-22B Palpatory route used by the examiner

Frontomaxillary Suture

Located at the bridge of the nose, the frontomaxillary suture makes up the lateral aspect of the nasion (Fig. 2-23A). Palpation commences by placing the index fingers against the right and left frontomaxillary junctions medial to the eye sockets (under the ledge of the superior frontal orbital ridge). The suture is traversed by following its course medially to its termination with the nasal bone (Fig. 2-23B). *Note:* The average suture is 7 to 8mm in length.

Normal findings: The suture's lateral seam begins superomedially to the medial canthus and runs anteriorly as it courses medially toward the lateral border of the nasal frontal suture. The articular seam is tucked into a fold created by the rostral-projecting maxillary frontal process as it perpendicularly inserts into the underbelly of the inferior rim of the glabella. Consequently, the articular seam is often unremarkable and is frequently perceived as merely a fold in the bone.

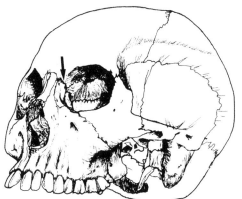

Fig. 2-23A Location of the frontomaxillary suture

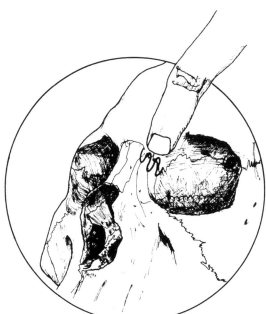

Fig. 2-23B Palpatory route used by the examiner

Frontonasal Suture

Located at the bridge of the nose, the frontonasal suture makes up the medial half of the nasion (Fig. 2-24A). Palpation extends from the end of the frontomaxillary suture's junction with the nasomaxillary suture and traverses medially under the frontal nasion ledge until the opposite frontonasal suture at the center of the nasion (Fig. 2-24B). *Note:* The average suture is 5 to 6mm in length.

Normal findings: Like the frontomaxillary suture, this suture is usually tucked into the anteroinferior fold of the frontal glabella. Consequently, it is often perceived as a fold in the bone, and the suture itself is unremarkable.

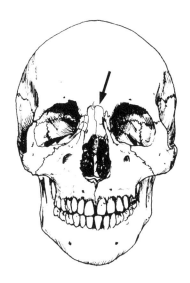

Fig. 2-24A Position of the frontonasal suture

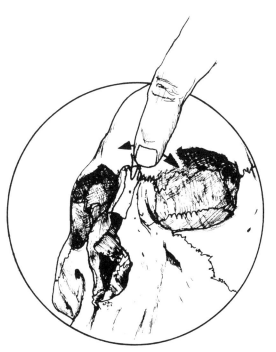

Fig. 2-24B Palpatory route used on the frontonasal suture

References

1. Pritchard JJ, Scott JH, Girgis FG. The structure and development of cranial facial sutures. *J Anat* 1956;90:73–85.
2. Herring SW. Sutures-a tool in functional cranial analysis. *Acta Anat* 1972;83:222–247.
3. Markens IS, Oudhof HAJ. Morphological changes in the coronal suture after replantation. *Acta Anat* 1980;107:289–296.
4. Oudhof HAJ. Sutural growth. *Acta Anat* 1982;112:58–68.
5. Hicks E. Slow maxillary expansion. a clinical study of the skeletal versus dental response to low magnitude force. *Am J Orthod* 1978;73:121–141.
6. Cotton L. Slow maxillary expansion: skeletal versus dental response to low magnitude force in macaca maulatta. *Am J Orthod* 1978;73:1–23.
7. Blum C. The effects of movement, stress, and mechanoelectric activities within the cranial matrix. *Int J Orthod* 1987;25:1–2.
8. Meikle MC. et. al. Rabbit cranial sutures in vitro: a new experimental model for studying the response of fibrous joints to mechanical stress. *Cal Tissue Int* 1979;28:137–144.
9. Meikle MC, Sellers A, Reynolds JJ. Effects of tensile mechanical stress on the synthesis of metalloproteinases by rabbit coronal sutures in vitro. *Cal Tissue Int* 1980;30:77–82.
10. Baker EG. Alteration in width of maxillary arch and its relation to sutural movement of cranial bones. *J Am Osteopathic Assoc* 1971;70:559–564.
11. Kostopoulos DC, Keramidas G. Changes in elongation of falx cerebri during craniosacral therapy techniques applied on the skull of an embalmed cadaver. *J Cranialmandibular Practice* 1992;10:9–12.
12. Berry AC. Factors affecting the incidence of nonmetrical skeletal variants. *J Anatomy* 1975;120: 519–35.
13. This is available from Tempur-Pedic, Inc., Lexington, KY. 1-800-878-8889.

CHAPTER THREE

Active Kinetic Sutural Palpation

Theory and Purpose

IN ACTIVE KINETIC palpation, the procedures described by DeJarnette, who often used mandibular motion during cranial motion analysis,[1] are employed. However, in active kinetic palpation, the palpatory emphasis is placed on the articular seams of the sutures. Although the assumption is that the sutures are directly palpated, the examiner is actually perceiving the motion of the epicranial muscles or aponeurotic fascia and is using their responses as a window through which to detect the suture's probable mobility. In support of this procedure, it should be noted that the masticator muscles are rooted in the skull's periosteum. Pritchard et al. observed that the outer cranial periosteum penetrates the suture's articular seam to join with the dura intercranially.[2] Consequently, it is highly likely that intersutural-engendered motion can be caused by the muscle's tugging on the periosteum. I have observed that the amount of muscular activity directly over a suture often reflects its degree of articular aberrance. This may be due to interarticular protein accumulation generated by increased biosynthetic activities from myotonically induced articular stress, as noted by Meikle et al.[3] Alternatively, it can arise from reduced trigeminal motor output causing diminished muscular activity and therefore decreased sutural tugs.

The examination then becomes an investigation into the symmetrical motion created along sutural articular seams during mandibular motion. Abnormal intracranial meningeal tension is usually expressed by increased muscle tension or decreased amplitude of motion either along the suture or when one suture is compared relative to its contralateral counterpart. Therefore, the practitioner is encouraged to check for both the smoothness of the motion and its amplitude during this analysis. The activity found by the examiner on the side of mandibular deviation depicts the suture's capacity to *reengage*, while the activity found on the opposing side depicts the suture's ability to *disengage.*

Other than direct trauma or local infection, the midline sutures, such as the sagittal or intermaxillary, are not subject to the same influences that govern sutures with direct muscular connections. Primary aberrant movement caused by the presence of acute trauma or infection can be identified by accompanying heat, swelling, and pain. The finding of traumatic or infectious changes can be confirmed by the patient's case history coupled with the presence of aberrant fibroid development, bony degeneration, or hypertrophic infiltration. However, I have often found that midline aberrations without a history of trauma or infection are often associated with aponeurotic strains emanating from increased or decreased muscular contractile activity in a distal area of the skull. Neurological abnormalities from perimeter sutures associated with the osseous structures adjoining the midline suture can also contribute to the muscles' aberrant behavior. In the following example, aberrant neuromuscular activity results in fibroid formation in the anterior sagittal suture from compensatory abnormal obliteration of a perimeter suture of the parietal bone.

A patient was involved in a traumatic head injury in which the left temporalis muscle was damaged and the skull fractured across the left sphenoparietal suture. The time of examination was five years postinjury. As a consequence of this injury, the area around the fracture underwent hypertrophic osseous regeneration that resulted in the partial obliteration of the injured suture. The injury to the left temporalis muscle coupled with its lack of use during the fracture's recovery caused tissue scarring and, undoubtedly, atrophic proteolytic degenerative changes of the fibroelastic elements. With the passing of time, the subject would chew food on his right side to avoid headaches evoked from exceeding the capacity of the left temporalis muscle. However, the increased right-sided chewing eventually led to myotonic and hypertrophic changes within the right temporalis and increased its contractile force on the cranial periosteum and gala aponeurosis. Meikle et al. found increased interarticular protein synthesis from stress.[3] The resulting asymmetrical tug generated by the temporalis' decreased left and increased right contractions indirectly led to the sagittal suture's aberrant behavior and eventual anterior interarticular fibrous development.

Therefore, the development of aberrant formations in a midline suture without a history of trauma or infection is usually a result of a compensatory reaction to associated articular abnormalities. These associated aberrations, which can arise as a result of distorted contractile activity in distant cranial muscles, are found around the perimeter of the osseous structures next to the midline suture. Alternatively, an aberration generated through association with other sutural distortions could cause a fixation of the entire midline suture. However, the presence of an aberration generated through association with other sutural distortions frequently manifests as partial aberrant mobility, that is, portions of the sutural seam will fixate and other regions will remain free and uninhibited.

To investigate this possibility, the examiner should expand the palpation beyond the seam of the midline suture to include the adjoining osseous formations. As an example, the parietal bones should be palpated when checking the sagittal suture. In this way, the practitioner is able to create a window through which to observe the indirect action of the bone upon the aponeurotic fascia, which should influence the midline suture aberration.

The following exercise is designed to show the aforementioned phenomenon as it relates to the sagittal suture. The subject is seated facing the examiner. The examiner is seated on an elevated stool, or stands in front of the subject, with both hands interlocked along their distal phalanges. The interlocking fingertips are placed in full contact with the subject's sagittal suture to guarantee a comprehensive monitoring of the suture's activities. The following steps are taken:

1. The examiner applies working-level pressure evenly into the tissue above the suture and holds this level of pressure for the entire duration of the exercise.
2. The subject moves his or her jaw from side to side while the examiner feels for motion along the articular seam. The examiner should observe for motion and mentally note its degree of amplitude.
3. While maintaining side-to-side mandibular motion, the subject is instructed to apply compressive force with the left hand into the antero-inferior region of the left parietal bone. The examiner should now perceive a decrease in amplitude of the motion at the anterior sagittal suture with no change in posterior sagittal activity.
4. Still applying side-to-side mandibular motion, the subject removes the compressive contact while the examiner continues to monitor activity changes. The examiner should now note that the amplitude of anterior sagittal motion returns to the level found before the application of the compressive force.
5. The subject continues to apply side-to-side mandibular motion while administering compressive force to the right posteroinferior angle of the parietal bone. The examiner should now perceive a decrease in posterior sagittal amplitude with preservation of the anterior suture's activity.
6. The subject is instructed to remove the posterior compression while continuing to move the mandible from side to side. The examiner should now feel the amplitude of the posterior sagittal motion return to its original level.

This exercise demonstrates that the inhibition of motion in a specific region associated with a bone adjacent to the sagittal suture will probably affect inhibitory control over a specific portion of the suture. The exercise shows that although part of the suture's motion was inhibited, the remaining articular seam retains normal functional activity. Therefore, aberrant formations or behaviors in midline sutures can be divided into those caused by direct stimuli and those caused by indirect stimuli. Local site infection or trauma are classified as direct causative agents, while aberrations in various sutures associated with the osseous structures adjacent to the midline sutures serve as indirect causative agents.

Note: The optimum time to apply this procedure is during the static examination. Therefore, upon completion of each suture's static analysis, the practitioner is encouraged to carry out an active kinetic examination before investigating the next suture.

Cranial Vault Palpation

The hand postures and pressure codes used in this section were described in the Introduction (see Fig. I-2 and Table I-1).

Coronal Suture

CONTACTS

Right hand: Use hand posture three with the four fingers contacting the surface area over the subject's left coronal suture (Fig. 3-1).

Left hand: Use a mirror-image contact over the right coronal suture.

MOBILIZATION

Both hands apply W-level pressure caudally, and the contacts simultaneously monitor the suture's motion (Fig. 3-1).

PATIENT PARTICIPATION

The subject's jaw moves from side to side.

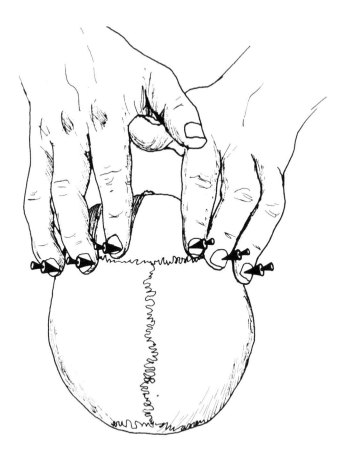

Fig. 3-1 Coronal suture: contact points and applied direction of sutural monitoring

Sphenofrontal Suture

CONTACTS

Right hand: Use hand posture three while the index finger contacts the suture's articular surface anterior to the coronal suture (Fig. 3-2).

Left hand: Use a mirror-image contact.

MOBILIZATION

Both hands apply W-level pressure toward the midsagittal plane of the vault, and the contacts monitor for sutural motion (Fig. 3-2).

PATIENT PARTICIPATION

The subject's jaw moves from side to side.

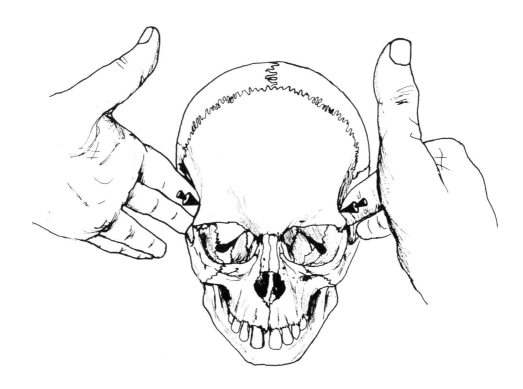

Fig. 3-2 Sphenofrontal suture: contact points and applied direction of sutural monitoring

Sphenoparietal Suture

CONTACTS

Right hand: Use hand posture three while the index finger contacts the suture's articular surface posterior to the coronal suture (Fig. 3-3).

Left hand: Use a mirror-image contact.

MOBILIZATION

Both hands apply W-level pressure toward the midsagittal plane of the vault, and the contacts monitor for sutural motion (Fig. 3-3).

PATIENT PARTICIPATION

The subject's jaw moves from side to side.

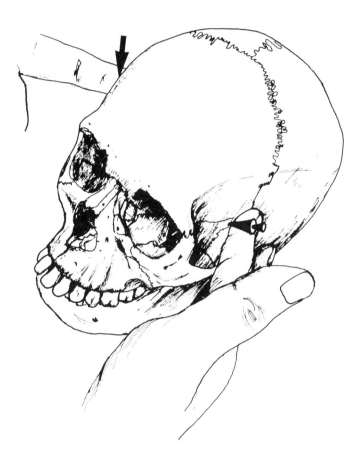

Fig. 3-3 Sphenoparietal suture: contact points and applied direction of sutural monitoring

Sphenosquamous Suture

CONTACTS

Right hand: Use hand posture three while the index and middle fingers contact the suture's articular seam (Fig. 3-4). The index finger contact is inferior to the sutural junction of the sphenoparietal and the squamoparietal sutures. The middle finger contacts the sutural seam superior to the zygomaticotemporal arch.

Left hand: Mirroring the right hand, the hand's contacts are applied to the sutural seam of the sphenosquamous suture.

MOBILIZATION

Both hands apply W-level pressure toward the midsagittal plane of the vault, and the contacts monitor for sutural motion (Fig. 3-4).

PATIENT PARTICIPATION

The subject's jaw moves from side to side.

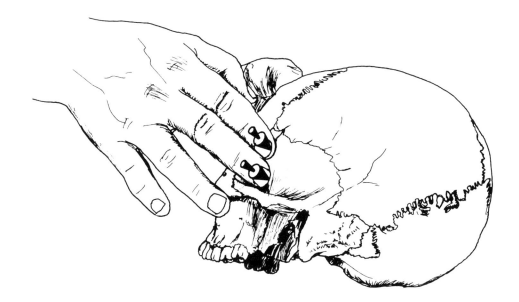

Fig. 3-4 Sphenosquamous suture: contact points and applied direction of sutural monitoring

Squamoparietal Suture

CONTACTS

Right hand: Use hand posture four while the index, middle, and ring fingers contact the suture's articular seam (Fig. 3-5). The fingers are spread to aid in the monitoring of the entire articular surface.

Left hand: Use a mirror-image contact.

MOBILIZATION

Both hands apply W-level pressure toward the midsagittal plane of the vault, and the contacts monitor for sutural motion (Fig. 3-5).

PATIENT PARTICIPATION

The subject's jaw moves from side to side.

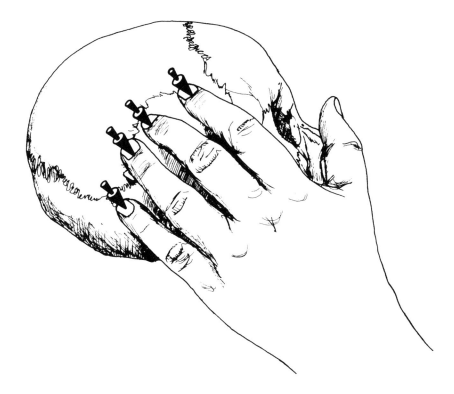

Fig. 3-5 Squamoparietal suture: contact points and applied direction of palpatory pressure

Parietomastoid Suture

CONTACTS

Right hand: Use hand posture three while the suture's articular junction is monitored with the middle finger (Fig. 3-6).

Left hand: Use mirror-image contact.

MOBILIZATION

Both hands apply W-level pressure toward the midsagittal plane of the vault, and the contacts monitor for sutural motion (Fig. 3-6).

PATIENT PARTICIPATION

The subject's jaw moves from side to side.

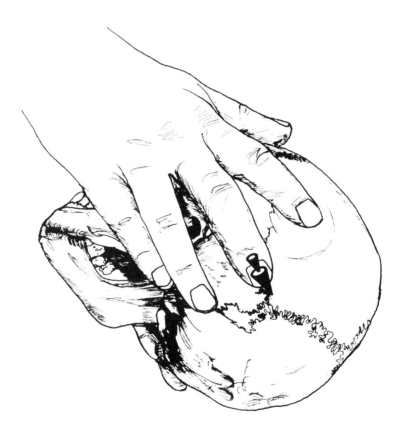

Fig. 3-6 Parietomastoid suture: contact points and applied direction of palpatory pressure

Occipitomastoid Suture

CONTACTS

Right hand: Use hand posture three while the index, middle, and ring fingers contact the suture's articular surface (Fig. 3-7).

Left hand: Use a mirror-image contact.

MOBILIZATION

Both hands apply W-level pressure in an anteromedial direction toward the sagittal midline of the sphenobasilar junction, and the contacts monitor for sutural motion. (Fig. 3-7).

PATIENT PARTICIPATION

The subject's jaw moves from side to side.

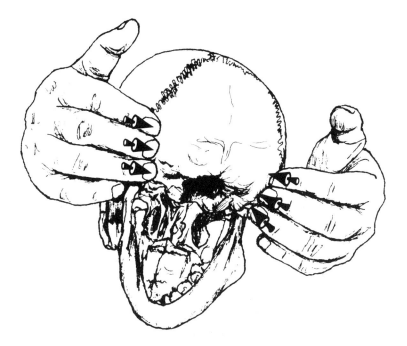

Fig. 3-7 Occipitomastoid suture: contact points and applied direction of palpatory pressure

Lambdoid Suture

CONTACTS

Right hand: Use hand posture three while the index, middle, and ring fingers contact the suture's articular surface (Fig. 3-8).

Left hand: Mirrors the right hand. The index finger is placed on the suture's articular seam immediately lateral to the lambda. The ring finger contacts the suture medial to the asterion, and the middle finger is positioned midway between the index and ring fingers.

MOBILIZATION

Both hands apply W-level pressure on the suture's external seam, and the contact areas are monitored for sutural motion (Fig. 3-8).

PATIENT PARTICIPATION

The subject's jaw moves from side to side.

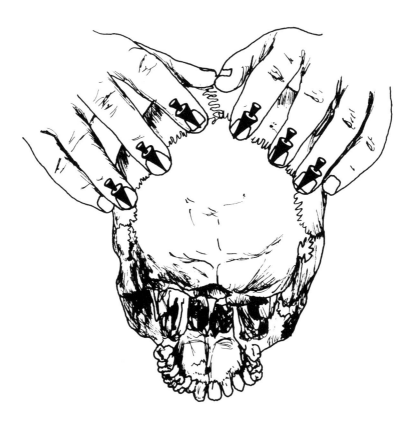

Fig. 3-8 Lambdoid suture: contact points and applied direction of palpatory pressure

Sagittal Suture

CONTACTS

Right hand: Use hand posture four while the four fingers spread out along the suture's entire articular surface (Fig. 3-9).

Left hand: Interlace with the right hand's contacts. The distal finger tips contact the suture's articular surface.

MOBILIZATION

Both hands apply W-level pressure in a caudal direction on the suture's articular surface, and the contact areas are monitored for sutural motion (Fig. 3-9).

PATIENT PARTICIPATION

The subject's jaw moves from side to side.

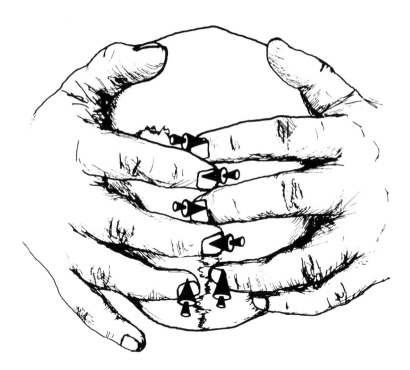

Fig. 3-9 Sagittal suture: contact points and applied direction of palpatory pressure

Facial Palpation

Remember that these procedures are applied to a suture following the suture's static palpatory examination. The examiner is now seated at the head of the examining table throughout the entire facial examination.

Zygomaticotemporal Suture

CONTACTS

Right hand: Use hand posture two while the index finger contacts the suture's articular seam (Fig. 3-10).

Left hand: Use a mirror-image contact.

MOBILIZATION

Both hands apply W-level pressure toward the sphenoid's greater wing, and the contacts monitor for sutural motion (Fig. 3-10).

PATIENT PARTICIPATION

The subject's jaw moves from side to side.

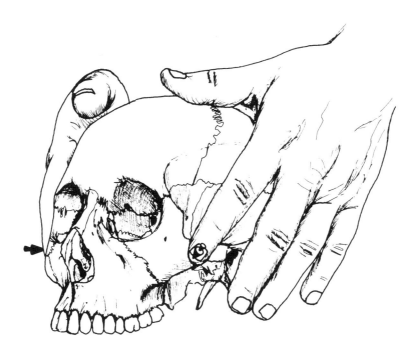

Fig. 3-10 Zygomaticotemporal suture: contact points and applied direction of palpatory pressure

Zygomaticomaxillary Suture

CONTACTS

Right hand: Use hand posture two while the index and middle fingers contact the right suture's articular surface (Fig. 3-11).

Left hand: Use a mirror-image contact.

MOBILIZATION

Both hands employ posterior W-level pressure on the contact areas to monitor for motion (Fig. 3-11).

PATIENT PARTICIPATION

The subject's jaw moves from side to side.

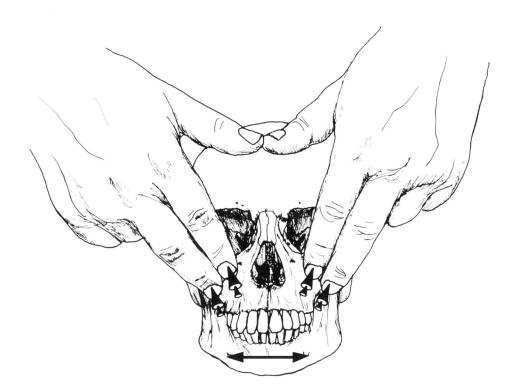

Fig. 3-11 Zygomaticomaxillary suture: contact points and applied direction of sutural monitoring

Intermaxillary Suture

CONTACTS

Right hand: The index finger is inserted inside the mouth and contacts the anterior aspect of the suture's articular seam (Fig. 3-12).

Left hand: Similar to the right hand, the index finger is placed inside the mouth. However, its contact is on the suture's articular seam posterior to the right index finger.

MOBILIZATION

Both hands employ W-level pressure in a rostral direction on the contact area to monitor for motion (Fig. 3-12).

PATIENT PARTICIPATION

The subject holds the mouth open while shifting the mandible from side to side.

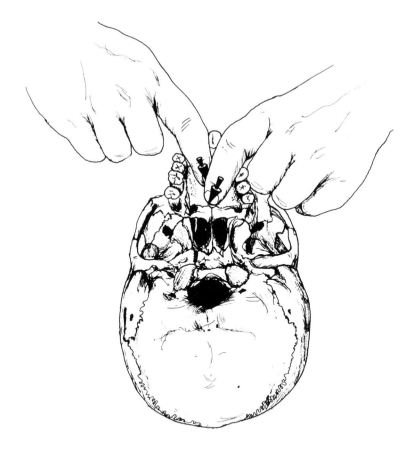

Fig. 3-12 Intermaxillary suture: contact points and applied direction of sutural monitoring

Interpalatine Suture

CONTACTS

Right hand: The index finger contacts the suture's articular seam, posterior to the transverse intersection of the palatomaxillary suture with the intermaxillary suture (Fig. 3-13).

Left hand: Has no contacts.

MOBILIZATION

The right hand employs W-level pressure in a rostral direction on the contact area to monitor for motion (Fig. 3-13).

PATIENT PARTICIPATION

The subject holds the mouth open while shifting the mandible from side to side.

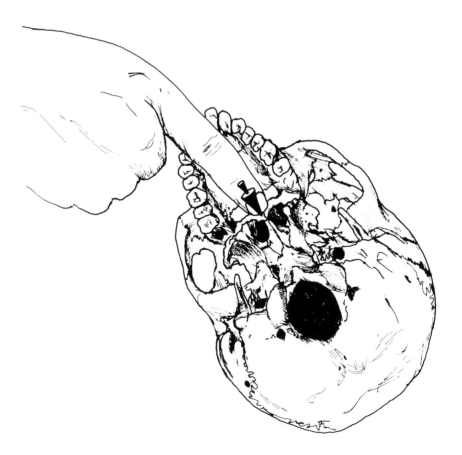

Fig. 3-13 Interpalatine suture: contact points and applied direction of sutural monitoring

Palatomaxillary Suture

CONTACTS

> *Right hand:* The index and middle fingers contact the palatomaxillary suture left and right of the sagittal midline (Fig. 3-14).
>
> *Left hand:* Has no contacts.

MOBILIZATION

> The right hand employs W-level pressure in a rostral direction to the contact areas to monitor for sutural motion (Fig. 3-14).

PATIENT PARTICIPATION

> The subject moves the mandible from side to side.

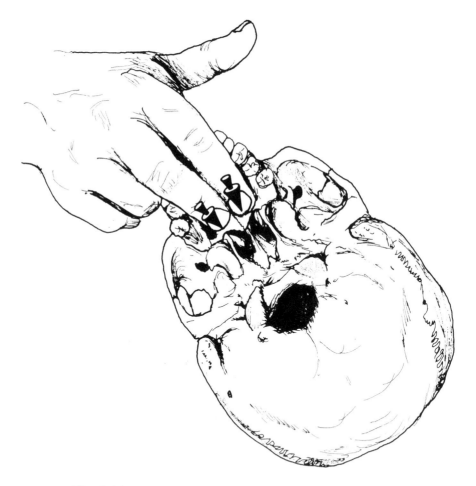

Fig. 3-14 Palatomaxillary suture: contact points and applied direction of sutural monitoring

Frontozygomatic Suture

CONTACTS

Right hand: Use hand posture two while the index finger contacts the suture's articular surface (Fig. 3-15).

Left hand: Use a mirror-image contact.

MOBILIZATION

Both hands employ medial W-level pressure to the contact areas to monitor for sutural motion (Fig. 3-15).

PATIENT PARTICIPATION

The subject moves the mandible from side to side.

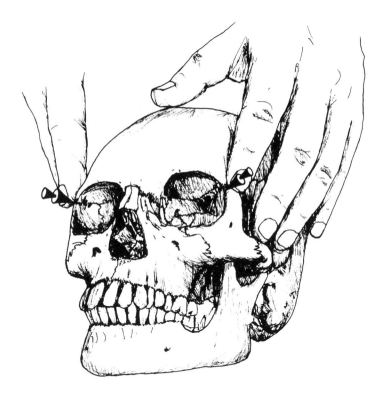

Fig. 3-15 Frontozygomatic suture: contact points and applied direction of palpatory pressure

Nasomaxillary Suture

CONTACTS

Right hand: Use hand posture three while the index finger contacts the suture's articular surface (Fig. 3-16).

Left hand: Use a mirror-image contact.

MOBILIZATION

Both hands employ posterior W-level pressure to the contact areas to monitor for sutural motion (Fig. 3-16).

PATIENT PARTICIPATION

The subject moves the mandible from side to side.

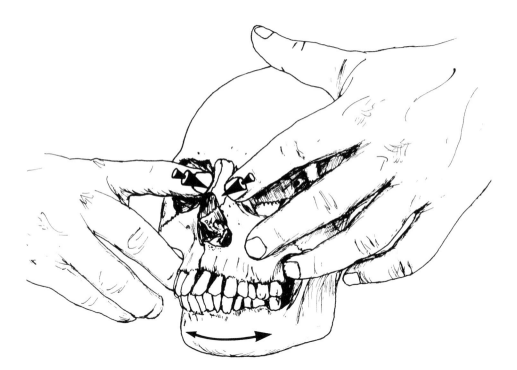

Fig. 3-16 Nasomaxillary suture: contact points and applied direction of palpatory pressure

Internasal Suture

CONTACTS

Right hand: The thumb or index finger contacts the suture's articular surface (Fig. 3-17).

Left hand: Has no contacts.

MOBILIZATION

The right hand employs W-level force in a posterocaudal direction on the contact area to monitor for motion (Fig. 3-17).

PATIENT PARTICIPATION

The subject moves the mandible from side to side.

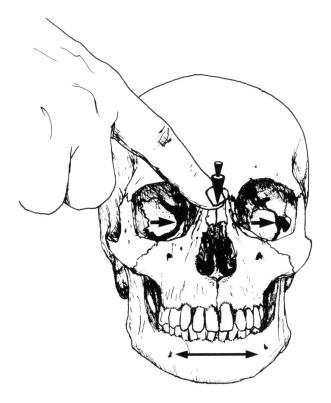

Fig. 3-17 Internasal suture: contact points and applied direction of palpatory pressure

Frontomaxillary Suture

CONTACTS

Right hand: Use hand posture three while the index finger contacts the suture's articular surface (Fig. 3-18).

Left hand: Use a mirror-image contact.

MOBILIZATION

Stabilize the contacts with W-level pressure while monitoring for sutural motion (Fig. 3-18).

PATIENT PARTICIPATION

The subject holds the mouth slightly open while moving the mandible from side to side.

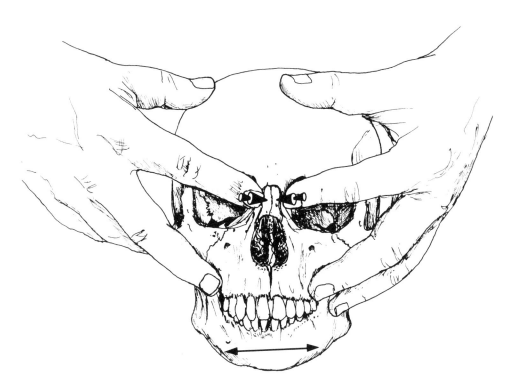

Fig. 3-18 Frontomaxillary suture: contact points and applied direction of palpatory pressure

Frontonasal Suture

CONTACTS

Right hand: Use hand posture three while the index finger contacts the suture's articular surface (Fig. 3-19).

Left hand: Use a mirror-image contact.

MOBILIZATION

Employing W-level pressure, both hands stabilize the contacts while monitoring for sutural motion.

PATIENT PARTICIPATION

The subject holds the mouth slightly open while moving the mandible from side to side.

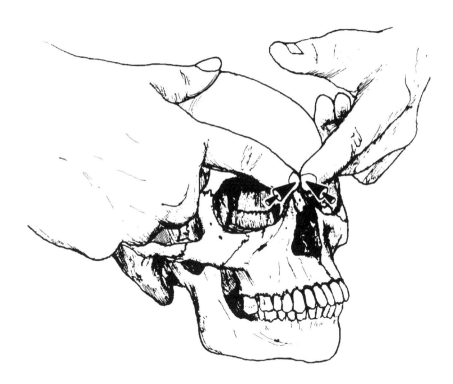

Fig. 3-19 Frontonasal suture: contact points and applied direction of palpatory pressure

References

1. DeJarnette MB. *Cranial Manual*. Nebraska City, NE: Sacro-Occipital Technique Organization, 1979–1980:39–40.
2. Pritchard JJ, Scott JH, Girgis FG. The structure and development of cranial facial sutures. *J Anat* 1956;90:73–85.
3. Meikle MC, Sellers A, Reynolds JJ. Effects of tensile mechanical stress on the synthesis of metalloproteinases by rabbit coronal sutures in vitro. *Cal Tissue Int* 1980;30:77–82.

Chapter Four

Passive Kinetic Sutural Palpation

Theory and Purpose

ALTHOUGH THE OSSEOUS structure of a suture can move independently, the network of interlocking bevels, corrugations, and gliding planes creates a communal interplay of sutures throughout the skull. However, as noted in Chapter 3, this communal interplay between the sutures may cause distortion and interfere with the practitioner's investigation when the subject's head is placed in a recumbent posture during static or active kinetic palpation. This distortion arises because of the effect of gravity on the intercranial structures as well as the low-level aberrant interactions between sutures that are created by the resistance to the headpiece. Since the goal of the practitioner is to determine the nature of the sutural interarticular seams, these factors will likely skew the results and lead to incorrect diagnoses. However, with passive kinetic palpation, the examiner uses pressure that exceeds the low-level forces exerted by gravity and resistance to the headpiece. Consequently, the examiner can bypass the factors that confuse static and active kinetic palpation. In passive kinetic analysis, the examiner can position the subject's head in any convenient posture without concern for low-level reactions.

In passive kinetic palpation, the patient is instructed to relax and breathe normally. The patient is passive while the practitioner creates motion within the sutural system by applying force to the maxilla through the crown surface of the posterior molars, since this region can be easily accessed. Close observation of the maxilla shows that it itself has little or no *direct* effect on the sutures of the cranial vault. However, because of its associated structures, it can influence other sutures, and it therefore becomes clear why it is chosen. The maxilla directly articulates with the frontal bone along its frontal process at the nasion. The maxilla indirectly associates with the sphenoid via the vomer, ethmoid, and zygomatic bones, and with the temporal bone along the zygomatic arch. Consequently, this latter association may influence the remaining vault sutures since the temporal bone directly articulates with all cranial vault structures except the frontal bone. As for the facial system, the maxilla has a direct association with all the facial bones. Because of all of these connections, this bone is the most obvious choice for use in passive kinetic palpation.

To apply this procedure, the maxilla is torqued in four directions—left to right, right to left, anterior, and posterior—while the sutures are individually palpated for their reactions. Although the sutures move in multidirectional planes, my observations have shown that each maxillary maneuver results in a single identifiable response. *Side-to-side* movements create identifiable inward rotation with the closing of the suture on the side that the maxilla is drawn toward, and outward rotation with the opening of the suture on the side from which the maxilla is drawn away. *Anterior* and *posterior* movements cause associated flexion and extension of the osseous structures and promote gliding along the suture's articular seams.

However, if we look at the sutures' multidirectional capacity for movement, gliding is apparently not the only motion that results from anterior and posterior movement of the maxilla. An example of this can be seen in the associated motions of the sphenofrontal and squamoparietal sutures. As the maxilla is directed posteriorly, the sphenoid bone is coerced in an anterosuperior direction into the frontal bone's inferior articular margin, and the superior border of the temporal squama is shifted in a posterosuperior direction against the parietal bone's inferior margin. Consequently, it may be noted that while the two sutures move in diametrically opposite directions, both glide in a superior direction along their articular seams. This is also seen when the maxilla is drawn in an anterior direction, causing the sphenoid bone to shift in a posteroinferior direction while the temporal squama moves in a anteroinferior direction. Here again the two sutures appear to oppose each other while they perform a similar movement—gliding. In summary, the maxilla is the most obvious cranial structure to use when performing passive kinetic palpation because of its association with all the cranial bones, and because the interlocking sutural network can carry the motion of the maxilla to a wide area.

However, when sutural aberrations are present, the remaining sutures respond by increasing their metabolic activity, resulting in the deposition of articular protein and, eventually, in interarticular tension. This compensatory reaction dampens interarticular mobility and can mislead the examiner concerning the health of the sutures. However, since the level of pressure used in passive kinetic palpation exceeds the level of sutural interarticular tension, the examiner can focus on the affected sutures and bypass the remaining sutures. For example, fixation or aberrant behavior of the sphenofrontal suture may lock these two bones. Thus, during the passive kinetic examination, the frontal and sphenoid bones will respond in unison as the maxilla is drawn to any one of the four primary examining directions. I have noticed that the remaining sutures, in contrast, are not subject to the same degree of stress. Consequently, since the force that is applied during passive kinetic palpation exceeds the level of tension found in the remaining sutures, they respond independently and will not affect the analysis of the primary aberration.

When to Apply Passive Kinetic Palpation

Although this examination may be performed at any time, it is recommended that it be done following the static and active kinetic palpation procedures discussed in Chapters 2 and 3, respectively. Because of the nature of this examination, examine one side of the skull at a time. The following procedures refer to the examination protocol for one side only. To examine the opposite side, simply switch sides and perform mirror-image procedures.

Practitioner-Patient Examining Posture

The patient is supine. The head rests on a supportive pillow and is turned to expose the side to be examined. The practitioner stands or sits, facing the patient's face. The hand closest to the patient's feet is used to move the maxilla (Fig. 4-1). The hand postures and pressure codes used in this section were described in the Introduction.

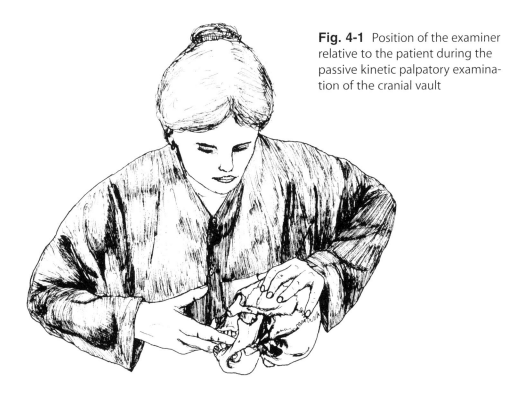

Fig. 4-1 Position of the examiner relative to the patient during the passive kinetic palpatory examination of the cranial vault

Note: Many treatment tables contain a bifurcating head support. Although the supports are built to aid in the comfort of the patient when prone, they may prove to be harmful when the patient is supine. This is due to the uneven surface and is true even when the head support is able to close, as found in most chiropractic adjusting tables. Even when the head supports are fully closed, the surface still dips where the two pieces come together. This dip creates a wedged furrow into which the head may sink. Should this occur while the patient is supine, the net result may be compression along the lateral borders of the occiput or the temporal mastoids. This could conceivably overextend the occiput and lock the vault, as discussed in the Theory and Purpose section in Chapter 2. To avoid this problem, the practitioner is encouraged to use a small support pillow such as the ones supplied on airplanes, or the Tempur-Pedic™ pillow, also noted in that chapter.

Cranial Vault Palpation

Passive kinetic palpation cannot be done simultaneously bilaterally. Unlike the bilateral comparative method used during static palpation, passive kinetic palpation requires that the practitioner use one hand for palpation and the other to generate motion. For all the bilateral sutures discussed here, the procedure given is for the left sutures. To examine the right half, the examiner reverses hands and performs the mirror-image actions.

Coronal Suture

Because of the average length of this suture, palpation is often cumbersome when the practitioner attempts to analyze the entire surface area with one hand. Thus the examiner is encouraged to divide the suture into right and left halves and examine each side separately.

CONTACTS

Right hand: The index and middle fingers bilaterally grasp the crown surface of the maxilla's posterior molars (Fig. 4-2a).

Left hand: Use posture two while the index finger palpates the entire left articular marginal surface of the suture. The middle finger parallels the index finger and occupies the entire parietal border posterior to the suture (Fig. 4-2b).

MOBILIZATION

Right hand: Use W⅓R-level pressure to gently rock the maxilla from side to side and anterior to posterior.

Left hand: Use W-level pressure to monitor the shifting motion along the suture's margins.

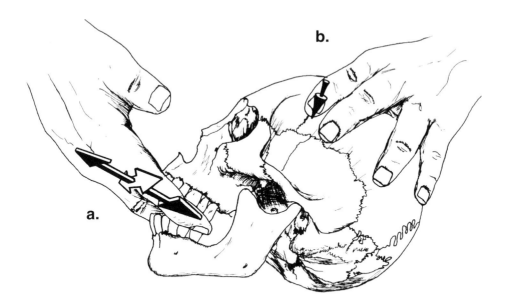

Fig. 4-2 Coronal suture: passive kinetic palpation

Sphenofrontal Suture

CONTACTS

Right hand: The index and middle fingers bilaterally grasp the crown surface of the maxilla's posterior molars (Fig. 4-3a).

Left hand: Use hand posture two while the index finger contacts the articular surface of the suture (Fig. 4-3b).

MOBILIZATION

Right hand: Use W⅓R-level pressure to gently rock the maxilla from side to side and anterior to posterior.

Left hand: Use W-level pressure to monitor the shifting motion along the suture's margins.

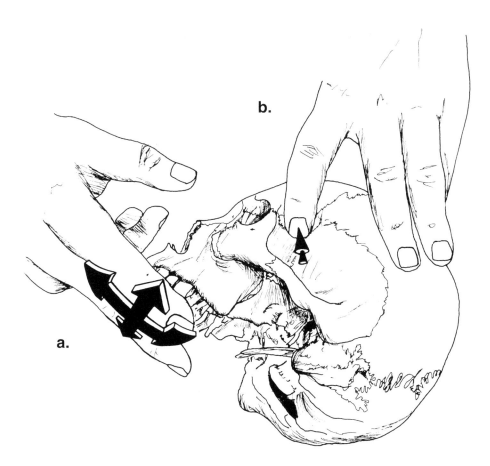

Fig. 4-3 Sphenofrontal suture: passive kinetic palpation

Sphenoparietal Suture

CONTACTS

Right hand: The index and middle fingers bilaterally contact the inferior crown surface of the maxilla's posterior molars (Fig. 4-4a).

Left hand: The distal phalangeal tip of the middle finger contacts the suture's articular surface (Fig. 4-4b).

MOBILIZATION

Right hand: Use W⅓R-level pressure to gently rock the maxilla from side to side and anterior to posterior.

Left hand: Use W-level pressure to monitor the shifting motion along the suture's margins.

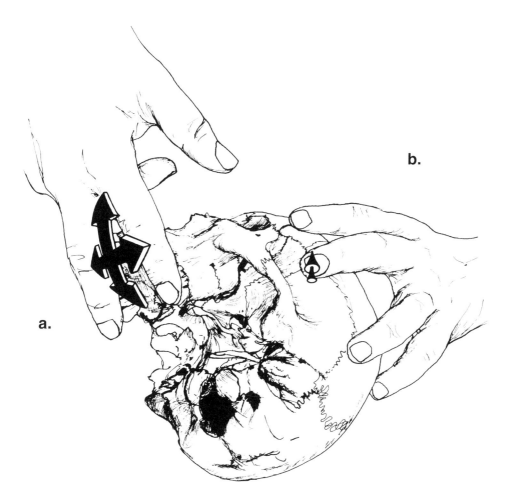

Fig. 4-4 Sphenoparietal suture: passive kinetic palpation

Sphenosquamous Suture

CONTACTS

Right hand: The index and middle fingers bilaterally grasp the crown surface of the maxilla's posterior molars (Fig. 4-5a).

Left hand: Use hand posture two while the middle finger contacts the entire longitudinal line of the suture's articular surfaces (Fig. 4-5b).

MOBILIZATION

Right hand: Use W⅓R-level pressure to gently rock the maxilla from side to side and anterior to posterior.

Left hand: Use W-level pressure to monitor the shifting motion along the suture's margin.

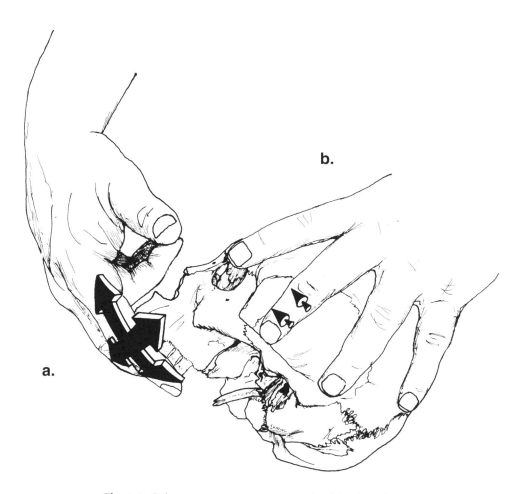

Fig. 4-5 Sphenosquamous suture: passive kinetic palpation

Squamoparietal Suture

CONTACTS

Right hand: The index and middle fingers bilaterally grasp the crown surface of the maxilla's posterior molars (Fig. 4-6a).

Left hand: Use hand posture two while the pads of the index, middle, and ring fingers contact the suture's articular surface (Fig. 4-6b).

MOBILIZATION

Right hand: Use W⅓R-level pressure to gently rock the maxilla from side to side and anterior to posterior.

Left hand: Use W-level pressure to monitor the shifting motion along the suture's margins.

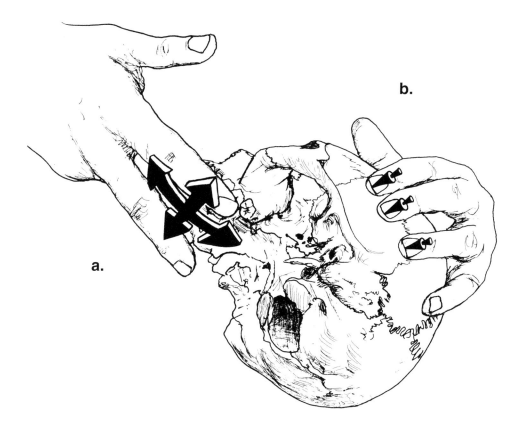

Fig. 4-6 Squamoparietal suture: passive kinetic palpation

Parietomastoid Suture

CONTACTS

Right hand: The index and middle fingers bilaterally grasp the crown surface of the maxilla's posterior molars (Fig. 4-7a).

Left hand: Use hand posture two while the index finger contacts the suture's articular surface (Fig. 4-7b).

MOBILIZATION

Right hand: Use W/R-level pressure to gently rock the maxilla from side to side and anterior to posterior.

Left hand: Use W-level pressure to monitor the shifting motion along the suture's margins.

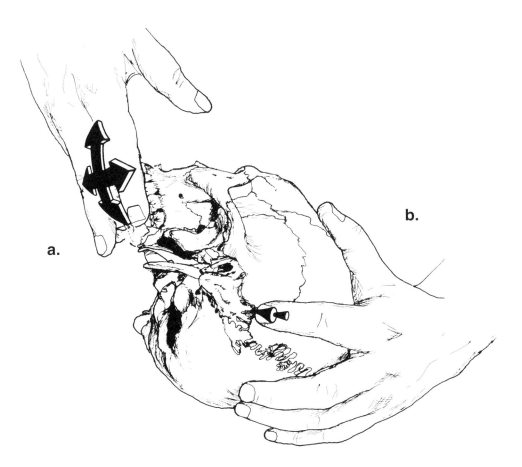

Fig. 4-7 Parietomastoid suture: passive kinetic palpation

Occipitomastoid Suture

CONTACTS

Right hand: The index and middle fingers bilaterally grasp the crown surface of the maxilla's posterior molars (Fig. 4-8a).

Left hand: Use hand posture one while the thumb extends caudally down the suture's articular surface (Fig. 4-8b).

MOBILIZATION

Right hand: Use W/R-level pressure to gently rock the maxilla from side to side and anterior to posterior.

Left hand: Use W-level pressure to monitor the shifting motion along the suture's margins.

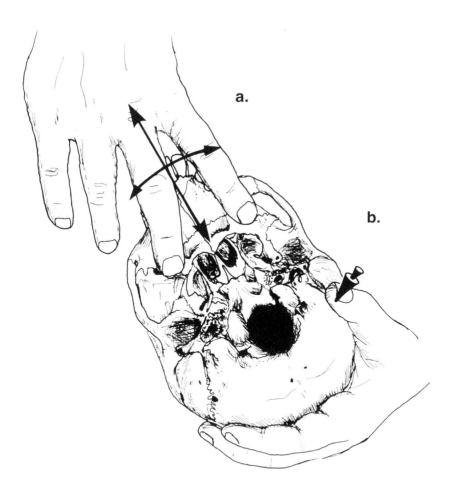

Fig. 4-8 Occipitomastoid suture: passive kinetic palpation

Lambdoid Suture

CONTACTS

Right hand: The index and middle fingers bilaterally grasp the crown surface of the maxilla's posterior molars (Fig. 4-9a).

Left hand: Use hand posture one. The hand rests over the parietal bone while the index, middle, and ring fingers contact the suture's articular surface (Fig. 4-9b).

MOBILIZATION

Right hand: Use W/R-level pressure to gently rock the maxilla from side to side and anterior to posterior.

Left hand: Use W-level pressure to monitor the shifting motion along the suture's margins.

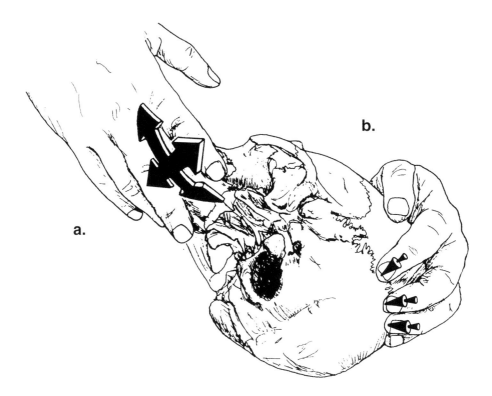

Fig. 4-9 Lambdoid suture: passive kinetic palpation

Sagittal Suture

For the sagittal suture, the examiner must approach the subject from a more caudal to rostral direction. For optimum inspection, the examiner is encouraged to divide the suture into anterior and posterior halves. Each half should be inspected separately.

CONTACTS

Right hand: The index and middle fingers bilaterally grasp the crown surface of the maxilla's posterior molars (Fig. 4-10a).

Left hand: Use hand posture four. Approach the sagittal suture over the temporal squamous bone and ascend over the parietal bone where the finger pads of the index, middle, and ring fingers contact the suture's articular surface (Fig. 4-10b).

MOBILIZATION

Right hand: Use W⅓R-level pressure to gently rock the maxilla from side to side and anterior to posterior.

Left hand: Use W-level pressure to monitor the shifting motion along the suture's margins.

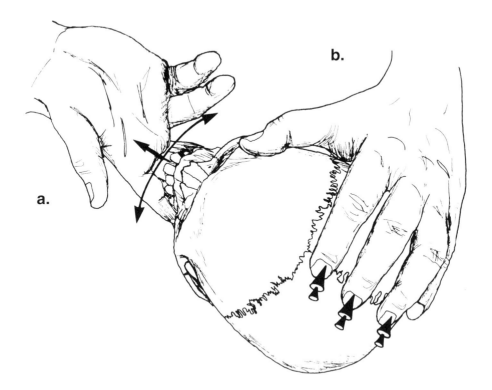

Fig. 4-10 Sagittal suture: passive kinetic palpation

Facial Palpation

Because of the close proximity of the facial sutures, the paired sutures can be simultaneously examined, and this practice is encouraged. The only exception is the zygomaticotemporal suture, because of its geographical location. This suture is still palpated as described above for the cranial vault sutures.

Practitioner-Patient Examining Posture

The subject's head faces the ceiling while the examiner approaches from a superior-lateral-rostral direction above the subject's right ear (Fig. 4-11).

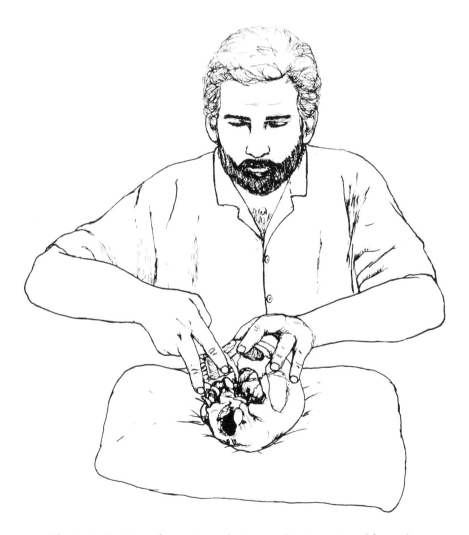

Fig. 4-11 Position of examiner relative to subject as viewed from above

Zygomaticotemporal Suture

CONTACTS

Right hand: The index and middle fingers bilaterally grasp the crown surface of the maxilla's posterior molars (Fig. 4-12a).

Left hand: Use hand posture two to support the lateral cranium while the index finger contacts the suture's articular surface (Fig. 4-12b).

MOBILIZATION

Right hand: Use W⅓R-level pressure to gently rock the maxilla from side to side and anterior to posterior.

Left hand: Maintain S¾W-level pressure. However, the index finger administers W-level pressure to monitor the shifting motion along the suture's margins.

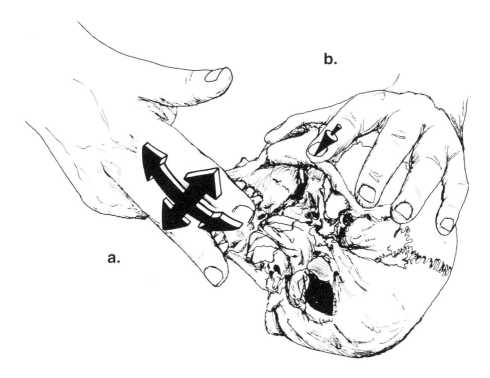

Fig. 4-12 Zygomaticotemporal suture: passive kinetic palpation

Zygomaticomaxillary Suture

CONTACTS

Right hand: The index and middle fingers bilaterally grasp the crown surface of the maxilla's posterior molars (Fig. 4-13a).

Left hand: Use hand posture one while the thumb contacts the right suture's articular surface and the index finger contacts the left suture's articular surface (Fig. 4-13b).

MOBILIZATION

Right hand: Use W⅓R-level pressure to gently rock the maxilla from side to side and anterior to posterior.

Left hand: Use W-level pressure to monitor the shifting motion along the suture's margins.

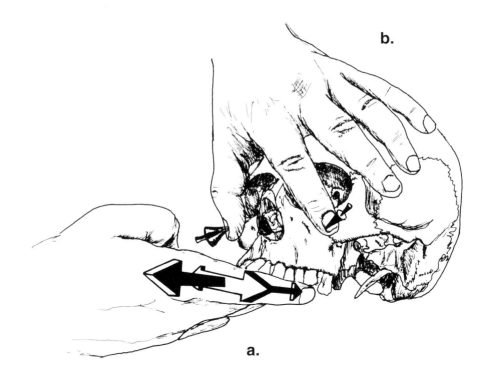

Fig. 4-13 Zygomaticomaxillary suture: passive kinetic palpation

Intermaxillary Suture

CONTACTS

Right hand: The thumb contacts the suture's articular seam (Fig. 4-14a).

Left hand: Use hand posture one; contacts the anterior squamous of the frontal bone (Fig. 4-14b).

MOBILIZATION

Right hand: Vary pressure W to W¾R to W and apply in a rostral direction. The action is performed over the suture's articular surface, and the contact is monitored for pliability.

Left hand: Stabilize the frontal squamous bone with W-level pressure.

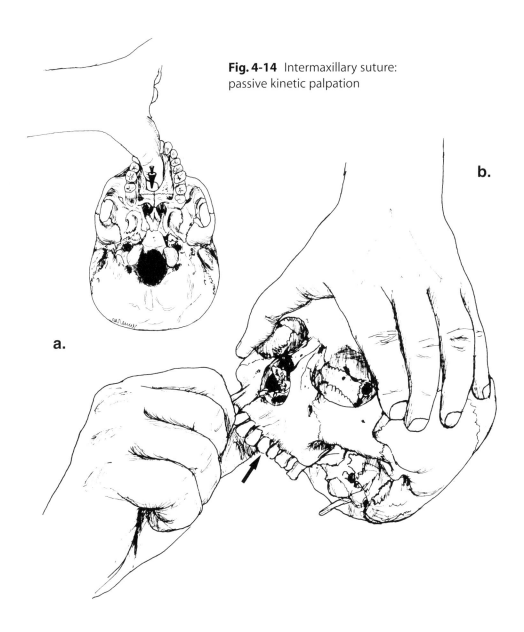

Fig. 4-14 Intermaxillary suture: passive kinetic palpation

Interpalatine Suture

CONTACTS

Right hand: The thumb or index finger contacts the suture's articular seam (Fig. 4-15a).

Left hand: Use hand posture one and contact the anterior squamous of the frontal bone (Fig. 4-15b).

MOBILIZATION

Right hand: The level of pressure varies from W to W⅓R to W and is applied in a rostral direction. The action is performed over the suture's articular surface and the contact is monitored for pliability.

Left hand: Stabilize the frontal squamous bone with W-level pressure.

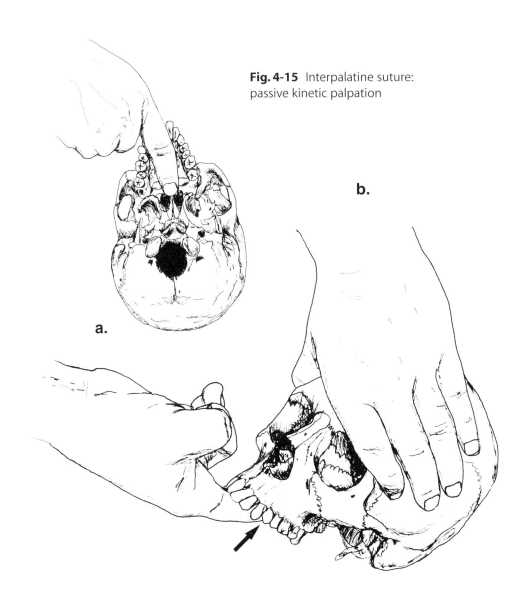

Fig. 4-15 Interpalatine suture: passive kinetic palpation

b.

a.

Palatomaxillary Suture

CONTACTS

Right hand: The index finger contacts the suture's left articular seam while the middle finger contacts the suture's right articular seam (Fig. 4-16a).

Left hand: Use hand posture one; contacts the anterior squamous of the frontal bone (Fig. 4-16b).

MOBILIZATION

Right hand: Vary the level of pressure intermittently from W to W⅓R. The action is performed over the suture's articular surface, and the contact is monitored for pliability.

Left hand: Stabilizes the frontal contact with W-level pressure.

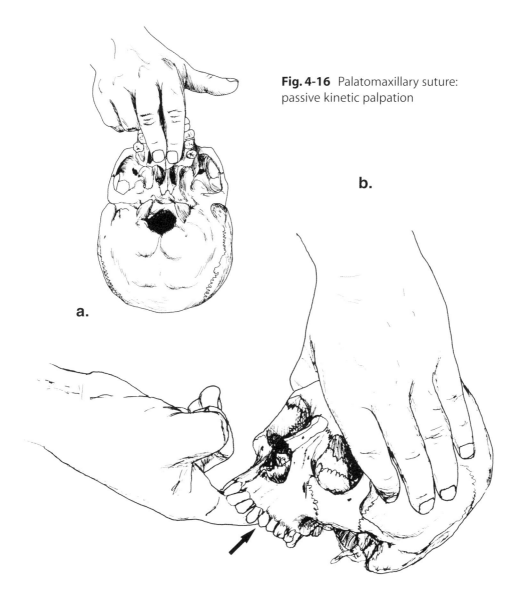

Fig. 4-16 Palatomaxillary suture: passive kinetic palpation

b.

a.

Frontozygomatic Suture

CONTACTS

Right hand: The index and middle fingers bilaterally grasp the crown surface of the maxilla's posterior molars (Fig. 4-17a).

Left hand: Use hand posture one over the frontal squama. The index finger contacts the left suture's articular surface and the thumb contacts the right suture's articular surface (Fig. 4-17b).

MOBILIZATION

Right hand: Use W-level pressure to gently rock the maxilla from side to side and anterior to posterior.

Left hand: Use W-level pressure on the suture's articular surfaces to monitor the shifting motion along the suture's margins.

Fig. 4-17 Frontozygomatic suture: passive kinetic palpation

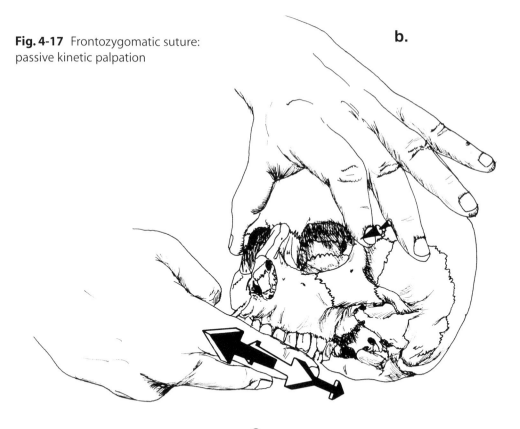

Nasomaxillary Suture

CONTACTS

Right hand: The index and middle fingers bilaterally grasp the crown surface of the maxilla's posterior molars (Fig. 4-18a).

Left hand: Use hand posture one while the index finger contacts the left suture and the thumb contacts the right suture (Fig. 4-18b).

MOBILIZATION

Right hand: Use W-level pressure to gently rock the maxilla from side to side and anterior to posterior.

Left hand: Use W-level pressure on the suture's articular surfaces to monitor for motion.

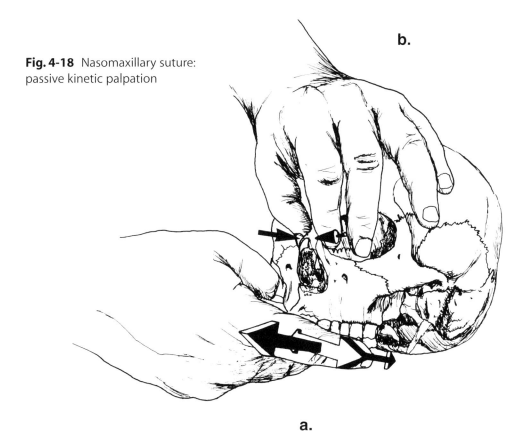

Fig. 4-18 Nasomaxillary suture: passive kinetic palpation

Internasal Suture

CONTACTS

Right hand: The index and middle fingers bilaterally grasp the crown surface of the maxilla's posterior molars (Fig. 4-19a).

Left hand: The index finger contacts the suture's articular surface (Fig. 4-19b).

MOBILIZATION

Right hand: Use W-level pressure to gently rock the maxilla side to side and anterior to posterior.

Left hand: Use W-level pressure on the suture's articular surfaces to monitor the shifting motion along the suture's articulating margins.

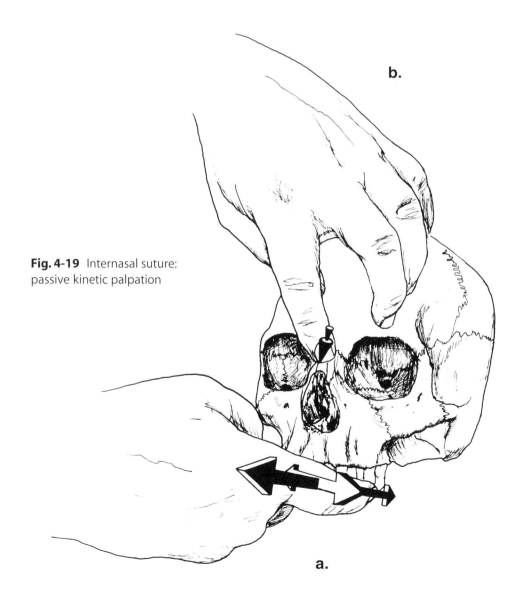

Fig. 4-19 Internasal suture: passive kinetic palpation

Frontomaxillary Suture

CONTACTS

Right hand: The thumb and index finger grasp the external surface of the maxilla above the alveolar processes of the teeth (Fig. 4-20a).

Left hand: The thumb and index finger contacts the right and left sutural articular surfaces, respectively (Fig. 4-20b).

MOBILIZATION

Right hand: Use side-to-side, rotational W-level pressure.

Left hand: Use W-level pressure to monitor the reciprocating motion between the articulating surfaces of the sutures.

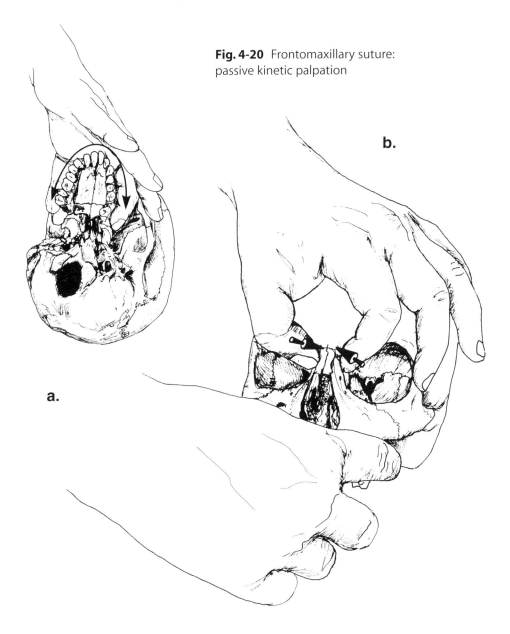

Fig. 4-20 Frontomaxillary suture: passive kinetic palpation

Frontonasal Suture

CONTACTS

Right hand: The thumb and index finger grasp the external surface of the maxilla above the alveolar processes of the teeth (Fig. 4-21a).

Left hand: The thumb and index finger contact the right and left sutural articular surfaces, respectively (Fig. 4-21b).

MOBILIZATION

Right hand: Use side-to-side, rotational W-level pressure.

Left hand: Use W-level pressure to monitor the reciprocating motion between the articulating surfaces of the sutures.

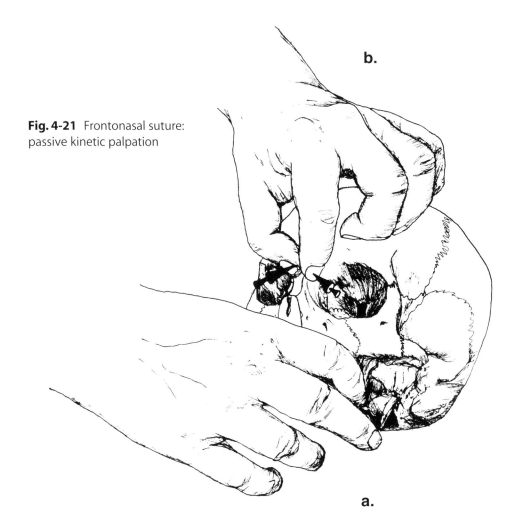

Fig. 4-21 Frontonasal suture: passive kinetic palpation

PART TWO

Sutural Morphology and Manipulative Strategies

Although many sutures exist within the human skull, not all are directly accessible. Therefore, to aid the reader in comprehending the subject matter, this section of the text has been divided into two primary subsections: *accessible* and *inaccessible* sutures. Chapter 5 addresses the palpably accessible sutures of the cranial vault, and Chapter 6 those of the face. Chapter 7 addresses the sutures that are inaccessible to direct palpation; that chapter has also been subdivided into the face and vault. Within each chapter, the morphological attributes, mobilizing behavioral characteristics, and manipulative strategies are presented for each suture. In addition, the suture's motion is described, and then illustrated in a set of paired images.

CHAPTER FIVE

Accessible Sutures of the Cranial Vault

A S SUTURES MATURE, they develop an elaborate interlocking communal network of overlapping bevels, corrugations, and gliding planes. Although conventional theories of sutural development arduously reject the notion of sutural motion, there have been numerous studies, in addition to those noted in the Introduction, that support the contention that sutures mature to allow for independent osseous mobility.[1-4] It is this inherent mobility that the practitioner needs to understand and use. Chapters 5, 6, and 7 present the reader with the necessary basic material for doing so.

Many cranial disciplines have evolved to address disorders of the human cranium, and each discipline has developed its own techniques, as outlined in the textbooks noted in the references to the Introduction. To date, I am aware of only one cranial technique, the SacroOccipital Technique (SOT), that includes a systematic exploration of the sutures as part of its analysis.[5] It appears that most techniques are more concerned with cranial rhythms or dural distortions and are less aware of the possible effects that sutural aberrations may have upon the treatment's outcome. Although the practitioner may frequently find patients who manifest the classic textbook conditions, many patients fall outside the standard text paradigms. These patients consequently require an approach that is individually tailored to their inherent needs. Therefore, to better equip the practitioner to address any aberrant conditions that may interfere with cranial manipulations, this text provides a comprehensive review of the following three areas:

1. The internal structural characteristics of each suture.
2. The pattern of motion of each suture as dictated by its morphological construction.
3. The contact areas and pressure that have the greatest probability of releasing or engaging the suture; these are based upon the suture's inherent motion patterns, which in turn are dictated by the suture's internal morphology.

Overview and Terminology

Morphology

Chapters 5, 6, and 7 begin with a morphologic description of each suture. Here, the reader is presented with a brief review of sutural morphology and terminology.

Sutures are the articular margins that exist between the bones of the skull. Separated by connective tissue, the articular junction of sutures appears to be inundated by an uncomplicated avascular ligamentous sheet of tissue. However, in 1956, Pritchard et al. uncovered five distinct layers in sutural interarticular junctions and defined their complex interarticular distribution.[6] They found that the interarticular bony surfaces are initially covered by a thin layer of flat osteogenic cells known as the cambium. Overlaying the cambium is a lamella of fibrous tissue known as the capsular layer. Both layers are part of the periosteum at the suture's outer marginal surface; they course through the suture as its periosteal layers until they reach the suture's inner marginal surface, where they integrate with the dura. A middle layer of loosely arranged fibrous connective tissue fills the gap between the two capsular layers; this middle layer contains thin-walled blood vessels deeply entrenched within its fibrous matrix. Branches from the veins in this region connect to the diploic vessels of the cranial bones, intercranial venous sinuses, and external venous supply to the scalp.

Primarily classified as juncturae fibrosae or synarthroses, sutures are divided into the following eight basic subcategories:

1. *Serrated sutures.* These sutures are noted for their sawtooth projections that cover the bony marginal edges along their articular seams. For example, the sagittal suture's serrated pointed ends allow for freedom of movement along the suture's articular junctions (Fig. 5-1).

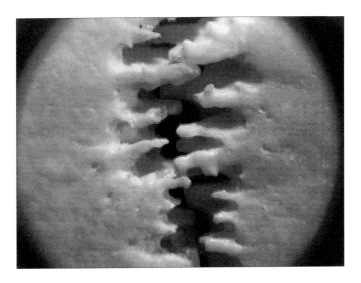

Fig. 5-1 Typical serrated articular seam in which the suture has been disarticulated to enhance the exposure. Note the exchange of sawtooth projections that extend from the suture's articular borders.

2. ***Denticulate sutures.*** These sutures are covered with teeth-like projections that characteristically widen as they approach their terminal end. This pattern is often found in the lambdoid suture; the widening serves to interlock the articular seam, stabilizing the suture from disarticulation (Fig. 5-2).

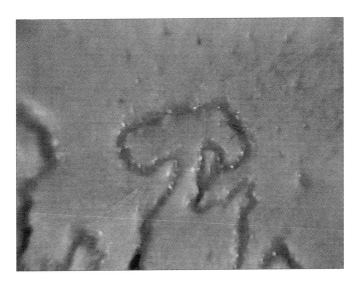

Fig. 5-2 Denticulated articular formation in the lambdoid suture. Note the widened terminal end of the serrated projection as it forms an interlocking union between the articular surfaces.

3. *Squamous sutures.* These sutures are characterized by overlapping articular surfaces as seen between the parietal and temporal bones (Fig. 5-3).

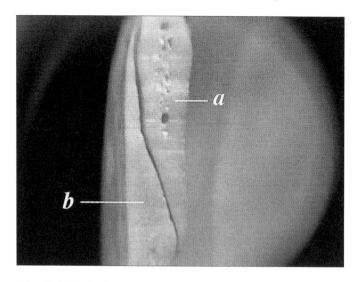

Fig. 5-3 Typical squamous articular union

    a. Internal bone with its smooth overlapped external beveled surface
    b. Outer overlapping bone with its beveled internal surface. Note that the
       articular union is basically smooth and absent of projecting structures.

4. *Limbous sutures.* These sutures are noted for their overlapping beveled
surfaces that are covered with serrated projections, as found along the articular junction of the coronal suture (Fig. 5-4).

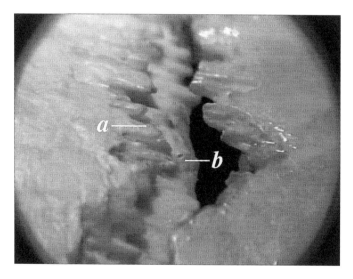

Fig. 5-4 Example of a limbous articulation as found in the
coronal suture

    a. Serrated projection extending from the frontal suture's
       articular margin
    b. Underlying continuation of the margin's beveled surface

5. *Plane sutures.* These sutures have junctures with simple apposition of contiguous surfaces. However, the surface is rarely smooth and is often covered by rough or irregular formations to provide protection against torsional forces that might produce articular shearing, for example, as found along the intermaxillary suture (Fig. 5-5).

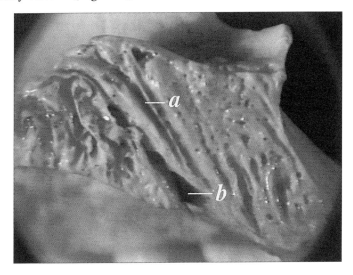

Fig. 5-5 Plane-type articular surface. Note that the general surface is flat but covered with irregular grooves, ridges, and sockets.

a. Groove and ridge formation
b. Grooved socket

6. *Schindylesis.* A schindylesis is characterized by a grooved bone which accommodates a ridged countersurface, for example, as found between the rostrum of the sphenoid and the vomer (Fig. 5-6).

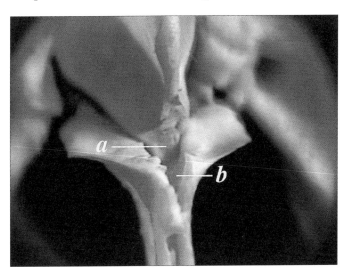

Fig. 5-6 Schindyletic articulation

a. Sphenoid's rostrum projection
b. Vomer's corresponding articular groove

7. *Gomphosis.* These articulations are characterized by a fibrous peg-and-socket type union. They are found primarily in the articular association between the teeth with the maxilla and mandible (Fig. 5-7).

Fig. 5-7 Partially sliced gomphotic articulation, exposing the typical peg-and-socket formation

a. Maxilla's socket bony surface
b. Projecting molar root peg

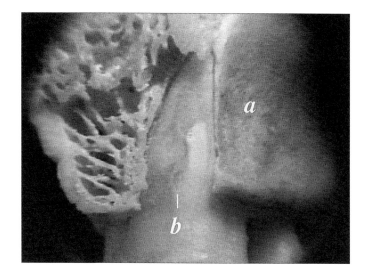

8. *Synchondroses.* These articulations are characterized by cartilaginous unions. Found in the chondrocranium, this articulation is associated with the sphenobasilar symphysis and fails to meet the interlocking criteria that would classify it as a true suture (Fig. 5-8).

Fig. 5-8 Lateral view of the synchondrosis articular union found between the sphenoid and occiput sutures. The cartilaginous tissue has been removed to expose the joint's articular seam. Note that this articulation is usually ossified in individuals in their late twenties.

a. Occiput
b. Sphenoid

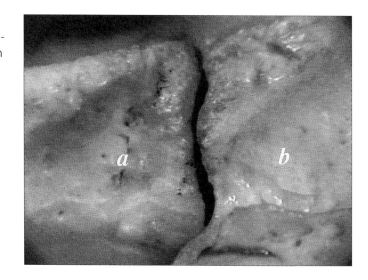

Visual Images Motion Review

The section on the morphology of each suture is followed by a discussion of the dynamics of the articular motion as dictated by the suture's structure(s). This description is then followed by a set of paired images. When viewed on their own, most images appear to be very similar, and distinguishing between them will be difficult. However, if the reader quickly looks back and forth between the images, the composite image will come alive, and the suture's motion will be discernible. An example of this can be seen in Figs. 5-11A and B. To observe the motion, first look at Fig. 5-11A and simply fix your eyes upon a chosen target along the suture's articular seam. Once the target has been selected, flip back and forth between this figure and the second image, Fig. 5-11B. This rapid movement between images will create an optical illusion that visually simulates the suture in motion.

Manipulative Strategies

For each suture, the discussion of motion is followed by a section on manipulative strategies. When addressing a suture's manipulative strategies, the reader will be given recommendations as to the optimal contact points and manipulative maneuvers to disengage or reengage the suture's articular seam.

Although the terms *disengaging* and *reengaging* are used within the confines of this text to describe the outcome of the recommended manipulative maneuvers, these terms do not actually imply that the practitioner is grossly disarticulating or rearticulating a suture. The term disengaging is used to depict the release of a suture from an aberrant locked behavior to one of mobile pliability, and the term reengaging is used to depict compressive articular stabilization of a suture's interarticular juncture.

Unlike the palpation sections in previous chapters, in which the specific finger contacts were indicated for the practitioner's systematic examination of the sutures, the reader will find that explicit finger placements and hand postures are not included in this section of the text. *The palpation sections in previous chapters were designed to give the practitioner a regimented protocol to ensure continuity in the sutural examination. However, the manipulative sections of Chapters 5, 6, and 7 do provide the optimal contact points and forces for disengaging or engaging sutures.*

As mentioned earlier, these maneuvers are based upon the sutures' patterns of motion, which in turn are dictated by their internal morphology. Because the choice of a particular hand postural application is dependent upon a suture's aberration, the text *could* provide the typical hand positions and finger locations for each suture's individual manipulative procedure. However, most cranial procedures appear to involve a variety of aberrant sutural combinations and are rarely restricted to one isolated aberrant suture. Thus, to give a specific hand posture for each suture's manipulation would be too restrictive, and often inappropriate, owing to the multitude of aberrant combinations. For example, the practitioner may find it necessary to release the coronal and sphenofrontal sutures simultaneously, or the practitioner may wish to release the coronal suture, stabilize the sphenofrontal suture, and close the squamoparietal suture. While both procedures include releasing the coronal suture, they also are concerned with other sutures as well. This means that the practitioner will use the same coronal contact points during both procedures to release the coronal suture. However, the means by which the practitioner can reach the key contact points vary as the hands alter their postures to adapt to the two aberrant combinations mentioned in the example above.

From the information presented in Chapters 5, 6, and 7, the practitioner will gain a broader understanding of the interarticular and associated articular functional dynamics of sutures. Therefore, should aberrant articular formations or behaviors interfere with a cranial maneuver, the practitioner can use this information to devise a method using associated articular maneuvers to address or bypass the aberration. Consequently, in such cases, the practitioner is released from the rigid constraints of individual techniques and liberated to alter the therapeutic approach to fit each patient's needs.

Tactical Applications

Tactical applications represent the methods for executing the manipulations. Although these tactics frequently vary from vibratory to rhythmic and from constant exertion to recoil, each tactical approach is compatible with the manipulative strategies offered in this manual. However, the use of each tactical approach is governed by the patient's inherent metabolic ability to sustain the maneuver's application. An example of this can be seen in two individuals possessing the same cranial lesion. One individual has a large frame, is very athletic, and possesses a strong metabolic capacity. The other is frail and small framed, and has a weak metabolic capacity. Whereas the larger and stronger individual may respond favorably to an aggressively forceful recoil maneuver, the smaller framed individual may metabolically fail to adapt and consequently undergo exacerbation of the condition upon aggressive treatment.

As implied by the aforementioned example, the practitioner should be aware of ascertaining the patient's metabolic potential. In addition, the practitioner should ensure that any contemplated manipulative techniques comply with the following rules of contraindication:

1. Vibratory or recoil maneuvers should not be performed on a hypotensive or frail subject. These procedures are frequently too aggressive for the subject's metabolic capacity and often result in adverse repercussions.
2. Consistently firm maneuvers should not be performed on subjects that are hypertensive, myotonic, or anxious; this will save the subject from excessive exacerbation of their condition due to aggravated metabolic irritation.

If the practitioner's tactics comply with these rules, the practitioner will find that the approach used in this text is compatible with a wide variety of technique styles.

Degree of Applied Pressure

The degree of pressure that should be applied is primarily dictated by the sutural articular formations and, in this text, is incorporated within the sections on manipulative strategies; the descriptions represent generic guidelines. However, depending on the type of aberration encountered and on the patient's metabolic or structural constitution, the suggested degree of force may vary. Therefore, in accordance with my observations of sutural manipulative responses, the recommended levels of force prescribed in this text reflect the most benign levels that will move the sutural articular unions.

Identification of Aberrations

The subject of identifying aberrations is not covered in the manipulative strategies' portion of this text. However, the reader is reminded that the palpable distinctions used to identify sutural aberrations are given in the text's palpation section. Therefore, the reader should refer to Chapter 1 for information concerning the palpatory assessment of aberrant formations and articular manifestations. For information about the sutures' normal topographical location and unique distinguishable characteristics, see Chapter 2; Chapter 3 should be referenced for information on examining protocols for detecting the flexibility of sutures. Unfortunately, palpatory methods for the inaccessible sutures of the vault and face are not covered in this text because of their inaccessibility. Consequently, readers are referred to the various cranial techniques cited in references 16~22 in the Introduction. These references contain information for diagnosing the presence of lesions and their locations according to symptomatic and functional presentation. However, if aberrant lesions are deemed to be present and if the subject fails to respond to the recommended conservative maneuvers, the practitioner can obtain further information about the presence of inaccessible aberrant formations through radiographic and magnetic imaging studies. In such cases, the morphological descriptions presented in this text can be used to aid the practitioner in identifying the aberrant lesions, and the manipulative strategies may consequently help in developing an alternate treatment approach.

Pressure Variations between Disengaging and Reengaging Sutures

Throughout my many years of sutural manipulation I have frequently noticed that the force necessary to generate sutural disengagement and reengagement did not always match. In fact, the force amplitude was primarily dictated by the suture's articular morphology and metabolic capacity. An example of this can be seen in the following section on the coronal suture where the pressure used to disengage the suture is not identical to the pressure needed to reengage it. In this example, the morphology of the suture is such that its rostral overlapping articular surface and serrated interdigitations are shallower than those found in the inferolateral regions. Consequently, the amplitude of force needed to reengage the suture's rostral portion is dictated by the shallowness of the suture's superior articular surface; thus, less pressure is required than is need when disengaging. To help the reader better understand the reasons behind the various forces used during each manipulative maneuver, it is suggested that the reader refer to the section "Pressure Application Techniques" in the Introduction, where the levels of applied pressure are described and their functional purposes are given.

  As just noted, the level of applied pressure needed for disengagement and reengagement can vary for most sutures. Therefore, many of the sections on manipulative strategies in Chapters 5, 6, and 7 are divided into the contacts and manipulations needed for articular disengagement and reengagement. This makes the different approaches clear.

Vault Sutures

Coronal Suture (Singular)

MORPHOLOGY

  Located posterior to the frontal bone's squamous and anterior to the two parietal bones, the coronal suture crosses over the top of the vault and shifts slightly in an anterior direction as it descends toward the superior aspect of the sphenoid's greater wings. The suture is beveled to interlock the frontal bone's articular junction with the parietal bones and is covered with anteroposterior serrations, embellished with pin-to-socket couplings.

  Traditionally, the entire suture has been divided into three equal portions (Fig. 5-9A). The upper medial third (around the bregma) consists of the region where the frontal bone overlaps the parietal bones, and the lower lateral third consists of the region where the parietal bones overlap the frontal bone. However, this division can be misleading and may obstruct attempts to disengage the suture's articular tension.

  A more accurate division requires a gross bisection of the suture into right and left halves. Each half is then further subdivided into thirds (Fig. 5-9B). With this new divisional concept, the superior third (nearest to the bregma) consists of the region where the frontal bone, beveled along its internal articular surface, overlaps the parietal bones (Fig. 5-10A). In the

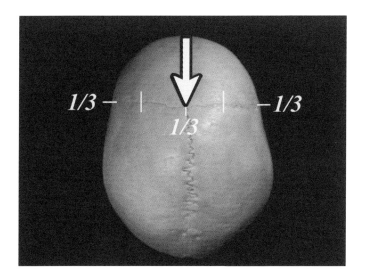

Fig. 5-9A Superior view of the coronal suture, illustrating its topographic location and the original three divisions

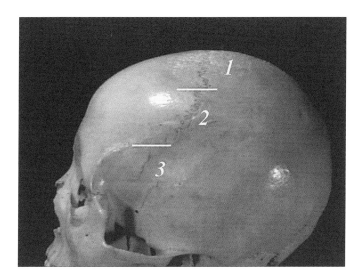

Fig. 5-9B Lateral view, illustrating the left half of the coronal suture and its partition into three distinct subdivisions

second third, the beveled articular surfaces undergo a transition whereby they alternate overlaps, creating a region of marginal interlocking (Fig. 5-10B). *Note:* Because of the interlocking nature of the surfaces in this region, surface contacts here are discouraged as they tend to inhibit or abort most attempts at releasing coronal tension. In the final inferior third, the suture undergoes a complete articular reversal as the frontal bone is fully overlapped by the parietal bones (Fig. 5-10C).

Fig. 5-10A Sagittal slice, illustrating the superior third of the coronal suture

a. Overlapping beveled surface of the frontal bone
b. Internal beveled articular surface of the parietal bone, which is overlapped by the frontal bone

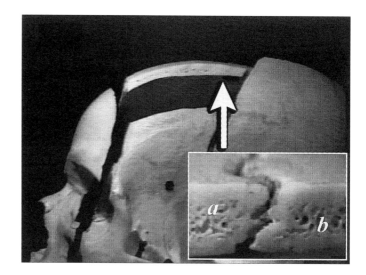

Fig. 5-10B Axial slice as viewed from the superior direction: the middle third of the coronal suture, depicting the alternating articular overlaps

a. Frontal bone
b. Parietal bone

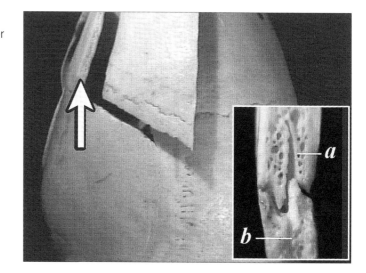

Fig. 5-10C Axial slice as viewed from the superior direction: the inferior third of the coronal suture, depicting the external overlap of the parietal bone onto the frontal bone's articular surface

a. Frontal bone
b. Parietal bone

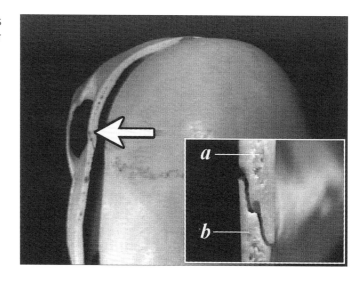

MOTION

Because of the suture's morphology, that is, the anteroposterior configuration of the suture's serrations, gliding along its articular margins occurs in an anteroposterior direction (Fig. 5-11).

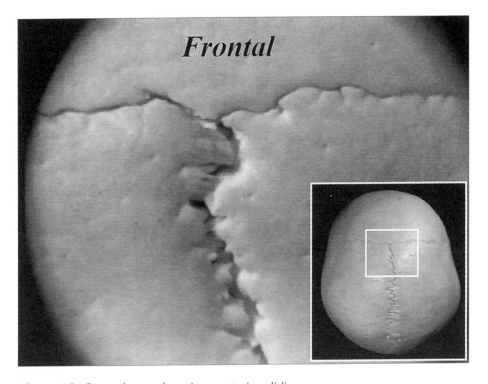

Fig. 5-11A Coronal sutural motion: posterior gliding

Compare with next photo ➡

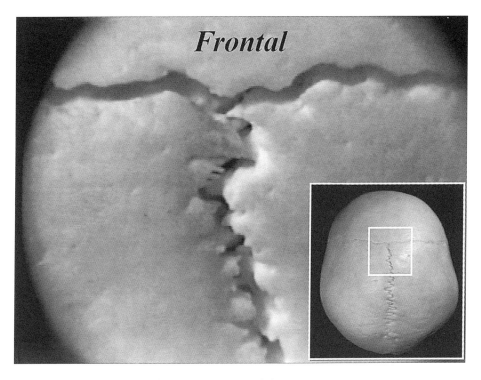

Fig. 5-11B Coronal sutural motion: anterior gliding

Articular Disengagement

CONTACTS

The optimal contacts to release the coronal suture are located along the right and left inferolateral surface of the frontal bone, anterior to the suture and above the medial sagittal region of the parietal bones (posterior to the bregma) (Fig. 5-12).

MANIPULATION

W⅓R-level force on the frontal bone's contacts coerces them in an anteromedial direction to disengage the inferolateral articular surface of the frontal bone from the overlapping beveled surface of the parietal bone. With W⅓R-level force, the parietal's contacts are simultaneously directed in a caudal-posterior direction, disengaging them from the underlying beveled articular surface (Fig. 5-12). *Note:* Medial compression of the frontal bone's contacts will cause arching of the frontal bone's superior sagittal region, thus indirectly lifting the overlapping frontal bone from the parietal's articular surface. Coincidentally, the caudal pressure directed into the parietal contacts will indirectly cause the inferior overlapping articular surfaces of the parietal bones to disengage from the frontal bone.

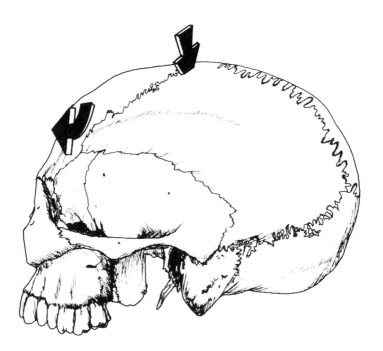

Fig. 5-12 Contact points and directions of manipulation (arrows) to release the coronal suture

Articular Reengagement

CONTACTS

The contacts are located along the right and left lateral parietal surface, no more than 2cm above the sphenoid's greater wings, and posterior to the coronal suture. The other contacts are anterior to the suture along the superomedial third of the frontal bone's squamous region (Fig. 5-13).

MANIPULATION

W-level pressure in a posterocaudal direction along the frontal bone's contact is used to engage the overlapping frontal-parietal articular surfaces. Simultaneous W/R-level force on the parietal contacts in an anteromedial direction compresses the articular surfaces together and reengages the joint's pin-and-socket couplings (Fig. 5-13). *Note:* Caudal pressure applied to the frontal bone's contact will flare the frontal bone's inferolateral borders externally and indirectly reengage the underlying articular surface of the frontal bone with the overlapping surface of the parietal bone. Similarly, medial compression of the parietal contacts will elevate the sagittal edges of the parietal bones and indirectly reengage the underlying parietal bones with the overhanging beveled edge of the frontal bone.

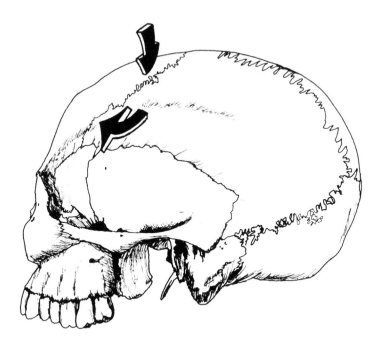

Fig. 5-13 Contact points and direction of manipulation (arrows) to reengage the coronal suture

Sphenofrontal Suture (Paired)

MORPHOLOGY

Located anterior to the coronal suture's junction with the sphenoid's greater wing, the sphenofrontal suture runs in an anterior direction along the superior rim of the sphenoid's greater wing and terminates at the junction of the zygomatic-frontal and zygomatic-sphenoid sutures (Fig. 5-14A). Observed externally, the suture appears to be superficial. However, upon disarticulation, the articular surface is noted to be triangular in shape with its broadest or deepest portion located along the suture's posterior aspect (Fig. 5-14B). The sphenoid's lateral articular surface is squamosal in nature and vertically descends (approximately 0.5cm) toward the suture's horizontal articular floor. Upon reaching the horizontal floor, the articular surface transforms into a dense field of serrated tongue-and-groove formations, extending obliquely from a posteromedial to anterolateral direction (Figs. 5-14B and C).

Figure 5-14A Location of the left sphenofrontal suture as viewed from the lateral plane of the vault (arrow)

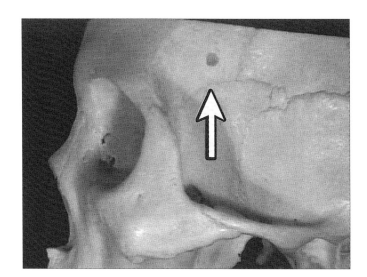

Fig. 5-14B Superior view of the sphenoid's right triangular articular surface: the arrow on the upper left image indicates the general posteromedial to anterolateral growth pattern of the suture's serrated projections

a. Lateral squamosal surface
b. Serrated articular surface

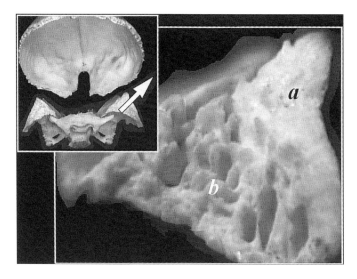

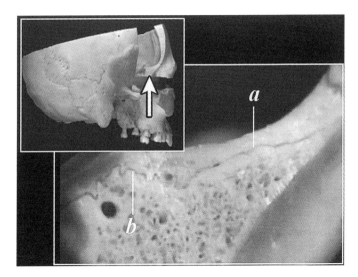

Fig. 5-14C Serrated articular junction of the right sphenofrontal suture when posteriorly exposed by a coronal slice through its articular seam

a. Lateral squamosal articular ledge
b. Internal serrated articular seam

MOTION

Because of the suture's morphology, gliding is encouraged in a posteromedial to anterolateral direction along its articular surface. However, the serrations' growth pattern also appears to discourage independent medial or lateral motion (Fig. 5-15).

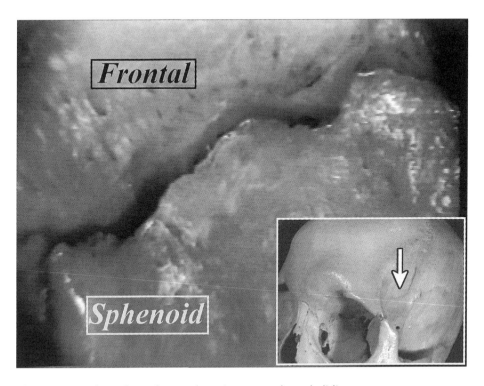

Fig. 5-15A Sphenofrontal sutural motion: anterolateral gliding

Compare with next photo ➡

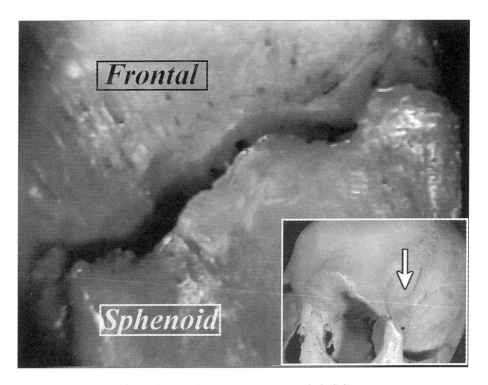

Fig. 5-15B Sphenofrontal sutural motion: posteromedial gliding

Articular Disengagement

CONTACTS

The contacts are located on the frontal bone in the depression posterior to the frontal zygomatic process and on the posterior aspect of the sphenoid's greater wing, crossing from the sphenosquamous suture to the anterior temporal squamous. *Alternative sphenoid contact:* The contact is located on the posteroinferior aspect of the pterygoid process, on the same side (ipsilateral) as the treatment (Fig. 5-16).

MANIPULATION

W-level force is employed on the frontal bone's contacts in an antero-cephalad direction while W⅓R-level force is used on the posterior sphenoid-temporal contact to stabilize the sphenosquamous suture in a postero-medial direction. *Note:* Care must be taken to avoid excessive pressure on the frontal bone's contact point. If excessive pressure is applied, it could bind the serrated articular surfaces and lock the suture. For this reason, the recommended pressure should never exceed W-level pressure.

Alternative manipulative procedure: The same frontal bone manipulative procedure is used in conjunction with W/R-anterolateral level pull on the posteroinferior region of the pterygoid process (Fig. 5-16). This procedure indirectly draws the sphenoid's greater wing in a posteroinferior direction and releases the sphenofrontal suture.

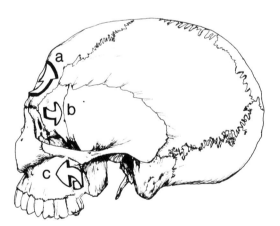

Fig. 5-16 Left posterolateral oblique view of the contact points used in disengaging the sphenofrontal suture (arrows depict direction of manipulation)

a. Frontal bone's contact superior to the sphenofrontal suture and anterior to the coronal suture
b. Contact is overlapping the sphenosquamous suture, supporting the posterior sphenoid's greater wing and anterior temporal's squamosal plate
c. Alternative sphenoid contact on the posteroinferior tip of the sphenoid's pterygoid process

Articular Reengagement

CONTACTS

The frontal bone's contact is the same as described for disengagement above. The practitioner can either contact the sphenoid over the center of its greater wing, or on the anteroinferior aspect of the pterygoid process, that is, the alternative approach described above (Fig. 5-17).

MANIPULATION

W-level pressure to the frontal bone's contact compresses the frontal bone's articular surface inferiorly toward the sphenoid's greater wing. W-level medial compression to the sphenoid's greater wing contact simultaneously unlocks the obliquely serrated tongue-and-groove formations of the suture. This allows the practitioner to then draw the sphenoid's greater wing in an anterosuperior direction, thus reengaging the suture's articular surface.

Alternative manipulative procedure: W/R-level pressure to the anteroinferior aspect of the pterygoid process elevates it in a superior-posterior direction (Fig. 5-17). This indirect procedure elevates the anterior portion of the sphenoid's greater wing and reunifies the sphenoid's serrations with the frontal bone's articular surface.

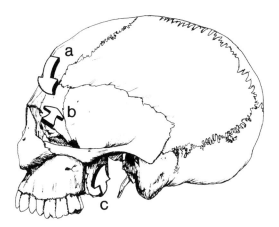

Fig. 5-17 Left posterolateral oblique view of the contacts on the sphenofrontal suture (arrows depict the direction of manipulation)

a. Frontal bone's contact superior to the sphenofrontal suture and anterior to the coronal suture
b. Contact on the center of the sphenoid's greater wing
c. Alternative sphenoidal contact on the anteroinferior aspect of the pterygoid process

Sphenoparietal Suture (Paired)

MORPHOLOGY

Like in the sphenofrontal suture, the parietal bone is overlapped along its externally beveled margin by the sphenoid's greater wing. Located posterior to the junction of the coronal suture with the sphenoid's greater wing (Fig. 5-18A), the sphenoparietal suture's articular surface is primarily squamosal and often contains wedges-to-trench projections deep within the suture's anteroinferior intracranial marginal surface. The wedge or ridge projections protrude from the articular surface of the parietal bone and extend in an anterior-caudal direction to insert within the shallow trenches along the sphenoid's adjacent surface (Figs. 5-18B~D).

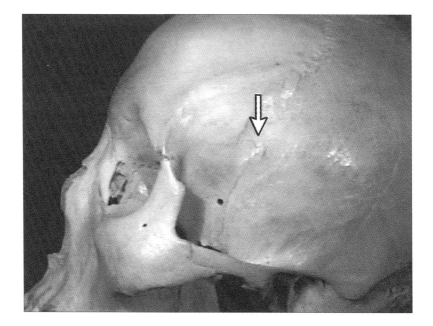

Fig. 5-18A Location of the sphenoparietal suture (arrow)

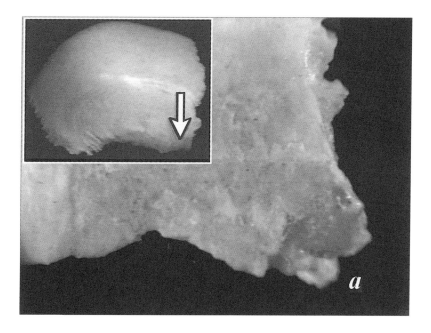

Fig. 5-18B Exposure of the parietal's articular surface when viewed from a lateral aspect

a. Parietal's anterocaudal wedge projections

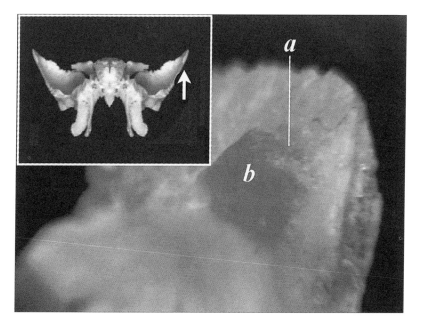

Fig. 5-18C Articular surface of the sphenoid's articular surface when viewed from a posterior aspect

a. Wedged shape trench that envelops the parietal's articular projections
b. Sphenoid's inner articular shelf that supports the parietal bone internally

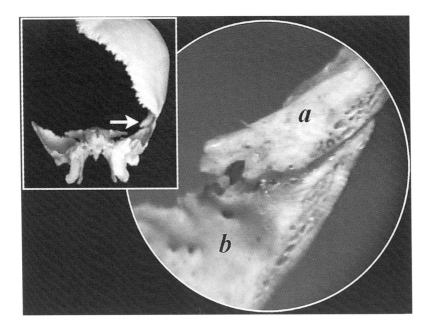

Fig. 5-18D Coronal slice of the right sphenoparietal suture, viewed from a posterior aspect

a. Parietal's articular surface
b. Sphenoidal articular surface

MOTION

Because of the presence and configuration of the suture's projecting wedge formations, the sphenoid's greater wing is restricted to anterosuperior or posteroinferior gliding over the parietal bone's articular surface. Although this movement is considered to be the suture's primary motion, the parietal bone can also glide independently in a posterosuperior direction under the sphenoid's greater wing. However, anterior, medial, and lateral motion would appear to interlock the suture's articular seam and thereby promote sphenoparietal articular stabilization (Fig. 5-19).

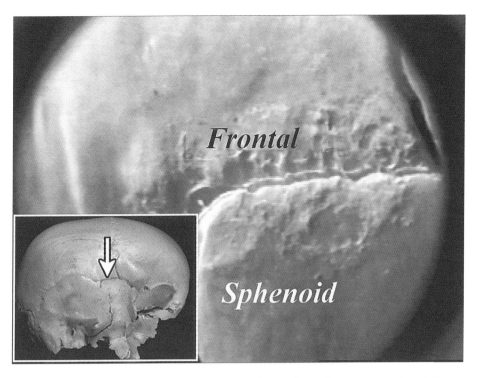

Fig. 5-19A Sphenoparietal sutural motion: sphenoid wing's anterosuperior gliding

Compare with next photo →

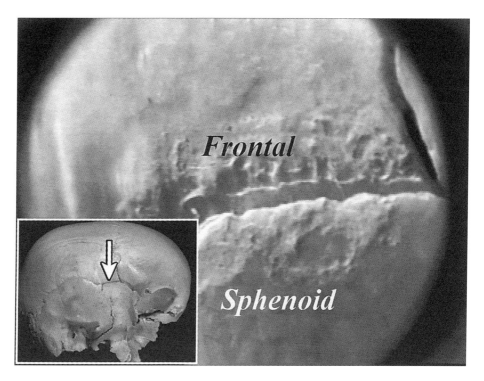

Fig. 5-19B Sphenoparietal sutural motion: sphenoid wing's posteroinferior gliding

Articular Disengagement

CONTACT

The contact is located on the parietal bone, posterior to the coronal suture's junction with the sphenoid's greater wing, and on the sphenoid's greater wing just superior to the zygomatic arch (Fig. 5-20).

MANIPULATION

W⅓R-level pressure on the parietal contact compresses the parietal's anterior angle medially to disengage the deeper wedged articular surfaces. The contact is then drawn in a superior direction to glide the parietal's internally beveled squamosal surface away from the sphenoid's articular border. The sphenoid's contact is simultaneously directed medially using W-level force to create an external flare of its superior articular border. This is followed by a caudal shift in the applied pressure to direct the sphenoid's parietal border away from the parietal's articular surface (Fig. 5-20). *Note:* This procedure is designed to disengage the suture's wedged borders first, permitting the practitioner to glide along the squamosal plates to separate the two suture's osseous borders.

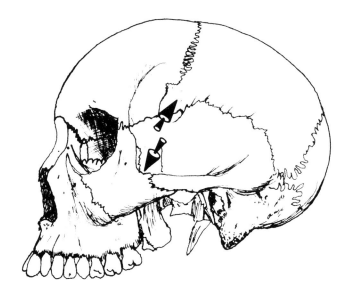

Fig. 5-20 Contact points and direction of manipulation (arrow) to release the sphenoparietal suture

Articular Reengagement

CONTACTS

Applied to the side of the involved suture, the optimal parietal contact is located posterior to the coronal suture, midway between the sagittal suture and the parietal's superior temporal line. The corresponding sphenoidal contact is applied below the involved sphenoparietal suture on the superior region of the sphenoid's greater wing (Fig. 5-21).

MANIPULATION

W⅓R-level pressure to the parietal contact is directed caudally toward the cerebral surface floor of the sphenoid's greater wing. This directional pressure will flare the lateral articular border of the parietal's sphenoidal angle and reengage the suture's wedged articular surface. Synchronous medial W-level force to the sphenoid's contact secures the sphenoid's greater wing against the bulging sphenoidal angle of the parietal bone. Maintaining W-level pressure, the practitioner then alters the sphenoid's contact in a superior direction. *Note:* The medial compression of the sphenoid's contact serves to resist the bulging force of the parietal bone and assists in reengaging the suture's wedged surface. The secondary superior force serves to realign and diminish the space along the suture's squamosal articular surface and thus completes the procedure (Fig. 5-21).

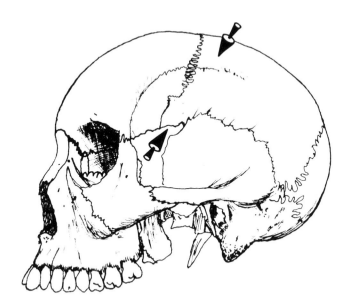

Fig. 5-21 Contact points and direction of manipulation (arrows) to reengage the sphenoparietal suture

Sphenosquamous Suture (Paired)

MORPHOLOGY

The sphenosquamous suture is located between the posterior articular margin of the sphenoid's greater wing and the anterior articular margin of the temporal bone (Fig. 5-22). Originating rostrally as a squamosal-type articular surface (Figs. 5-23A~C), the temporal bone externally overlaps the sphenoid's articular surface and descends caudally until it is adjacent to the superior rim of the zygomatic arch (Figs. 5-23A and B). As the suture exits the axial level adjacent to the arch's inferior border, the articulation is transformed from squamosal to serrated, and the temporal bone is caudally overlapped by the sphenoid's articular surface. This inferior portion of the suture continues its descent in a posteroinferior arc until its termination medial to the temporal mandibular joint (Figs 5-23B and D). Close observation of the serrated configuration reveals a posterolateral to anteromedial oblique pattern that runs parallel to the petrous portion of the temporal bone (Figs. 5-23E and F).

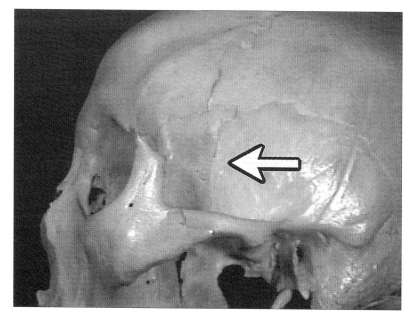

Fig. 5-22 Left lateral view of the left sphenosquamous suture (arrow)

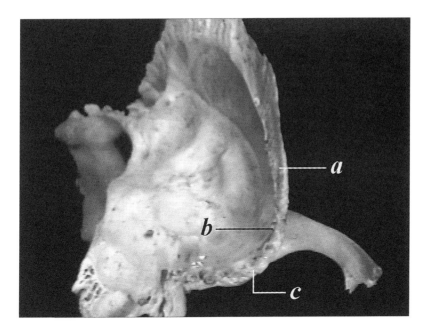

Fig. 5-23A Anteromedial view of the left temporal's articular border exposing the superior squamosal surface, the region of articular transition, and the inferior serrated surface. Note that the region of transition is level to the temporal's zygomatic process.

a. Squamosal articular surface　　　　c. Serrated articular surface
b. Articular transitional region

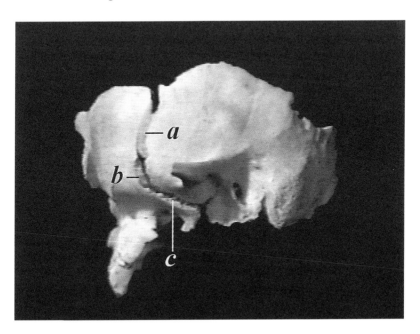

Fig. 5-23B Lateral view, exposing the temporal's superior external articular border, which overlaps the sphenoid above its zygomatic process, and the sphenoid's caudal external articular border, which overlaps the temporal from below

a. Squamosal articular surface　　　　c. Serrated articular region
b. Articular transitional region

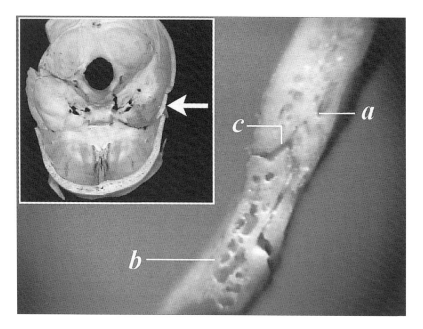

Fig. 5-23C Superior axial exposure of the left temporal-squamosal articular surface

a. Temporal bone

b. Sphenoid bone

c. Typical serrated projection extending from the sphenoid bone into the temporal's anterior articular border. Note that the single serrated projection extending from the sphenoid's articular margin is often developed by the third decade of life. Its growth pattern is parallel to that of the petrosal process and offers further evidence in support of the suture's anteromedial to posterolateral gliding motion.

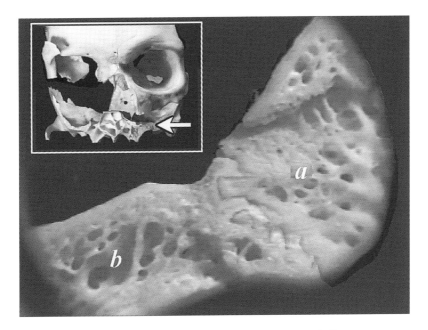

Fig. 5-23D Viewed from an anterior direction, a coronal slice exposes the inferior left sphenosquamous serrated articular junction as the sphenoid caudally externally overlaps the temporal bone

a. Temporal bone
b. Sphenoid bone

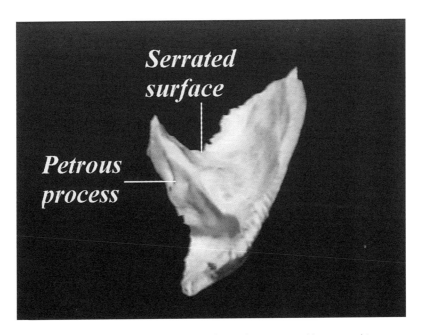

Fig. 5-23E Superior view, exposing the right temporal bone and its serrated articular surface relative to the temporal's petrosal process

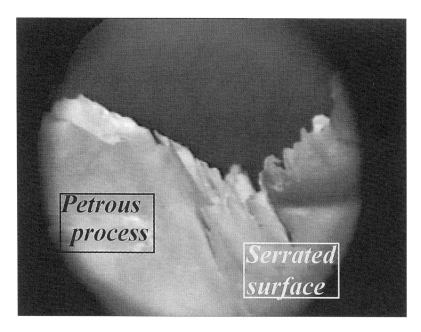

Fig. 5-23F Magnification of Fig. 5-23E. Note that the angle of the serrated teeth runs parallel to the petrosal process of the temporal bone.

MOTION

As often found in nature, a bone's development is usually dictated by its function. In the case of the serrated articular surface, the direction of serrated growth offers the least amount of resistance when the temporal bone is rocked obliquely in an anteromedial to posterolateral direction (parallel to the angular shape of the temporal petrous process). There is also some limited anteroposterior rotation (Figs. 5-24 and 5-25).

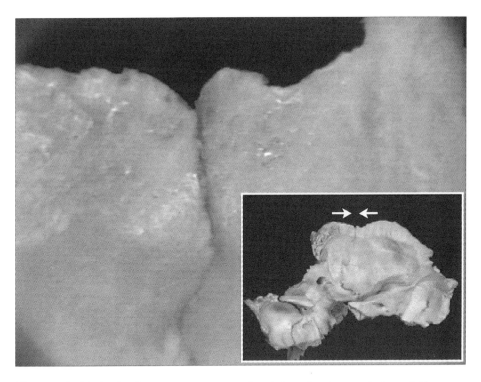

Fig. 5-24A Limited sphenosquamous rotation: internal anteroposterior rotation

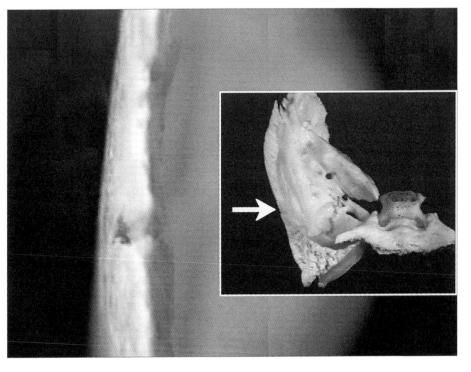

Fig. 5-25A Permitted sphenosquamous flaring: internal anteromedial flaring

Compare with next photos ➡

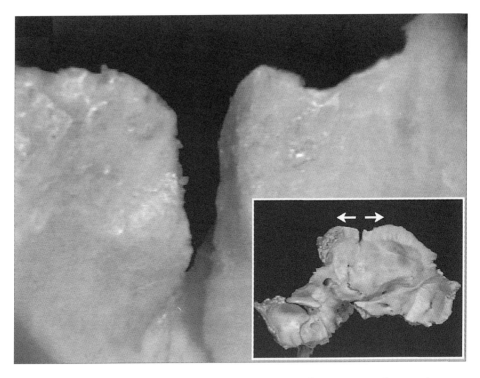

Fig. 5-24B Limited sphenosquamous rotation: external anteroposterior rotation

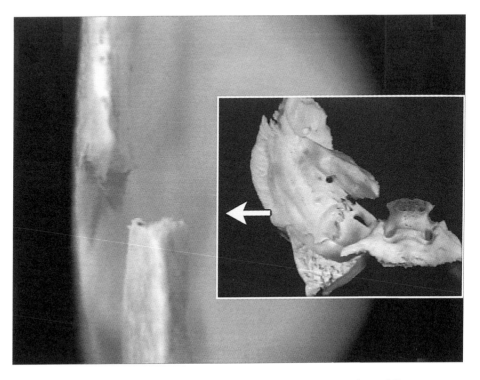

Fig. 5-25B Permitted sphenosquamous flaring: external posterolateral flaring

Articular Disengagement

CONTACTS

Because of the complex nature of this suture, the practitioner must first decide which portion of the suture to disarticulate. To open the entire articulation, the optimal contacts are anterior to the suture in the center of the sphenoid's greater wing above the zygomatic arch and anterior to the mastoid process of the temporal bone (Fig. 5-26).

MANIPULATION

W⅓R-level pressure is used to draw the sphenoid contact in an anterior direction as the mastoid's contact rolls into the mastoid; W/R-level force draws the temporal bone in a posterior direction (Fig. 5-26). This will create a general, full sutural spread, simultaneously opening the serrated and squamosal articular surfaces.

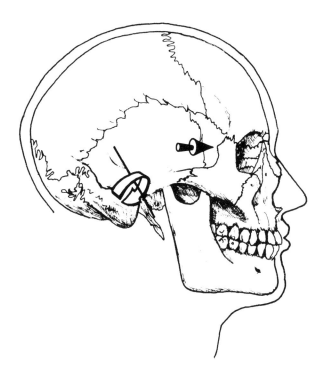

Fig. 5-26 Contacts on the sphenoid's greater wing and along the anterior surface of the mastoid process. Arrows depict the direction of manipulation used to release the suture

Disengaging-Reengaging Combination Procedures

Although this suture can completely disengage along its entire articular seam, it is likely that it disengages at one articular region while reengaging at another because of its rotational behavior (Fig. 5-27). This dual behavior is due to the shape of the sphenoid's lower serrated articular margin and its gear-like interdigitations with the temporal's inferior border.

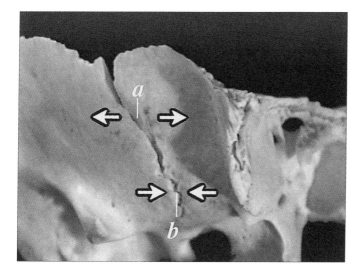

Fig. 5-27 Typical disengaging-reengaging pattern often seen with the sphenosquamous suture

a. Disengaged superior articular seam
b. Reengaged inferior articular seam

Consequently, an understanding of this suture's interarticular functional relationships will aid practitioners that need to manipulate this suture. The following disengaging-reengaging combination procedures address the suture's dual rotational pattern. With these procedures, the practitioner can make use of several effective contacts to open the superior squamosal articular surface or the inferior serrated articular surface.

To aid in the comprehension of the procedures, they have been divided into two strategies. In the first strategy the superior articular seam is disengaged with concomitant reengagement of the inferior seam, and in the second strategy the superior seam is reengaged with concomitant disengagement of the inferior seam. In both strategies the reader is given four basic maneuvers to achieve the desired articular response. Of the four basic maneuvers, two use the sphenoid bone and two use the temporal bone. To execute the required articular response successfully, the practitioner must choose at least two of the recommended contacts, one of which must be associated with the sphenoid bone and the other with the temporal bone. This combination of contacts and manipulative procedures gives the practitioner a variety of approaches to most effectively treat a given subject.

1. *Contacts and manipulative procedures to release the upper squamosal articular surface or close the inferior serrated articular surface (Fig. 5-28)*

a. The contact is found in the center of the sphenoid's greater wing. W⅓R-level pressure on the sphenoid bone draws the sphenoid's greater wing in a anterosuperior direction relative to the subject's skull.
b. The contact is the inferior tip of the sphenoid's pterygoid process. Manipulate the pterygoid in a cephalad-posterior direction with W/R-level pressure.
c. The contact is the posteroinferior aspect of the mastoid tip. Manipulate the contact with R^1-level force directed anteromedially toward the sphenobasilar junction.
d. The contact is the posterosuperior rim of the zygomaticotemporal process, anterior to its origin at the temporal squamosal plate. Manipulate the contact in a caudal direction with W¼R-level pressure.

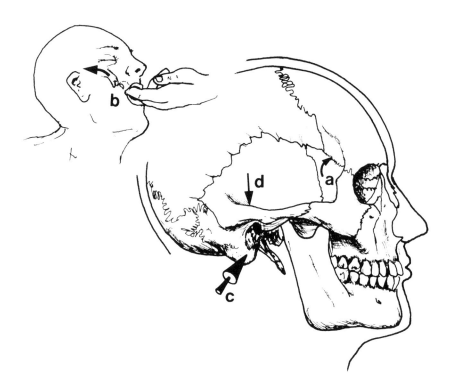

Fig. 5-28 Contact points and direction of manipulative pressure (arrows) used to release the superior squamosal articular surface or to close the inferior serrated articular surface of the spheno-squamous suture

2. *Contacts and manipulative procedures to release the lower serrated articular surface or close the upper squamosal articular surface (Fig. 5-29)*

a. The contact is the sphenoid's greater wing along its superior aspect anterior to the sphenosquamous suture. Manipulate the contact with W-level pressure in a posterocaudal direction toward the external auditory meatus.
b. The contact is the posterosuperior aspect of the mastoid process. Manipulate the contact in an anterosuperior-medial direction using R^1-level force.
c. The contact is the anterior aspect of the mastoid tip. Manipulate the contact in a posterolateral-superior direction with W/R-level pressure.
d. The contact is the posterior tip of the sphenoid's pterygoid process. Manipulate the contact with $W\frac{1}{3}R$-level pressure to draw the process in an anterolateral direction.

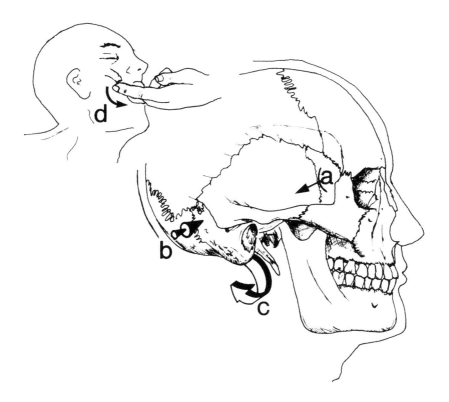

Fig. 5-29 Contact points and direction of manipulative pressure (arrows) used to release the inferior serrated articular surface or to close the superior squamosal articular surface of the spheno-squamous suture

Articular Reengagement

CONTACTS

To close the entire articulation, the optimal contacts are anterior to the sphenosquamous suture on the sphenoid's greater wing and posterior to the mastoid body and process (Fig. 5-30).

MANIPULATION

Closure can be obtained by applying W⅓R-level pressure to the sphenoid's contact in a posteroinferior direction, as the posterior mastoid's contact is pushed in the opposite direction toward the sphenoid contact point with W⅔R-level pressure (Fig. 5-30). The motion generated by the sphenoid's maneuver aligns and compresses the squamosal articular surfaces along the anterior side of the suture. In contrast, the motion generated by the mastoid's maneuver acts as a counterpressure to squamous infiltration while reducing (from a posterior to anterior direction) the suture's inferior serrated articular surfaces. *Note:* An alternative approach is to substitute the mastoid contact with one along the anterior wall of the internal auditory canal. In this approach the practitioner simply applies W¼R-level pressure anteriorly to the canal wall and W-level pressure to the sphenoid's contact to draw the sphenoid's greater wing in a posteroinferior direction (Fig. 5-30).

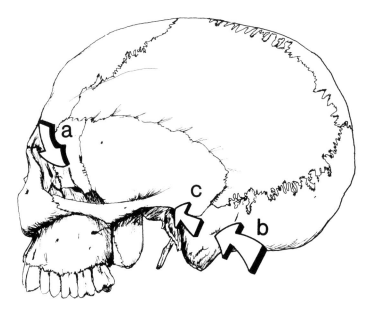

Fig. 5-30 Contact points and direction of manipulative pressure (arrows) used to close the entire sphenosquamous suture

a. Sphenoid contact
b. Mastoid contact
c. Alternative auditory canal contact

Squamoparietal Suture (Paired)

MORPHOLOGY

Bordered anteriorly by the junction of the sphenoparietal suture and the sphenosquamous suture and posteriorly by the parietomastoid suture, the squamoparietal suture, also known as the temporal (squamosal)-parietal suture, is made up of the temporal's superior squamosal border and the adjacent parietal's inferior articular surface (Fig. 5-31). The surface area where the temporal and parietal bones overlap is classified as squamosal and its internal articular surface is beveled, allowing the temporal to glide on the parietal's adjacent externally beveled seam (Fig. 5-32A). Caudal to cephalad ridges wedged within trench-like depressions often cover the suture's beveled articular surface. These may form as a result of chronic sutural stress (Fig. 5-32B~D).

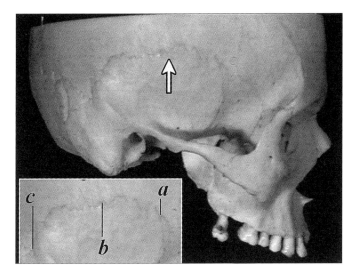

Fig. 5-31 Squamo-parietal suture's topographic location on the vault

a. Region of the pterion
b. Squamoparietal suture
c. Posterior junction of the squamoparietal suture with the parietomastoid suture

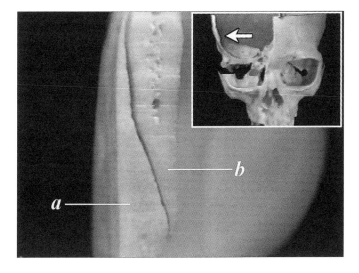

Fig. 5-32A Coronal slice exposing the right squamoparietal suture

a. Superior temporal squamous border beveled along its internal articular surface
b. Inferior parietal articular border beveled along its external articular surface

Fig. 5-32B Shelf formation often resulting from
an osseous response to
stress along the articular
seam

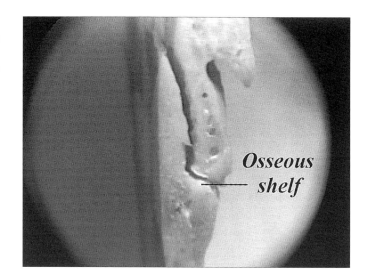

Fig. 5-32C Superior disarticulated view exposing
the temporal squamosal
suture's parietal surface.
Arrow depicts the area of
macroscopic enlarge-
ment in Fig. 5-32D

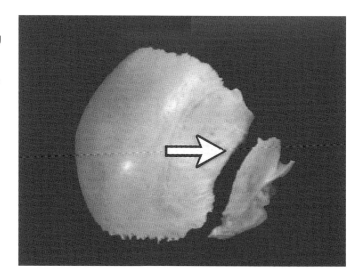

Fig. 5-32D Macroscopic
enlargement of the pari-
etal's squamosal articular
surface exposing the
series of ridges and
trenches that cover the
suture's articular surface

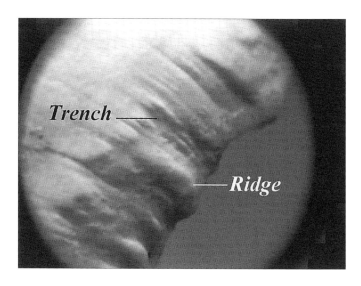

MOTION

Because of the presence of the ridges and their position, motion is easiest when the suture is maneuvered using posterosuperior external flaring and anteroinferior internal compression (Fig. 5-33).

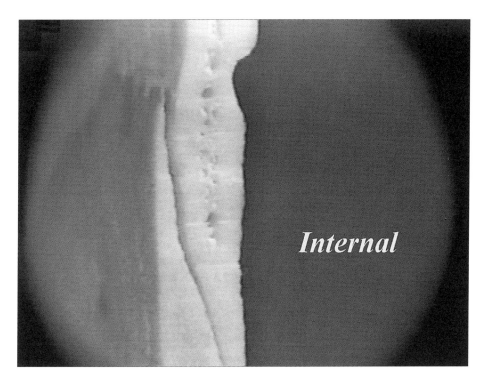

Fig. 5-33A Squamoparietal motion: anteroinferior internal compression

Compare with next photo →

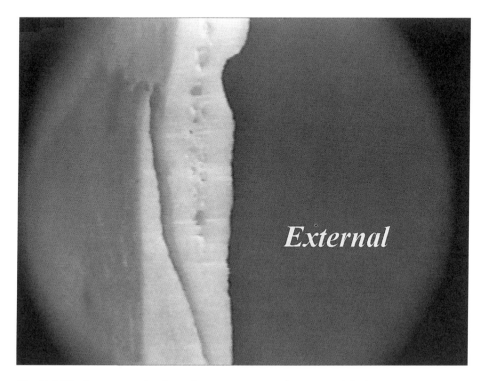

Fig. 5-33B Squamoparietal motion: posterosuperior external flaring

Articular Disengagement

As with the preceding articulation, the practitioner can use a variety of contacts and manipulative procedures to disengage the articulation.

CONTACTS AND MANIPULATION

1. *Use of the temporal bone (Fig. 5-34A).* To open this articulation, attention must be paid to the overlapping of the temporal bone onto the parietal articular surface. Because of this overlap, temporal contacts directly inferior to the suture should be *avoided*. The following are three possible contact points that may be used in conjunction with the parietal bone maneuver:

   a. Contact posterior to the mastoid tip. Manipulation is performed by applying W⅓R-level pressure anteromedially toward the sphenobasilar junction.
   b. Contact under the posterior angle of the mandible. Manipulation is performed by applying W¼R-level pressure toward the temporal mandibular joint.
   c. Contact on the posterosuperior edge of the zygomaticotemporal process. Manipulation is performed by applying W⅓R-level pressure caudally.

2. *Use of the parietal bone (Fig. 5-34B).* Applied simultaneously with one of the selected temporal maneuvers, the contact is located superior to the suture along the parietal's inferior border. Manipulation is performed by applying W⅓R-level force medially toward the vault's sagittal midline and in a cephalad direction toward the corpus callosum of the brain.

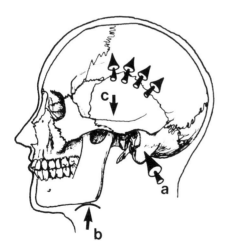
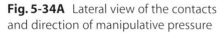
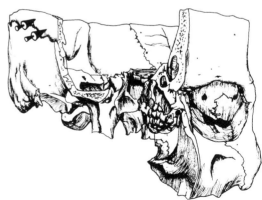

Fig. 5-34A Lateral view of the contacts and direction of manipulative pressure

Fig. 5-34B Coronal slice depicting the parietal's contacts and direction of manipulative pressure to release the squamoparietal articular surface

Articular Reengagement

CONTACTS AND MANIPULATION

1. *Use of the temporal bone (Fig. 5-35).* To close or reengage this articulation, temporal contacts directly inferior to the suture are *encouraged*.

   a. The contact is inferior to the suture along the superior rim of the temporal squamous. Manipulation is performed by applying W⅓R-level pressure in a medial-cephalad direction.
   b. The contact is inferomedial to the mastoid tip. Manipulation is performed by applying W/R-level pressure in a lateral-cephalad direction.
   c. The contact is inferior to the zygomaticotemporal process. Manipulation is performed by applying W⅓R-level pressure in a cephalad direction toward the superior temporal line of the parietal bone.

2. *Use of the parietal bone (Fig. 5-35).* The contact is located along the superior sagittal margin of the parietal bone, perpendicular to the area along the temporal margin that is most obviously flared. Manipulation is simultaneously performed with the selected temporal maneuver by applying W/R-level force directed caudally toward the foreman magnum at the base of the vault.

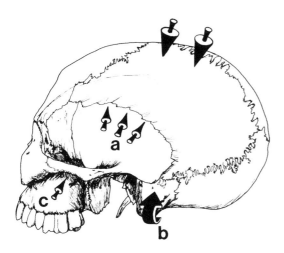

Fig. 5-35A Left posterolateral view of closure contacts and direction of manipulative pressure

Fig. 5-35B Posterior coronal slice depicting the direction of manipulative pressure to close the squamoparietal articular surface

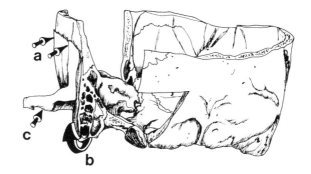

Parietomastoid Suture (Paired)

MORPHOLOGY

Slightly serrated but primarily squamosal, the parietomastoid suture is an intricate combination of overlapping bevels located along the superior surface of the mastoid process and inferior to the parietal's posteroinferior angle (Fig. 5-36A). To accurately describe this suture, the articular surface must be divided into its anterior two quarters and posterior half. In the anterior quarter of this suture the parietal bone is wedged between the articular surface of the temporal squamous externally and the anterior quarter of the mastoid process internally (Fig. 5-36B). The external parietal-temporal portion is squamosal in nature, and the internal portion of parietal that overlaps the mastoid articular surface is minutely serrated (Fig. 5-36B). As the suture courses posteriorly over the mastoid process along its other anterior quarter, the parietal bone momentarily reaches the external surface of the skull and overlaps the mastoid. Upon reentry to the interior, the parietal bone is once again wedged in an anteromedial to posterolateral trench created by the internal and external lips of the mastoid articular surface (Fig. 5-36C). At the suture's midpoint there is often found a protrusion of the mastoid's articular surface, which is beveled into a wedge-shaped trench embedded within the parietal articular surface (Fig. 5-36C).

Once the suture is posterior to this point, that is, it is in its posterior half, the mastoid's articular surface is superficially overlapped by the parietal bone which arcs over the mastoid to descend along the mastoid's overlapping internal beveled edge (Fig. 5-36D). This edge appears to be primarily squamosal and sparsely laced with superficial serrations. Finally, the internal overlapping articular surface of the mastoid descends into the suture, terminating in a medial direction and creating a shelf for the parietal bone to rest upon (Fig. 5-36D).

Fig. 5-36A Posterior oblique view of the skull depicting the topographical location of the right parietomastoid suture

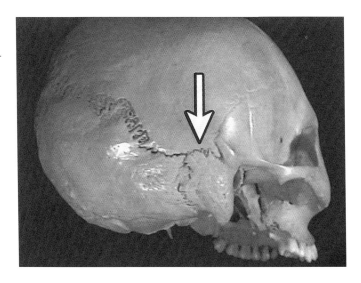

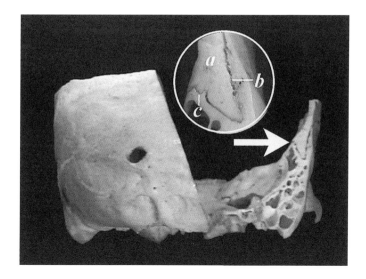

Fig. 5-36B Enlarged posterior view of a coronal slice through the anterior quarter of the parietomastoid suture

a. Parietal wedge
b. Temporal squamosal articular surface
c. Mastoid's serrated articular surface

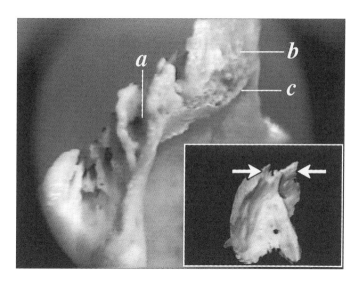

Fig. 5-36C Anterosuperior view exposing the series of beveled trenches and overlaps along the parietomastoid suture. Note the posterolateral angle as the trench formations extend from the inner edge of the mastoid to its outer edge.

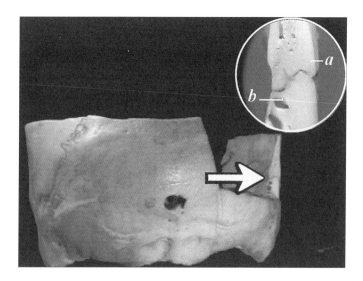

Fig. 5-36D Coronal slice exposing the posterior portion of the right parietomastoid suture

a. Parietal's articular surface that overlaps the mastoid's superior articular surface
b. Mastoid's internal shelf supporting the parietal's overlapped articular surface

MOTION

To fully understand the motions employed by this suture, the practitioner should focus on the suture's morphology as seen in coronal slices (Fig. 5-36B and D). The parietal bone is seen wedged between the outer temporal plate and the inner, sparsely serrated mastoid edge (Fig. 5-36B). Closer investigation of the parietal's temporal margin reveals that the surface exhibits a slight concavity in its articular margin. The parietal's inner articular border that faces the mastoid is convex, with articular serrations projecting in a superolateral direction. Based on these configurations, it appears that the parietal bone can be unlocked from the temporal and mastoid bones by gently compressing its inferior marginal border, that is, "rocking" it internally, as it is elevated from its seat in the anterior trench. Corroboration for this elevation of the parietal bone from its mastoid seat can be found in analysis of:

- The suture's posterior half (Fig. 5-36D), especially the internal inferior mastoid shelf and unobstructed superior parietal border
- The arched formations consistently found within the articular margins of this region

In conclusion, an examination of the morphological features suggests that lateral expansion of the parietal's inferior boundaries causes interlocking of the suture and generates internal to external rotational motion between the parietal and temporal-mastoid bones (Figs. 5-37 and 5-38). However, independent motion may be produced by gentle compression of the parietal bone toward the sagittal midline coupled with rostral elevation of the parietal from its mastoid trench.

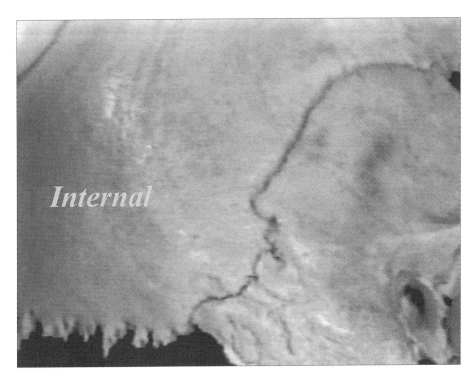

Fig. 5-37A Parietomastoid rotation: internal compression

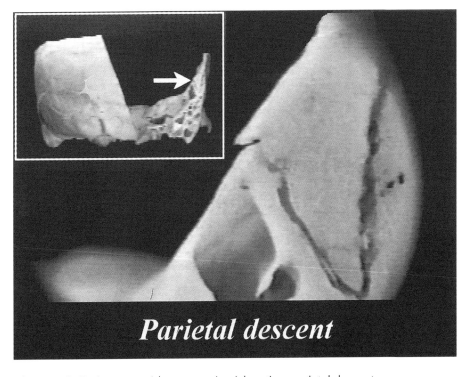

Fig. 5-38A Parietomastoid compression/elevation: parietal descent

Compare with next photos →

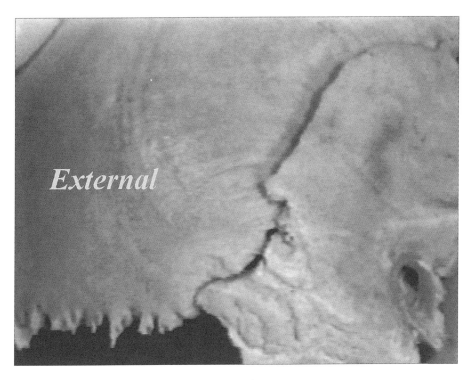

Fig. 5-37B Parietomastoid rotation: external expansion

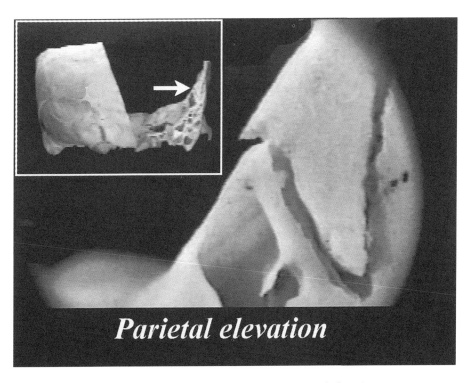

Fig. 5-38B Parietomastoid compression/elevation: parietal elevation

Articular Disengagement

CONTACTS

Because of the multiple interlocking beveled articular surfaces associated with the anterior half of this suture, anteroposterior rocking or gliding is structurally discouraged. However, lateral expansion and medial compression of the parietal bone are structurally encouraged, and cephalad elevation of the parietal's posterior angle offers the least resistance to disengagement. The optimal contacts for disengagement are on the parietal bone, cephalad to the parietomastoid suture, in axial alignment with the top of the ear, and inside the external auditory canal against its anteroinferior rim (Fig. 5-39). *Note:* Contacts close to the suture are to be avoided since their use could result in jamming of the articular surface along the alternating internally-beveled ridges.

MANIPULATION

Manipulative force applied to the parietal contacts should be directed in a cephalad direction toward the posterior quarter of the sagittal suture using W⅓R-level pressure. The disengaging force is applied simultaneously along the auditory meatus with W-level pressure caudally toward the posterior angle of the mandible (Fig. 5-39).

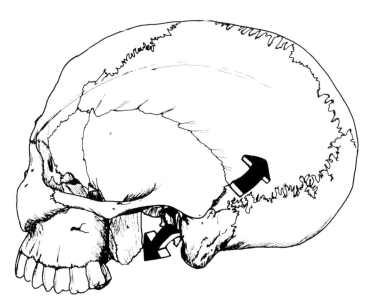

Fig. 5-39 Various contact points and manipulations used to release the left parietomastoid suture

Articular Reengagement

CONTACTS

The optimal parietal contact to reengage this suture is on the posterior parietal angle immediately above the suture; the use of this contact may be enhanced by the use of a second parietal contact superior to the parietal eminence (Fig. 5-40). The other contact is located on the body of the mastoid process, midway between the asterion and the mastoid tip.

MANIPULATION

W⅓R-level pressure on the contact above the suture is directed in a medial-caudal direction while the supporting contact above the parietal eminence is compressed with W⅓R-level pressure into the vault toward the parietomastoid suture (Fig. 5-40). *Note:* The medial compression of the parietal's posterior angle releases the parietal's articular borders, which are overlapped by the mastoid within the suture's trench system. The caudal compression of the region surrounding the parietal eminence generates an opposing lateral expansion of the parietal's posterior angle to release its overlapping articular surface along the inner lining of the mastoid trench. The two manipulative procedures are designed to align the parietal bone within the mastoid's trench since both contacts caudally compress the suture's articular surface into the mastoid's articular furrow. Concurrently, an opposing cephalad W⅓R-level pressure is applied through the mastoid contact toward the center of the suture (Fig. 5-40). This opposing force in the mastoid stabilizes it against the stress from the parietal contacts and completes the rearticulation process.

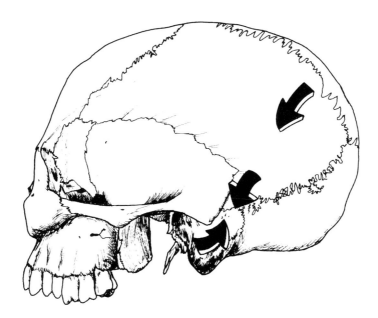

Fig. 5-40 Various contact points and manipulations used to close the left parietomastoid suture

Occipitomastoid Suture (Paired)

MORPHOLOGY

Lined with shallow serration's, the occipitomastoid suture may be considered more of a combined plane- and squamosal-type articulation. The suture originates at the asterion and descends along the posteromedial aspect of the mastoid process (Fig. 5-41A). As the suture descends caudally, dividing the occiput from the mastoid, it follows the contour of the occiput and wraps under the skull on an anterior route to terminate at the posterior border of the jugular foramen (Fig. 5-41B). The portion of the mastoid's articular surface that descend along the posterior aspect of the vault is internally beveled to laterally overlap the occiput's externally beveled articular surface (Fig. 5-41C and D). As the suture tucks under the skull on its anterior course to the jugular foramen, the mastoid's articular surface alters its position, directing it in a more medial-caudal direction,

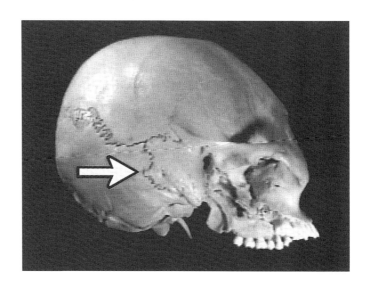

Fig. 5-41A Right posterior oblique view of the location of the occipitomastoid suture (arrow)

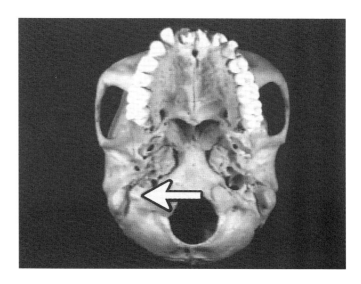

Fig. 5-41B Inferior view of the skull: topographical location of the occipitomastoid suture and its route to the jugular foramen (arrow)

Fig. 5-41C Macroscopic enlargement of the occiput's posterosuperior sutural surface

a. Superior beveled surface overlapped by the mastoid
b. Projecting border marking the occiput's transition to overlapping dominance

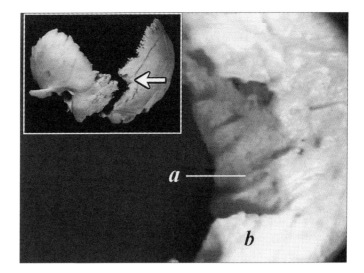

Fig. 5-41D Axial slice through the right upper occipitomastoid suture. Exposed from above, the mastoid's outer articular surface appears to initially tuck into a furrow along the occiput's articular margin. Nevertheless, in the main, the mastoid appears to externally overlap the occiput as the suture courses toward the inside of the vault.

a. Mastoid bone
b. Occipital bone

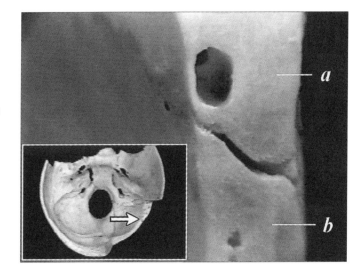

Fig. 5-41E Coronal slice through the right lower occipitomastoid suture. Viewed from the posterior, the mastoid's articular surface has changed to a medial-caudal direction as it is overlapped inferiorly by the occiput.

a. Occipital border
b. Mastoid's border

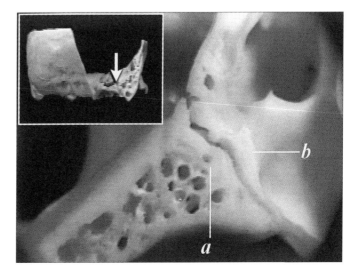

Fig. 5-41F

Anterosuperior exposure of the occiput's left mastoid articular surface revealing its anterior pseudocondylar articular surface posterior to the jugular foramen

a. Condylar surface
b. Inferior articular ledge to support the mastoid

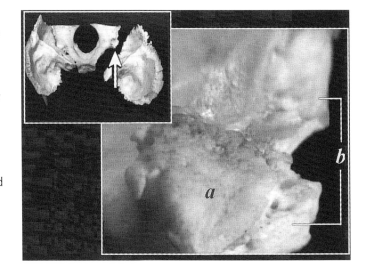

and the articular plane of the occiput transfigures into a diametrically supportive articulate ledge for the mastoid (Fig. 5-41E and F). This alteration in the suture's articular formation also reverses the overlapping process of the mastoid to the occiput, that is, the occiput's internal beveled surface now overlaps the external beveled articular surface of the mastoid (Fig. 5-41E). As the suture reaches its anterior terminus with the jugular foramen, the occiput's articular surface broadens and smooths out to form a pseudo-condylar surface (Fig. 5-41F).

MOTION

The morphological characteristics associated with this suture's beveled formations appear to support two predominant sequences of motion along its articular seam. The first generally glides the mastoid from anteromedial compression to posterolateral expansion along the occiput's articular border. This is not associated with flexion or extension of the cranial rhythmic impulse but rather with interarticular contraction and expansion. The second may best be described by relating to the overall motion of the temporal bone during its rotational activity. As the temporal bone rotates around its central axis *(in line with the petrous process)*, external rotation generates opening of the suture's posterosuperior marginal seam and compressive anteromedial closure of its anteroinferior seam. Consequently, during the temporal's internal phase of motion, the reverse occurs, and the suture closes along its posterosuperior seam and opens along its anteroinferior margin (Figs. 5-42 and 5-43).

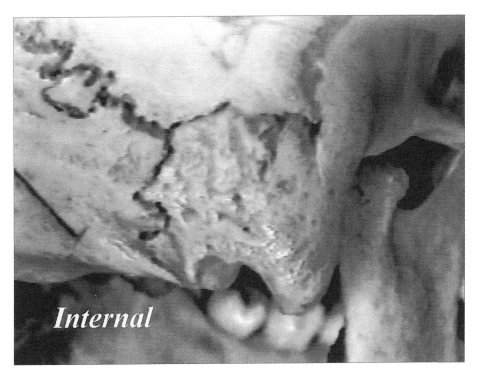

Fig. 5-42A Occipitomastoid gliding: anteromedial motion

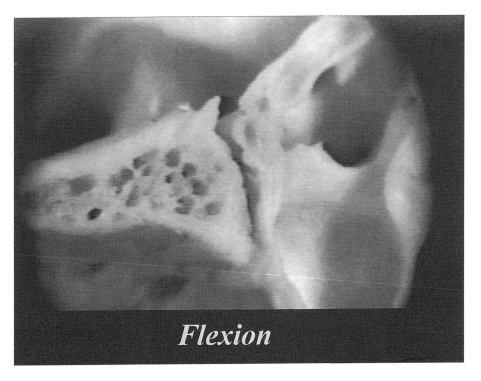

Fig. 5-43A Occipitomastoid rotation: flexion

Compare with next photos →

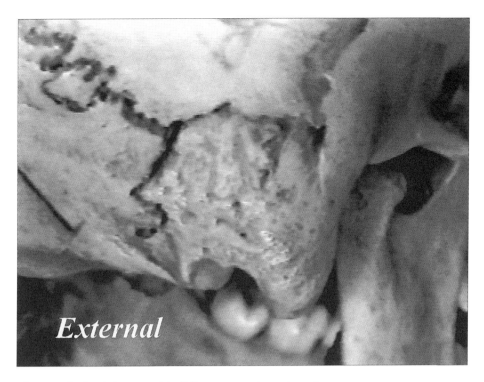

Fig. 5-42B Occipitomastoid gliding: posterolateral motion

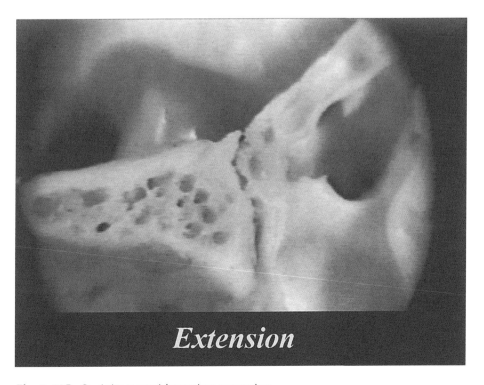

Fig. 5-43B Occipitomastoid rotation: extension

Articular Disengagement

CONTACTS AND MANIPULATION

The path of least resistance for releasing this articulation originates in the center of the sphenobasilar junction and extends in a posterolateral-oblique direction through the center of the mastoid body (Fig. 5-44). Unfortunately, this ideal approach for releasing this suture is impossible to access since it would require a contact inside the vault. This leaves several other practical contacts and manipulations.

One is the mastoid contact, which is found along the posteromedial surface of the process just superior to the mastoid's tip. Manipulative pressure using W/R-level force is directed in an anterolateral direction to the subject's vault (Fig. 5-45). This contact and manipulative procedure should be applied in conjunction with any of the following opposing methods.

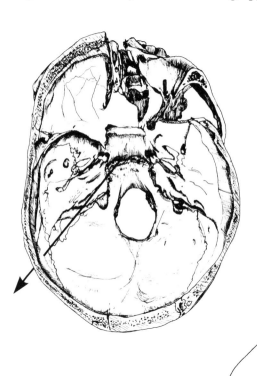

Fig. 5-44 Path of least resistance for releasing the occipitomastoid suture

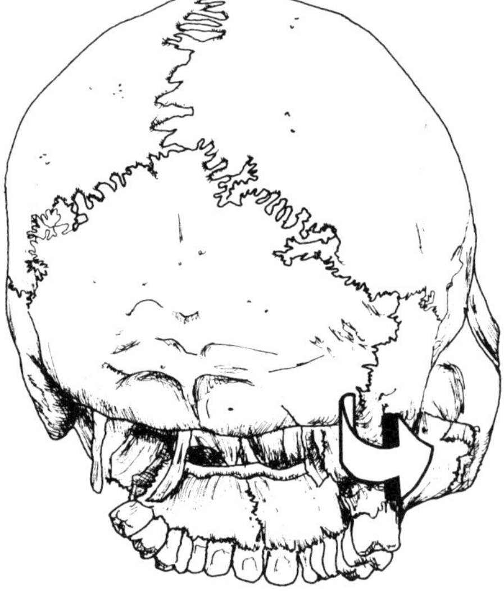

Fig. 5-45 Right mastoid contact and direction of manipulation

OPPOSING CONTACTS AND MANIPULATION

Opposing manipulative pressure is often applied to the occiput's squamous surface. However, contacts applied close to the suture may have the adverse effect of compressing the occiput into the mastoid's underlying articular surface, which may negate the practitioner's attempt to open the suture. For this reason a more distal contact is preferred. The following suggestions are alternative countercontacts that will achieve sutural release when combined with the mastoid procedure on the previous page.

1. The contact is on the posteroinferior-medial aspect of the opposite mastoid process, and manipulation is performed using opposing anterolateral W¼R-level pressure (Fig. 5-46).
2. The contact is on the ipsilateral anterolateral transverse process margin of the atlas, and manipulation is performed using W¼R-level posterior pressure (Fig. 5-47). *Note:* This procedure is *not* considered to be the most reliable and is contraindicated in conditions such as posterior basilar stroke, vertebral artery aneurysm, hypertension, and advanced atherosclerosis. Its inclusion in this text is more for the edification of the practitioner.
3. The contact is on the anterior third of the maxillary hard palate, and manipulation is performed using W/R-level pressure in a rostral-anterior direction (Fig. 5-48).
4. The contact is on or rostral to the superior nuchal ridge (midway between the occipitomastoid suture and the external occipital protuberance). W⅓R-level pressure is directed away from the suture toward the external occipital protuberance (Fig. 5-49).

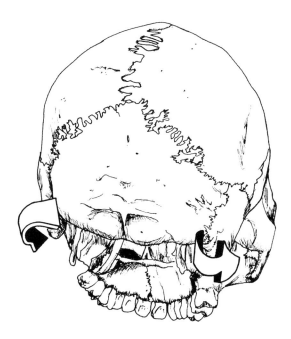

Fig. 5-46 Posterior view: bilateral mastoid procedure for opening the occipitomastoid suture

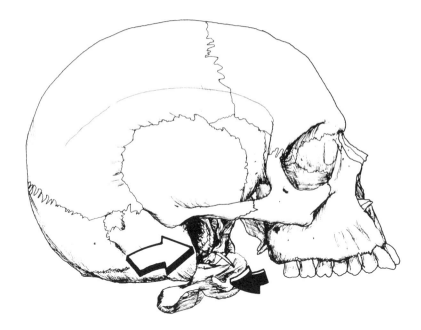

Fig. 5-47 Lateral view: mastoid-atlas procedure for opening the occipitomastoid suture

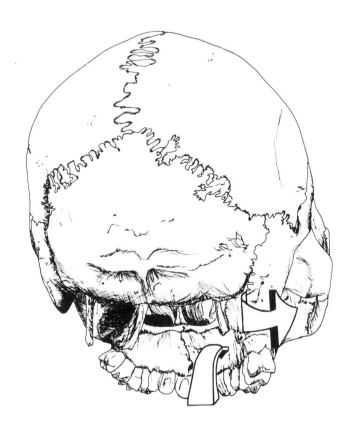

Fig. 5-48 Indirect release used in the maxillary anterior pull procedure

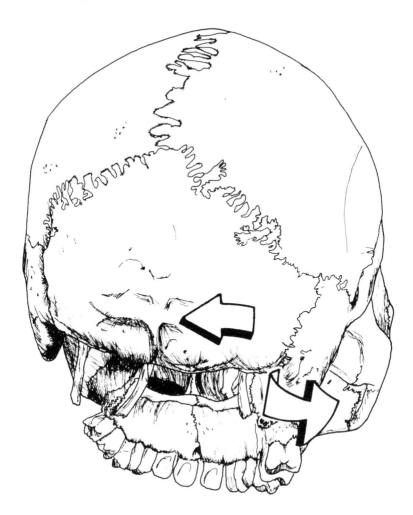

Fig. 5-49 Release used when drawing toward the occipital protuberance

Articular Reengagement

CONTACTS

Contact points to reengage this suture are much less complex and more direct than those used to release it. Since the direction which supports closure is through the center of the mastoid's body in line with the anterior-sagittal midpoint of the sphenobasilar junction, the practitioner will find these optimal contact points much more accessible than the disengagement points. The optimal contact points for the occipital portion of this procedure are located posterior to the suture and superior to the external occipital protuberance. The mastoid's contact is applied to the posterolateral center of the mastoid body, midway between the asterion and the mastoid's tip (Fig. 5-50).

MANIPULATION

W⅓R-level pressure is applied to the occipital region (posterior to the suture) and is directed anterolaterally into the suture's articular surface, while anterior compression applied superior to the external occipital protuberance simultaneously utilizes W/R-level pressure toward the sphenobasilar junction (Fig. 5-50). *Note:* Because of the overlapping nature of this suture's articular surface, care must be taken not to compress the occiput's posterior sutural contact medially. Such an application of pressure would only serve to release the articulation, resulting in further instability. During the occiput's maneuver, W⅓R-level pressure is placed on the mastoid's contact in a medial-anterior direction toward the sagittal midline of the sphenobasilar junction (Fig. 5-50). This creates a counterresistance along the mastoid articular margin to ensure rearticulation.

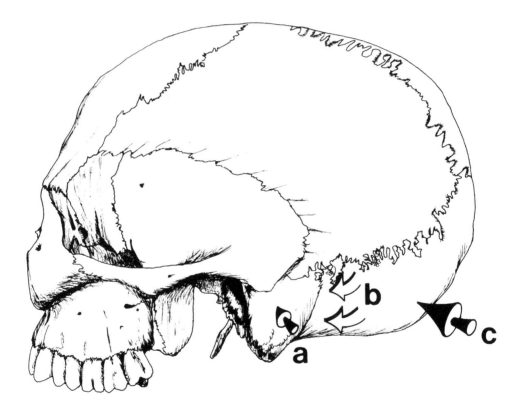

Fig. 5-50 Vault as viewed from the left posterior oblique showing the contact points and direction of manipulation (arrows)

a. Center of the mastoid body
b. Occipital contact points posterior to the suture
c. Occipital contact point superior to the external occipital protuberance

Lambdoid Suture (Paired)

MORPHOLOGY

The right and left lambdoid sutures are located between the asterion (the junction of the parietal, mastoid, and occipital bones) and the lambda (posterior terminus of the sagittal suture on the occipital bone) (Fig. 5-51A). The lambdoid and coronal sutures appear structurally similar upon gross inspection. Like the coronal suture, the lambdoid's combined articular surfaces can be divided into three primary regions delineated by the presence of beveled overlapping articular surfaces. In the medial-superior third, articular beveled surfaces of the occiput overlap the parietal's surfaces, while in the lateral two-thirds the parietal's surfaces overlap the occiput's (Fig. 5-51A).

To truly comprehend the intricate overlapping beveled system of this suture, the right and left lambdoid sutures should be considered as two separate sutures that mirror each other. In this way, a description of the right lambdoid suture will serve to define the left's articular surface. Although the suture is generally divided into thirds (Fig. 5-51B), an in-depth macromorphological investigation of the right lambdoid suture's articular beveled surface reveals the necessity of dividing the suture into fifths (Fig. 5-51C).

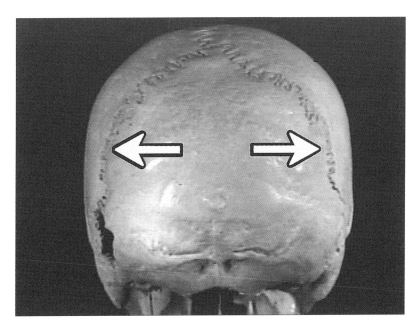

Fig. 5-51A Posterior view exposing the lambdoid suture's topographical location

Fig. 5-51B
Posteroinferior view of
the lambdoid's three
primary subdivisions

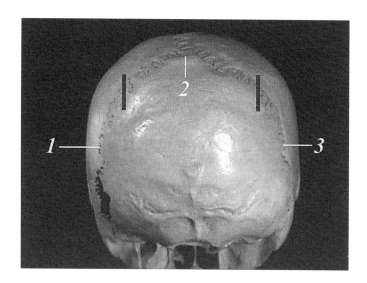

Fig. 5-51C Right posteroinferior oblique view
of the five subdivisions
of the right lambdoid
suture

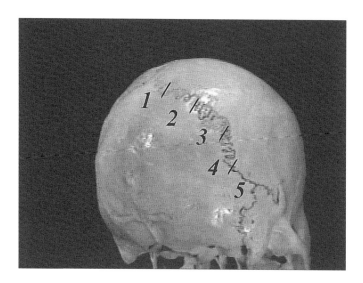

The superior one-fifth of this suture is mildly serrated and beveled to allow for overlapping of the occiput's internal beveled surface upon the parietal's externally beveled margin (Fig. 5-52). The middle articular surface comprises three-fifths of the suture's surface area. In this region, the serrations are very pronounced and set into deep interlocking pockets to discourage separation, via gliding, of the articulation's surfaces (Fig. 5-53).

Although the middle three-fifths of this suture is permeated with serrated projections, regions of nonserrated articular plates often cover the suture with interchanging beveled articular overlays. Because of this continuous series of alternating overlaps, the parietal and occiput bones incessantly alternate for external position (Fig. 5-54).

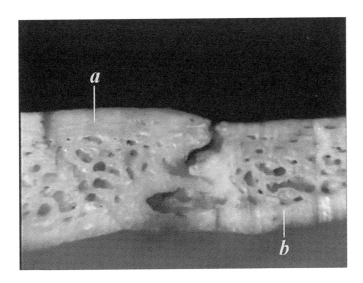

Fig. 5-52 Sagittal slice through the right lambdoid's superior one-fifth articular surface

a. Occipital bone
b. Parietal bone

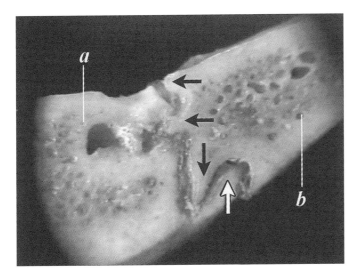

Fig. 5-53 Axial slice view of the interlacing pockets formed by the deep serrations along the medial three-fifths of the lambdoid suture

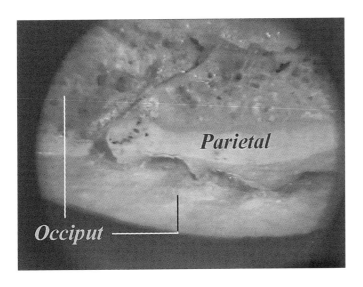

Fig. 5-54 Posterosuperior oblique macroscopic view of the lambdoid's middle three-fifths articular surface, exposing the typical alternating articular plate projections that cover this region of the suture

Looking at this suture from the surface, in the inferior one-fifth of this suture, the occiput initially appears to overlap the parietal's articular margin. However, when the suture is axially sliced, the occiput's overlap (if present) is only superficial and appears to be the external edge of a shallow furrow. In fact, the occiput's overall articular surface is externally beveled to permit general overlapping by the parietal bone. The interlocking formations of this region are not always apparent when viewed from a topographical view point. What may appear topically to be a simple wedge-and-groove may prove to have a second hidden wedge or bottleneck formation burrowed between the outer and inner surfaces of the bone (Fig. 5-55). Topographically, the suture may give the illusion that it can be disengaged by elevating the exterior articular serration from its seat in the inferior articular groove. However, the hidden wedge and bottleneck formation burrowed between the parietal's internal and external surfaces can actually inhibit the practitioner's efforts at disengaging the seam.

Fig. 5-55 Axial slice exposing the lambdoid's inferior one-fifth articular union

a. Parietal bone
b. Occipital bone

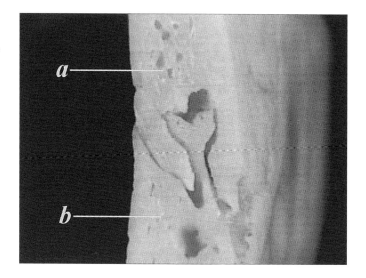

MOTION

The mobility of this suture is dictated by its fan-like morphological arrangement of serrations and the occiput's anterolateral articular marginal angle. Coupling these two properties, it becomes apparent that the suture's marginal seam will widen as the occiput's squamous region is drawn posteroinferiorly and the parietal bones are shifted anterolaterally (spreading apart the posterior aspect of the sagittal suture). Conversely, the suture is compressed, as the occiput's squamous region is drawn anterosuperiorly and the parietal bones are shifted posteromedially (Figs. 5-56 and 5-57). These two sets of images show the ability of the parietals to move within the confines of the denticular sockets and their inability to grossly disengage.

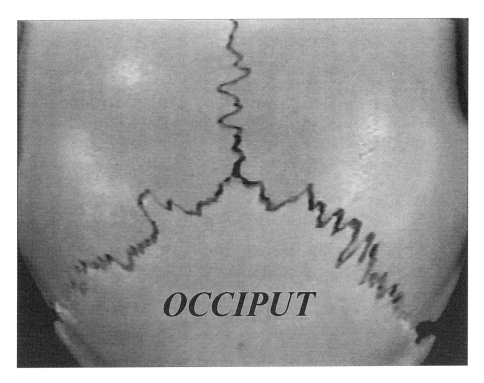

Fig. 5-56A Occipitoparietal motion 1: compression

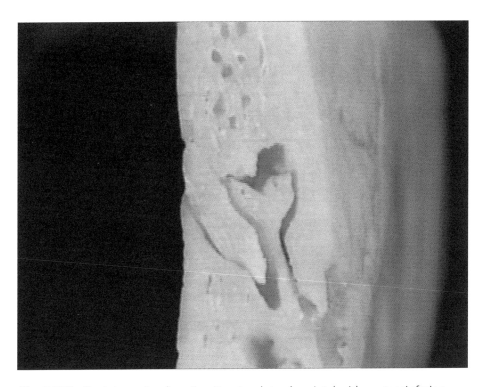

Fig. 5-57A Occipitoparietal motion 2: anterolateral parietal with posteroinferior occiput

Compare with next photos →

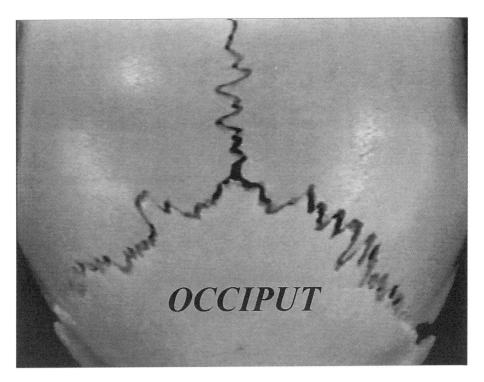

Fig. 5-56B Occipitoparietal motion 1: spread

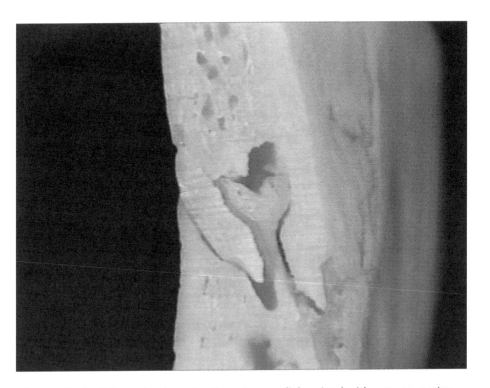

Fig. 5-57B Occipitoparietal motion 2: posteromedial parietal with anterosuperior occiput

Articular Disengagement

CONTACTS

Articular disengement is actually a misnomer when referring to this suture; because of its interlocking grooves and alternating beveled overlaps, the practitioner would find it necessary to literally break a few of the more intricate interlocking serrations in the neck to disengage this suture on an adult over the age of thirty (Fig. 5-58). However, the term *release* is still applicable, and loosening the suture to return functional pliability can still be considered appropriate if the practitioner confines the work within the suture's interarticular surface.

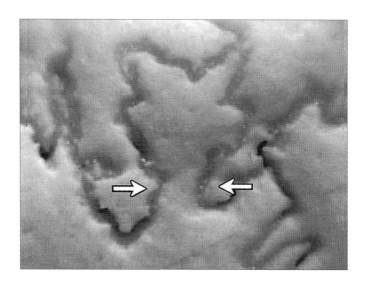

Fig. 5-58 Typical intrasutural trench-and-wedge formation. Arrows depict the bottleneck region that interlocks the suture.

Because of the interlocking nature of the occiput and the two parietal bones in the area surrounding the lambda, the practitioner must first open the posterior sagittal suture. In the superior third of the occiput's lambdoid articular surface, the occiput's serrated teeth extend superolaterally on both sides of the posterior sagittal suture (Fig. 5-59). This forms a key bone-locking device to the vault, which can only be released if manipulative pressure pulls all three bones away from the central junction of the lambda.

Again, because of the unusual nature of the lambdoid's interlocked serrated articular projections, this suture appears to resist direct occipital squamous manipulation to release its fixed position relative to the parietal bones. It appears that the anterolateral direction of the occiput's articular surface resists every kind of external pressure and tends to compress the suture's articular surfaces. For this reason, the practitioner is advised to manipulate this suture with a combination of osseous- and nonosseous-based contact postures. The optimal contact points for this maneuver are located over the anterior half of the sagittal suture, while grasping the occiput's hair and scalp posterior to the suture. Unfortunately, this approach is limited to individuals with enough regional hair to grasp.

Fig. 5-59 Posterior view of the angular growth pattern of the serrated teeth around the lambda. Arrows depict the directional force required to release this articular region.

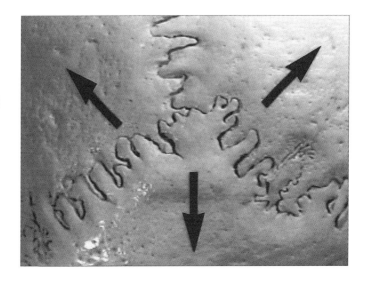

MANIPULATION

Compression applied with W⅓R-level force, directed caudally toward the sphenobasilar junction, will spread the posterior sagittal articulation. Simultaneously, W¼R-level force at the hair and scalp contacts draw the scalp in a posterocaudal direction from the suture's articular surface. This releases the three key locked bones around the lambda and disengages the tension within the suture's articular surface. *Note:* The optimal occipital contact for releasing this suture is located on the inner squamous surface of the vault and extends posteriorly through the occiput's osseous structure. For obvious reasons, this contact can only be reached by surgical intervention. However, the hair and scalp anchor into the external periosteal tissue of the skull, and the periosteum penetrates the suture to become the epidural membrane inside.[6,7] This allows the practitioner to effectively execute an external draw on the occiput (which infiltrates through the suture) to release the lambdoid suture's articular processes (Fig. 5-60).

Alternative Contacts and Manipulation

Although the preceding approach is the procedure of choice, its application is limited in cases of baldness or short hair. In such cases, the following two procedural approaches are recommended:

1. As in the preceding example, the parietal contact is applied to the anterior third of the sagittal suture. The accompanying occipital contacts are located bilaterally along the occipital margins of the occipitomastoid suture. W⅓R-level compression toward the sphenobasilar junction is applied to the anterior sagittal sutural contact. As mentioned in the previous approach, this manipulative maneuver lifts the parietal bones' inferolateral margins and encourages the posterior opening of the sagittal suture, unlocking the three-way bone-locking device of the lambda. Simultaneous bilateral application of W¼R-level compression into the occiput's mastoid

margins directs the margins medially toward the midsagittal plane, inducing extension in the occiput's squamous and releasing the occiput's lambdoid articular margins (Fig. 5-61.)

2. Although this strategy is suggested as an alternative method for bald or short-haired individuals, its application is most often recommended in cases where limited marginal fixations lock a specific region of the suture's articular junction. In the event that the suture is fixed on the right, contacts

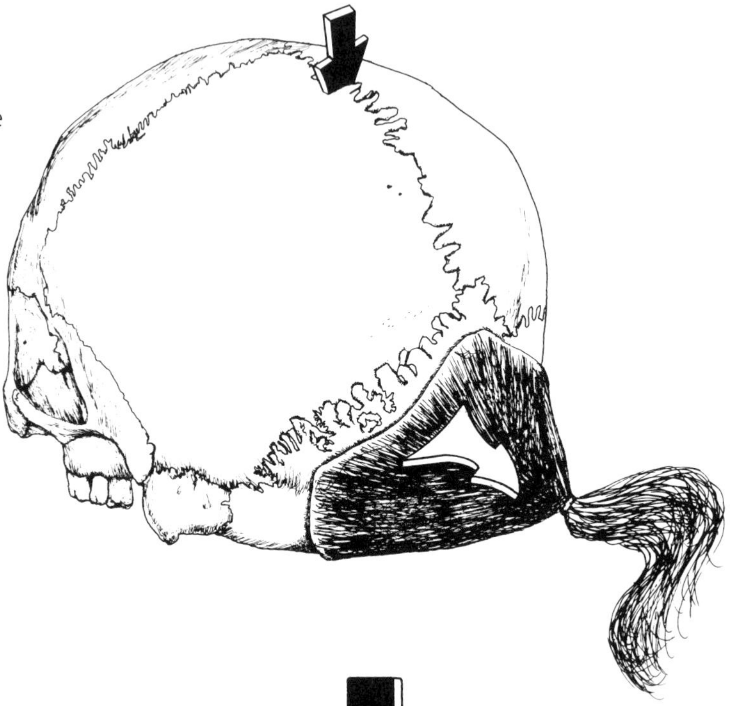

Fig. 5-60 Unusual osseous and non-osseous contacts used to release the lambdoid suture, and direction of manipulation (arrows)

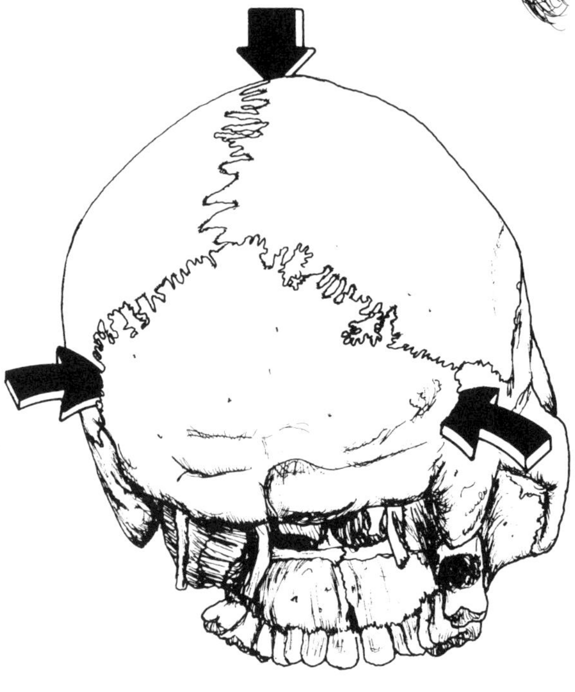

Fig. 5-61 First alternative occipital contact point and direction of manipulation

are applied on the right parietal and occipital articular margins adjacent to the region of greatest articular fixation (Fig. 5-62). *Note:* Care should be taken not to contact the suture's articular seam. To ensure against this mistake, the practitioner is reminded that the articular serrations may overlap the seam by 4 to 6cm. This means the adjacent sutural contact should be at least 6cm from the articular seam (Fig. 5-59).

The degree of manipulative pressure is governed by the contact's location along the suture's articular seam. This is due to the various overlapping beveled planes and their tendency to interlock when incorrect pressure is applied. Should the region of sutural jamming be located along the inferolateral margin of the suture, care must be taken since an incorrect level of compression of the parietal contacts can cause its overlapping bevels to lock the suture. *Remember:* When attempting to disengage this suture, manipulative pressure to the overlapping osseous margin should not exceed W level.

In contrast, pressure to the overlapped osseous margin may exceed W level but not exceed W/R level. Once the articulation has been disengaged, spreading the articular surface may be accomplished by securing the overlapping margin with W-level pressure and pulling the overlapped margin's contact in a perpendicular direction away from it using W/R-level pressure (Fig. 5-62).

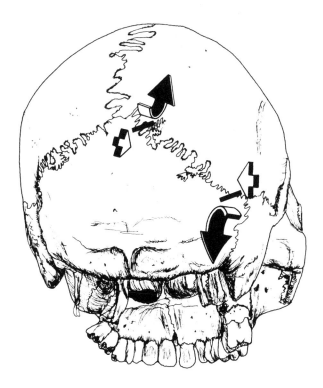

Fig. 5-62 Second alternative strategy for disengaging the lambdoid's articular junction. Slash marks depict the region of sutural jamming, while the arrows delineate the contact points and the direction of their manipulation.

Articular Reengagement

CONTACTS

Closure of this suture is more direct than the previous approach used to release the suture. Optimal contacts are located across the occipital squamous, inferior to the superior nuchal ridge, and on the superior third of the occiput posterior to the lambda. The associated parietal contacts are located on the posterior half of the parietal bones, with the primary contacts bilateral to the posterior sagittal suture and anterior to the involved lambdoid suture (Fig. 5-63).

MANIPULATION

Manipulation to the occipital contact is performed using W¼R-level pressure directed rostrally along the occiput's base and in an anterocaudal direction in the zone posterior to the lambda. Manipulation to the parietal's contact is performed using W¼R-level pressure posteriorly along the affected anterior lambdoid region as the bilateral posterior sagittal contacts compress the two parietal bones together (Fig. 5-63).

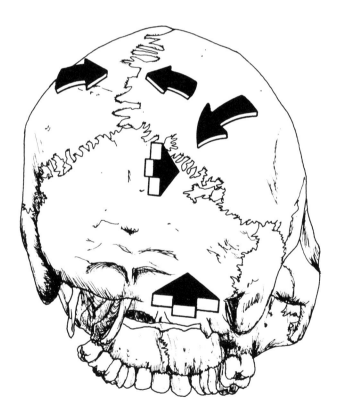

Fig. 5-63 Posterior oblique view of the occipital and parietal contacts used in closing the right lambdoid suture

Sagittal Suture (Singular)

MORPHOLOGY

Located over the superior midline of the cranial vault, the sagittal suture's anterior portion originates at the bregma and travels posteriorly to terminate at the cranial lambda (Fig. 5-64). The sagittal suture divides the two parietal bones and is classified as a serrated-type articulation. To look at this more closely, from 1990 through 1996 I conducted sutural dissections on the skulls of one-hundred twenty-five human cadavers at Cleveland Chiropractic College in Los Angeles. While the sagittal suture is in fact primarily serrated, our unpublished findings also consistently revealed a combination of plane, schindyletic, limbous, and denticulate patterns frequently integrated throughout the sutures articular surface. These patterns not only appeared frequently, but their location along the suture's seam was also found to be predictable.

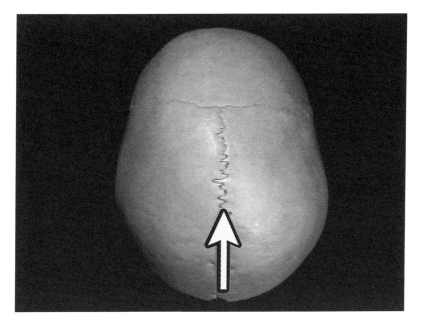

Fig. 5-64 Superior view depicting the topographic position of the sagittal suture in the vault

Therefore, in this text the suture is divided into three primary divisions. The anterior third is often similar to a plane-type articular surface but appears to have a shallow schindyletic wedge-and-groove quality that suggests hinged-like activity (Fig. 5-65A). The middle third is generally pure serration but often develops a shallow underlying beveled edge in its posterior aspect, giving it a slight limbous pattern (Fig. 5-65B). As the suture enters its posterior third, its interarticular surface remains predominantly serrated. However, the internal underlying edge that originated in the middle division takes on a more dominant ledge formation, making this division

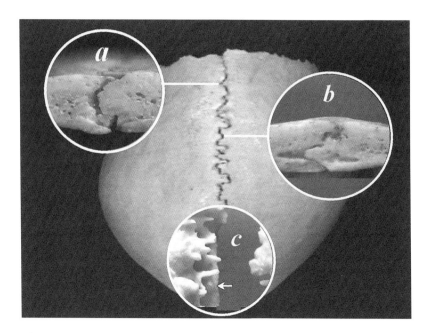

Fig. 5-65 The various alternating articular beveled surfaces within the sagittal suture

a. Coronal slice view showing wedge and trench articulations
b. Coronal slice view with serrated and beveled articulations
c. Superior view of a series of pins, sockets, and a supporting shelf

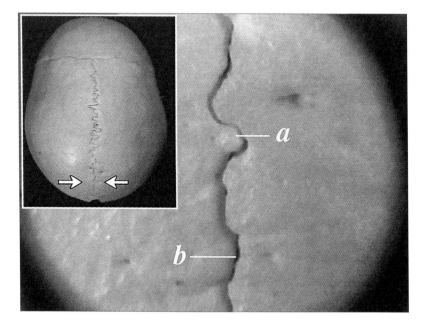

Fig. 5-66A Typical external seam of the sagittal suture's posterior third. Note the overall plane-like appearance.

a. Typical shallow serration that sparsely projects along this division's external edge
b. Division's typical plane-type edge

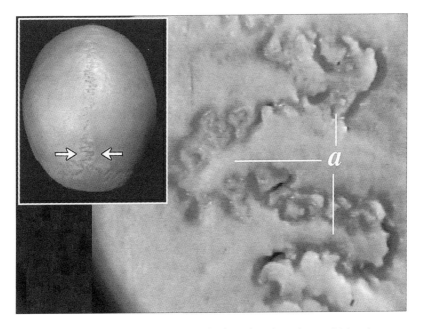

Fig. 5-66B Posterior third's external edge showing the multidenticulated projections

a. Three alternating denticulated projections. Note the multiple branches of denticulated formations that project from each main branch.

more limbous in nature along its internal edge (Fig. 5-65C). The posterior third's external edge is frequently noted for its almost plane-like appearance that is often sparsely covered with shallow serrations (Fig. 5-66A). However, some skulls have displayed multidenticulated projections, giving this division a combined serrated, limbous, denticulate configuration (Figs. 5-65C and 5-66B). Consequently, this entire suture is frequently inundated with alternating pins-to-socket serrations, wedge-to-groove hinges, overlapping ledges, planes, and occasional denticulate formations (Figs. 5-65 and 5-66).

MOTION

The intricate multifaceted shapes found along the suture's articular surface limit motion in this suture to two separate planes. The first is a uniform expansion (separation) and contraction (compression) of the suture along its transverse plane (Figs. 5-67 and 5-69). In the second, the suture takes on the role of a hinge joint, causing the elevation (external rotation) and descent (internal rotation) of the two parietal bones. This can be viewed as similar to the motion produced by a bird's wings while in flight (Figs. 5-68, 5-69, and 5-70). Unlike the first motion, which uniformly opens the entire sagittal suture, the second motion only partially opens the suture. During the act of elevation, the inferior parietal borders expand laterally and lift superiorly, creating the illusion of parietal external rotation as the suture descends caudally into the cranial vault. During this action, the anterior and posterior sixth of the suture separates. As the anterior and posterior articular surfaces separate, the remaining two-thirds of the suture (between the two points) spread along its internal edge and compress along its external articular margin (Fig. 5-70A). During internal rotation, the parietal plates descend, causing the bones' lateral inferior borders to shift in a medial-caudal direction. This motion results in the compression of the suture's anterior, posterior, and middle internal articular surfaces while the midexternal articular margin separates (Fig. 5-70B).

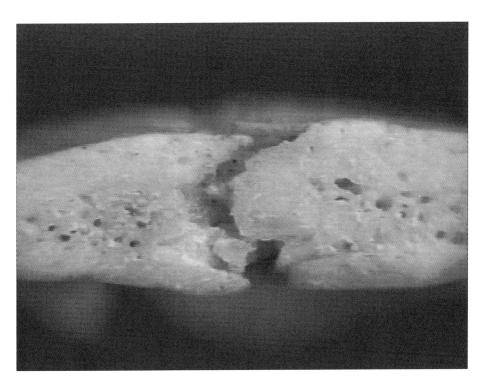

Fig. 5-67A Coronal slices of the sagittal suture showing lateral expansion

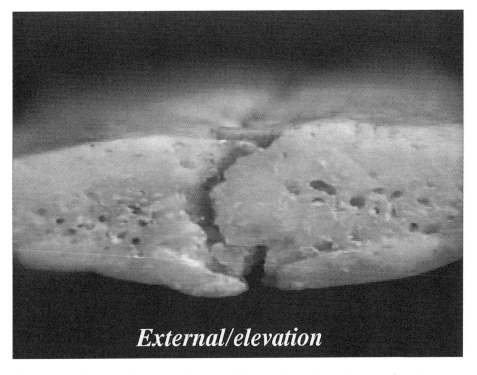

Fig. 5-68A Coronal slice magnification of the sagittal suture showing elevation

Compare with next photos →

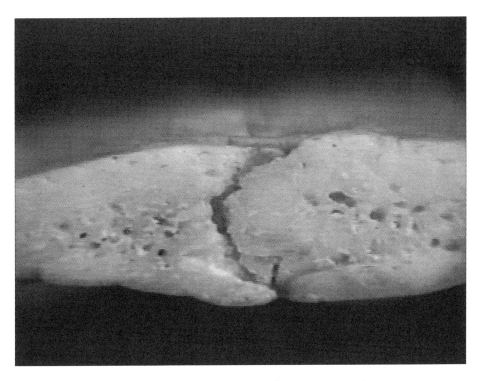

Fig. 5-67B Coronal slices of the sagittal suture showing contraction

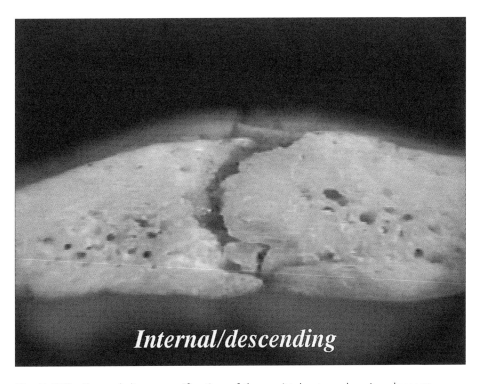

Fig. 5-68B Coronal slice magnification of the sagittal suture showing descent

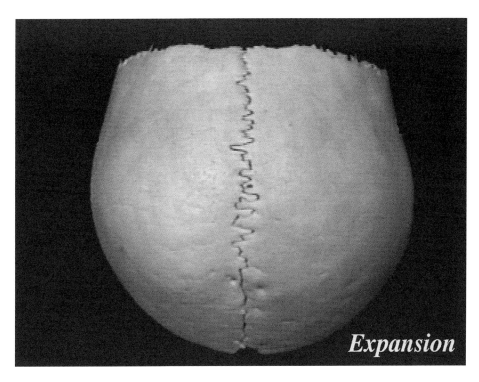

Fig. 5-69A Sagittal suture: expansion

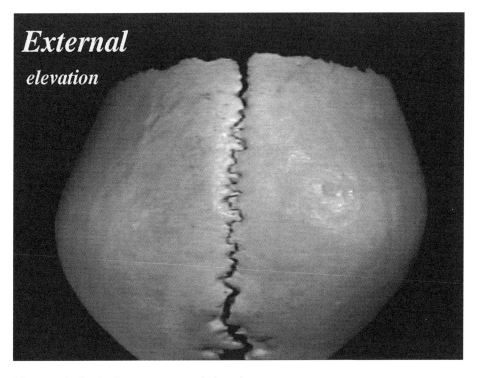

Fig. 5-70A Sagittal suture: external elevation

Compare with next photos ➡

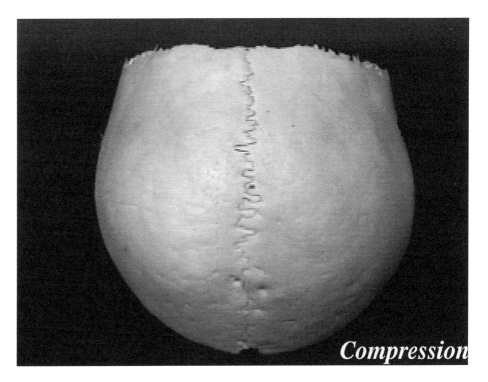

Fig. 5-69B Sagittal suture: compression

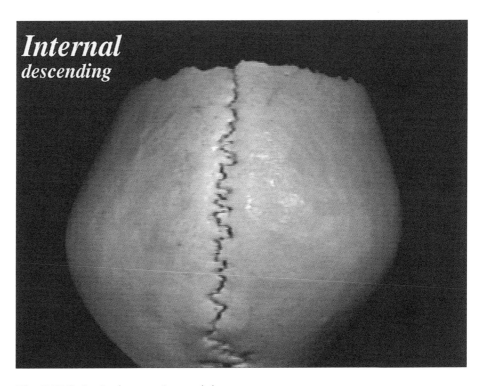

Fig. 5-70B Sagittal suture: internal descent

Articular Disengagement of the Entire Sagittal Suture

CONTACTS AND MANIPULATION

To release the entire articulation (lateral expansion), the optimal contact points are located bilateral to the jammed articular surface of the sagittal suture and along the inferior border of the parietal bones (superior to the lateral sutures of the skull). At the superior parietal contacts, W¼R-level force is directed at the suture's articular margins in a lateral direction away from the suture's articular junction. At the inferolateral contacts, W/R-level pressure draws the parietal's inferior articular surfaces in a medial-cephalad direction (Fig. 5-71). *Note:* Care must be taken to contact only the parietal bones and avoid all direct contact with sutures.

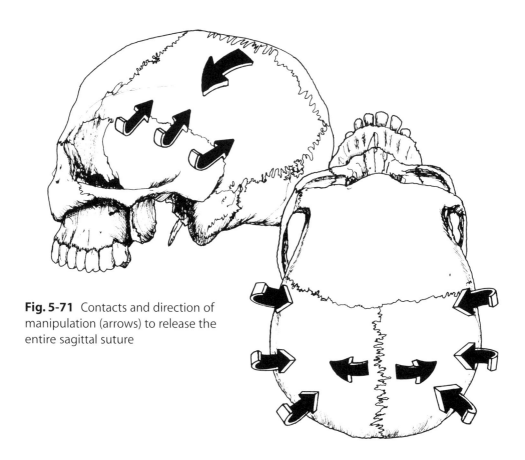

Fig. 5-71 Contacts and direction of manipulation (arrows) to release the entire sagittal suture

Combined Sutural Disengagement and Reengagement

Unobstructed cephalad and caudal hinge motion of the sagittal suture's articular seam is essential for the overall motions of the cranial bones. This is due in part to the integrated associations that the sutures create between the osseous cranial structures. An example of this can be seen between the articular association of the posterior sagittal suture and the lambda portion of the occipital bone. In this region, the occiput's articular surface projects anterolaterally into the parietal's articular border, and in order for the practitioner to disengage this portion of the occiput, the posterior sagittal suture must be released (Fig. 5-59). Although the practitioner may wish to release the posterior sagittal region, the subject may also require articular stability within the majority of the sagittal seam to protect the integrity of the underlying vascular system. By understanding the combination disengaging-reengaging methods, the practitioner can effectively address localized aberrations along the suture's articular seam and articular junctions that are dependent upon the suture's mobilization, as in the aforementioned example.

Disengaging the Anterior, Posterior, and Internal Articular Surfaces while Reengaging the Articular Surface of the External Middle Two-Thirds

Contacts are applied bilaterally against or on the sagittal suture's articular seam, approximately one-third of the way posterior from the bregma and along the parietal bones' inferolateral borders. Manipulative pressure employing W¼R-level force directs the superior sagittal contact points caudally through the cranial vault toward the anterior border of the foramen magnum. Simultaneously, W-level manipulative pressure to the contact points along the parietal's inferolateral borders compresses and lifts the outer parietal surface in a cephalad direction (Fig. 5-72).

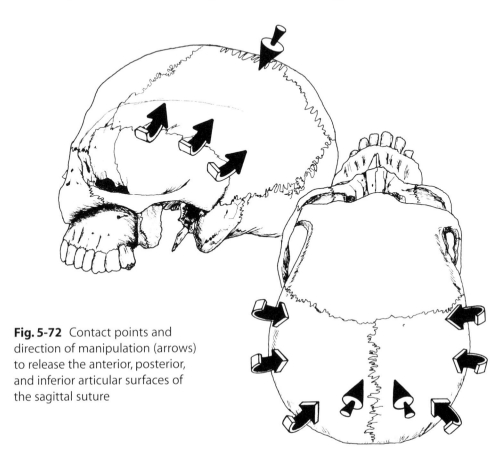

Fig. 5-72 Contact points and direction of manipulation (arrows) to release the anterior, posterior, and inferior articular surfaces of the sagittal suture

Reengaging the Anterior, Posterior, and Inferior Surfaces while Disengaging the Articular Surface of the Superior External Middle Two-Thirds

Optimal contacts are located on the inferolateral borders of the parietal bones. Manipulative pressure along the parietal's inferolateral border using W¼R-level force directs the contacting borders medially toward the sagittal center of the vault (Fig. 5-73).

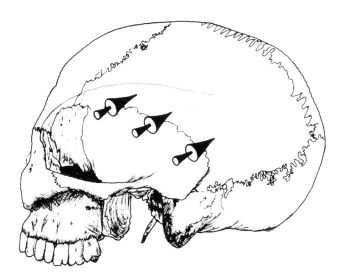

Fig. 5-73 Contact points and direction of manipulation (arrows) to close the sagittal suture's anterior and posterior articular surface, while releasing the articular surface of the superior external medial two-thirds of the suture

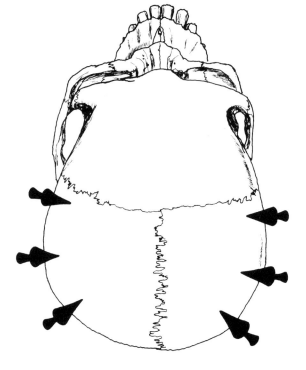

Reengaging the Entire Sagittal Suture

CONTACTS AND MANIPULATION

The optimal contact points to close the entire sagittal suture are located along the inferolateral borders of the parietal bones and bilateral to the sagittal suture. Manipulative pressure using W¼R-level force is directed in a cephalad direction through the parietal's inferior border contacts, while the contact points adjacent to the sagittal suture use W-level medial compressive force directed toward the suture's articular junction. *Note:* Care must be taken to avoid direct contact with the sagittal suture (Fig. 5-74).

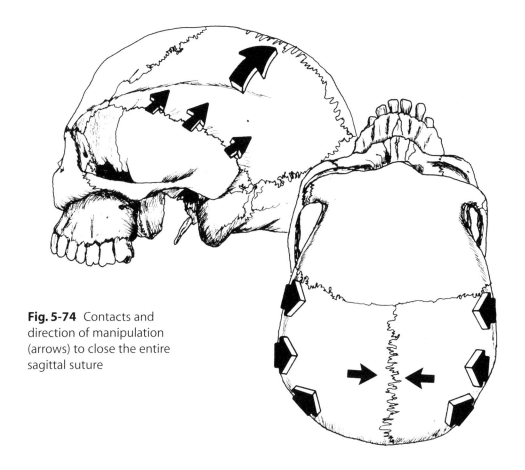

Fig. 5-74 Contacts and direction of manipulation (arrows) to close the entire sagittal suture

References

1. DeJarnette MB. *The History of Sacro-Occipital Technique.* Nebraska City, NE: Sacro-Occipital Technique Organization , 1958:23.
2. Michael DK, Retzlaff EW. A preliminary study of cranial bone movement in the squirrel monkey. *J Am Osteopathic Assoc* 1975;74:866–869.
3. Blum C. Biodynamics of the cranium, a survey. *J Craniomandibular Practice* 1985;3(2):164–171.
4. Pavlin D, Vukicevic D. Mechanical reactions of facial skeleton to maxillary expansion determined by laser holography. *Am J Orthod* 1984;85 (6):498–507.
5. SOT was founded by M. B. DeJarnette, a chiropractor and osteopath who began his investigations into cranial analysis and manipulation in 1933. Through his theory of departmentalizing analysis of the human condition he developed the "category system" of analysis and treatment. He enhanced the methodology of cranial manipulation by developing specific procedures according to the various types of categories. Some of these procedures were specific manipulations of the sutures.
6. Pritchard JJ, Scott JH, Girgis FG. The structure and development of cranial facial sutures. *J Anat* 1956;90:73–85.
7. Wood J. Dynamic response of human cranial bones. *J Biomechanics* 1971; 4:1–12.

CHAPTER SIX

Accessible Sutures
of the Face

THERE ARE thirty-nine different sutures within the facial region of the human skull. Of these, sixteen are paired sutures and seven are single. However, only six of the paired and three of the individual sutures are considered accessible for palpable examination. This section is devoted to the morphological description of the nine accessible sutures. Although the paired sutures' morphological structure may differ slightly on each side, it has been observed that their primary structural design remains basically the same. As in the previous chapter, the text material will be further subdivided to suggest optimal contact points and manipulative procedures for releasing and reengaging the suture's articular surfaces.

Zygomaticotemporal Suture (Paired)

MORPHOLOGY

Located along the zygomatic arch of the temporal and zygomatic bones, in a lateral view, the zygomaticotemporal suture resembles a child's playground slide. In order to fully comprehend the articular surface of this suture, it must first be divided into thirds, and the posteroinferior third must be further subdivided into halves. Extending from the suture's superior point of origin, the articulation sharply drops posterocaudally for approximately one-third of its articular surface length. In the posteroinferior third's anterior half the suture forms a plateau and courses posteriorly. Upon entering the remaining posterior half, the suture again alters its

course in an abrupt caudal descent to terminate along the inferior border
of the zygomaticotemporal arch (Fig. 6-1).

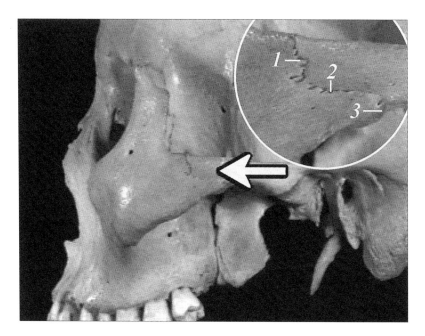

Fig. 6-1 Lateral view depicting the suture's topographic location along
the zygomatic arch. *Note:* The suture changes its course three times as it
extends from its anterior to posterior borders.

1. Anterior division (caudal descending)
2. Middle division (plateau)
3. Posterior division (caudal descending)

Serrated in nature, the anterior two-thirds of the zygomatic's articular surface is slightly beveled along its internal surface, thus making the zygomatic
surface the most lateral bone to the cranial vault (Fig. 6-2). However, when
the suture approaches its terminal third, the articular border of the temporal
process appears to cover a greater percent of the zygomatic's surface; in this
region the temporal process makes up a greater percent of the external overlapping surface (Fig. 6-3A). As the zygomatic's serrated surface extends into
the suture's remaining inferior third, its articular plane often deviates to face
in a cephalad-lateral direction, resulting in total external overlap by the temporal process. This is caused by a medial deviation of the zygomatic's inferior
osseous border as it tucks in the direction of the vault (Fig. 6-3B).

Fig. 6-2 Superior-medial view exposing the zygomatic's overlapping internally beveled articular surface and the adjacent externally beveled articular surface of the temporal process

a. Zygomatic surface
b. Temporal process's surface

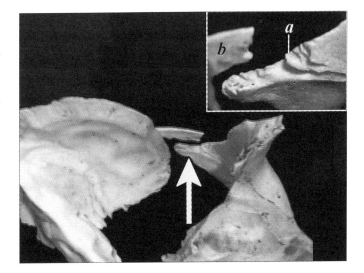

Fig. 6-3A Coronal slice of the articular union along the posterior aspect of the middle division, just before the suture enters it final one-third articular division. Note the shift of the temporal toward dominance of the external overlapping surfaces.

a. Temporal's zygomatic process
b. Zygomatic's temporal process

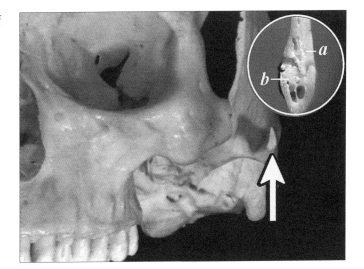

Fig. 6-3B Posterior view exposing the zygomatic's posterior one-third articular division. Note the cephalad-lateral deviation of the posterior third, meshing it with the temporal's complete external overlap.

a. Temporal's zygomatic process
b. Posterior third of the zygomatic's temporal process

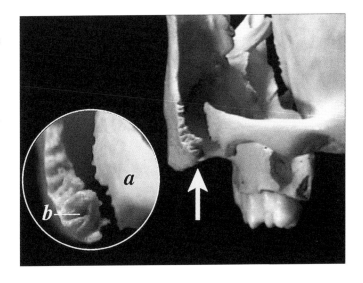

The articular serration's directional growth patterns are primarily anterior to posterior throughout the suture's articular surface. This pattern appears to run perpendicular to the suture's upper two-third's articular border and parallel to the suture's lower third margin (Fig. 6-4).

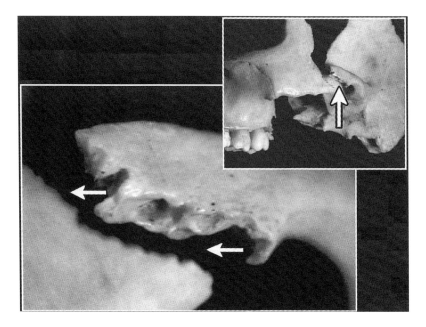

Fig. 6-4 Anteroinferior lateral view exposing the left temporal zygomatic suture. Arrows indicate the serrations' anteroposterior direction of projection.

MOTION

Dictated by the direction of the serrations' growth patterns and the angle of engagement of the articular surface, this suture appears to support two predominant motions. The first is anteroposterior gliding along the suture's serrated articular projections (Fig. 6-5). The second is more limited than the first and manifests as rotational pivoting. To aid in its conceptualization, the point of reference when addressing the zygomatic bone will be its posterior angular rim between its frontal and temporal processes. Rotation along this suture is generated by the anteroinferior-lateral flare of the zygomatic bone during temporal external rotation, and the posterosuperior-medial compression of the zygomatic bone during temporal internal rotation. Due to the zygomatic's general external articular overlap of the temporal's zygomatic process, the former motion opens the suture's superior articular seam and closes its inferior medial articular margin, while the latter closes the superior articular seam and opens the inferior medial articular margin (Fig. 6-6).

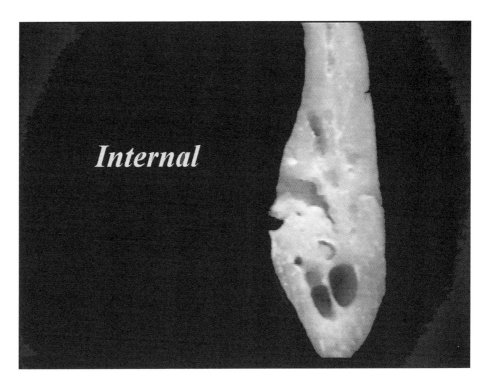

Fig. 6-5A Zygomaticotemporal rotation: internal rotation

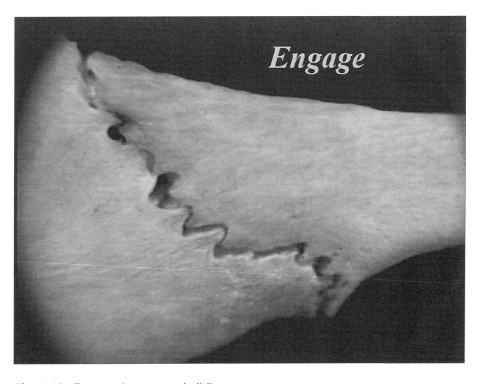

Fig. 6-6A Zygomaticotemporal gliding: engagement

Compare with next photos ➡

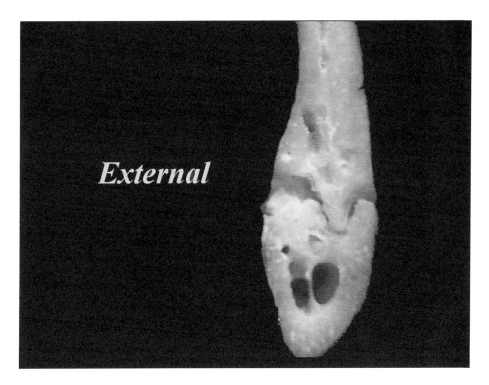

Fig. 6-5B Zygomaticotemporal rotation: external rotation

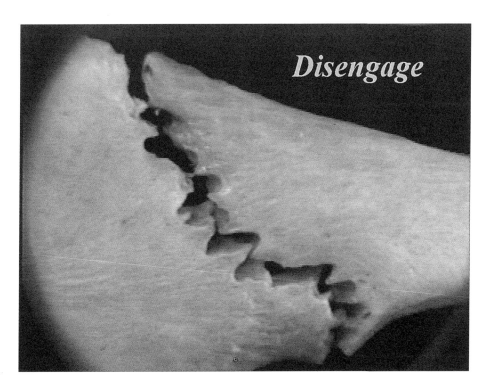

Fig. 6-6b Zygomaticotemporal gliding: disengagement

Articular Disengagement

CONTACT

The optimal contact points are located inside the mouth, posterior to the zygomatic anterolateral fossa surface and along the superior and inferior margins of the zygomaticotemporal process posterior to the suture.

MANIPULATION

W¼R-level pressure, administered inside the zygomatic fossa, is directed anteriorly to disengage the serrated teeth and laterally to separate the zygomatic's overlapping beveled surface. W-level pressure is synchronously applied to the contacts along the zygomaticotemporal process margins in a posterior direction to draw the temporal articular surface away from the zygomatic border (Fig. 6-7).

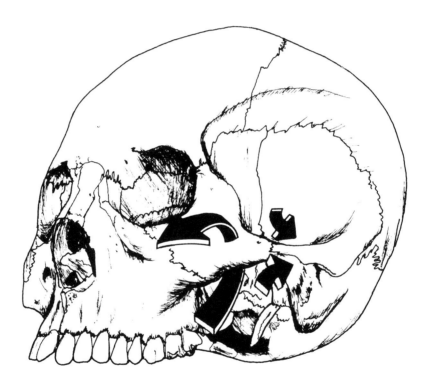

Fig. 6-7 Contacts and direction of manipulation (arrows) used to release the zygomaticotemporal suture

Articular Reengagement

CONTACTS

The optimal zygomatic contact is located inferior to the posterior zygo-maticotemporal margin, on the external posterolateral zygomatic surface. The temporal contact is applied superior to the anterior temporal process border (Fig. 6-8).

MANIPULATION

W¼R-level pressure to the zygomatic's contact is directed in three stages:

1. Posterior to engage the suture's lower third's serrated surface
2. Medial to close the zygomatic's overlapping beveled surface with the temporal process
3. Cephalad to stabilize the zygomatic bone against the temporal process contact's counterpressure.

Simultaneous W-level countercaudal force to the temporal contact secures the temporal process's position during the manipulation of the zygomatic's contact (Fig. 6-8).

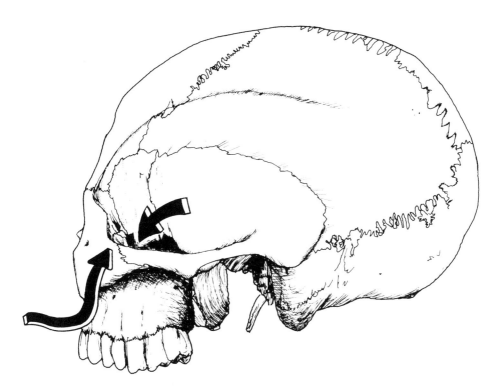

Fig. 6-8 Contacts and direction of manipulation (arrows) used to close the zygomaticotemporal suture

Zygomaticomaxillary Suture (Paired)

MORPHOLOGY

Located between the zygomatic bone and the maxilla, this suture runs in a lateral-caudal direction from the center of the inferior orbital rim to the inferior edge of the zygomatic bone (Fig. 6-9). The suture superficially appears to be shallow, and its articular characteristics would appear to be similar to those found in the superior portion of the coronal suture. However, when disarticulated, the exposed maxillary surface resembles an arrowhead with three distinct articular borders (Fig. 6-10A).

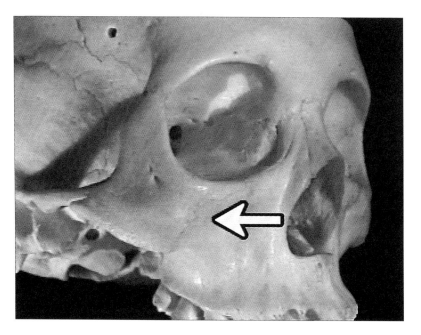

Fig. 6-9 Anterior topographic location of the zygomaticomaxillary suture depicting the suture's anterolateral articular margin

For descriptive purposes, the borders have been labeled as posterior, superomedial, and anterolateral. The posterior border (base of the arrowhead) originates along the superior-anteromedial aspect of the zygomatic fossa and descends in a lateral-caudal direction along the fossa's anterior wall to terminate at the zygomatic's inferior osseous edge. Upon macroscopic exposure, the posterior articular seam reveals a series of alternating beveled edges where the zygomatic and maxilla's articular margins vacillate in being externally dominant (Fig. 6-10B). Although the presence of these alternating edges appears to discourage anteroposterior gliding, it does seem to encourage a hinged-type of movement.

The arrowhead's superomedial articular border originates at the superomedial edge of the posterior articular border and traverses along the internal lateral surface of the inferior orbital floor to terminate anteriorly in the center of the inferior orbital rim. The anterolateral articular margin

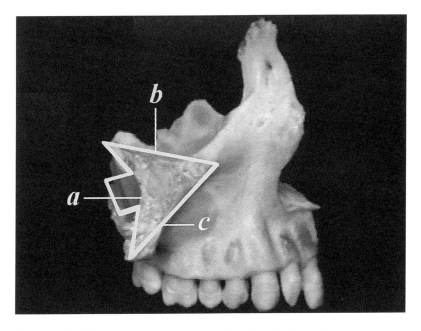

Fig. 6-10A The suture's exposed arrowhead articular surface.

a. Posterior border
b. Superomedial border
c. Anterolateral border

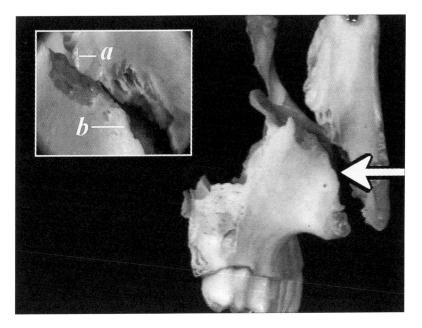

Fig. 6-10B Posterior border of the zygomaticomaxillary suture located along the anterior wall of the zygomatic fossa. The suture's laterally caudal course is clearly exposed and the arrow delineates the area of macroscopic exposure, depicting a typical alternation of sutural overlap along the posterior border.

a. Zygomatic's posterior overlapping articular margin
b. Maxilla's alternate posterior overlapping margin

emerges from the caudal-lateral edge of the posterior articular border and rostrally courses anteromedially to terminate as a pinnacle junction with the superomedial articular margin in the center of the inferior orbital rim (Fig. 6-10A).

The suture's maxillary floor is often paper-thin and elevated to form a small trihedral projection within the suture's internal articular surface (Fig. 6-11). The outer articular border circumvents the trihedron with internally beveled peripheral walls and serrated pinnacle corners. The presence of the external wall formations along the maxillary's three peripheral borders ensures the encasement of the zygomatic's wedged shape articular margins by creating an almost continuous enveloping trench between the maxilla's external edges and internal trihedron (Fig. 6-11).

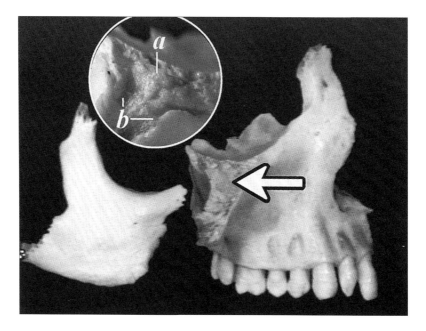

Fig. 6-11 The maxilla's arrowhead shape articular surface is exposed to display the trihedron and its surrounding trench formation. Note the external marginal wall formations which help to create the trenches' outer edges.

a. Trihedral formation
b. Trench formation

Upon closer observation, the lateral four-fifths of the maxilla's anterolateral and posterior articular walls are internally beveled to form a deep-seated articular trench for enveloping the zygomatic's wedge-shape articular surface. The trench's inferolateral apical junction is often covered with medial to lateral serrated projections which appear to support the zygomatic bone and discourage it from inferior or anteroposterior slippage (Fig. 6-12). The absence of an internally beveled peripheral wall projecting from the superomedial fifth of the maxilla's anterior articular border is consistently noted. This absence of external maxillary lipping (elevated external wall) allows the zygomatic's articular surface to reverse its position, from being overlapped to that of overlapping. Shallow serrations projecting superolaterally from the articulation's anterior-superomedial corner appear to mimic the lower lateral corner in protecting the suture from anteroposterior slippage (Fig. 6-12). The maxilla's posterosuperior-medial corner contains serrated projections which extend in a posterosuperior-lateral direction, following a course set by the maxilla's posterior fossa wall (Fig. 6-12).

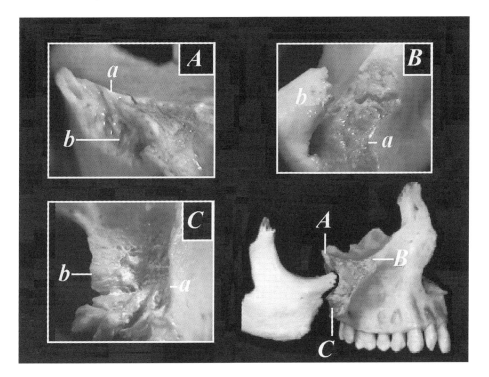

Fig. 6-12 Exposed maxillary surface revealing the articulation's arrowhead configuration. The three projecting surfaces are labeled and macroscopically enlarged to reveal their characteristic compositions

A. Posterosuperior-medial corner
  a. Superomedial articular edge
  b. Posterosuperior-medial articular surface. Note that the posterior articular surface is beveled to allow for the posterior external overlapping of the zygomatic's articular margin. The superior-posterolateral serrated projections are exposed.

B. Superior-anteromedial corner
  a. Maxilla's articular surface. Note the absence of external articular lipping and the raised arch configuration of the articular surface.
  b. Zygomatic's overlapping articular projection. Note the exposed shallow serrations that cover the articulation's marginal edge.

C. Inferior-anterolateral corner
  a. Anterolateral articular wall
  b. Posterior articular wall. Note the articular trench created by the wall's internal beveling.

MOTION

The suture's morphology appears to allow for hinged motion along the anterior articular seam. This is often noted as internal to external rotation. This motion may best be explained if the practitioner's focus is directed toward the posterior rim of the zygomatic's frontal orbital process. As the zygomatic bone hinges anteriorly, the posterior edge of its frontal process is drawn in an anteroinferior-lateral direction. This is considered synonymous with external rotation. During the posterior hinged motion of the zygoma, the posterior edge of its frontal process shifts in a posterosuperior-medial direction (Fig. 6-13). Synonymous with internal rotation, this motion produces narrowing of the posterior zygomatic fossa (the space between the sphenoid's greater wing and the posterior internal surface of the zygomatic bone).

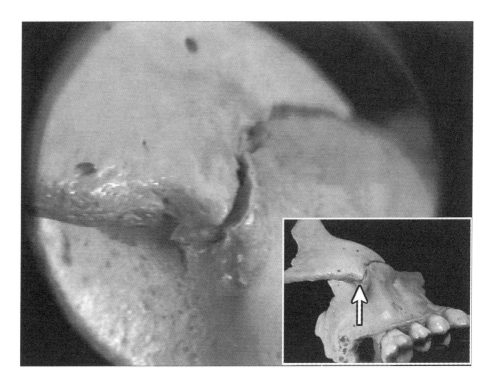

Fig. 6-13A Zygomaticomaxillary motion: internal rotation

Compare with next photo ➡

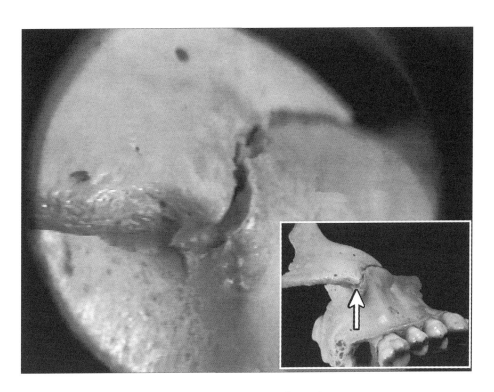

Fig. 6-13B Zygomaticomaxillary motion: external rotation

Articular Disengagement

CONTACTS

The optimal zygomatic contact points to disengage this suture are located posterior to the zygomatic bone in the zygomatic fossa and along the anterior zygomatic surface lateral to the anterior articular border of the zygomaticomaxillary suture (Fig. 6-14). The maxillary contact point is located medial to the anterior zygomaticomaxillary suture in a bony depression inferior to the infraorbital foramen.

MANIPULATION

W⅓R-level pressure applied to the zygomatic contacts are compressed into the osseous surface to grasp the bone and rotationally lift it laterally as simultaneous inferomedial W⅓R-level force is used to orient the maxillary contact to resist (Fig. 6-14).

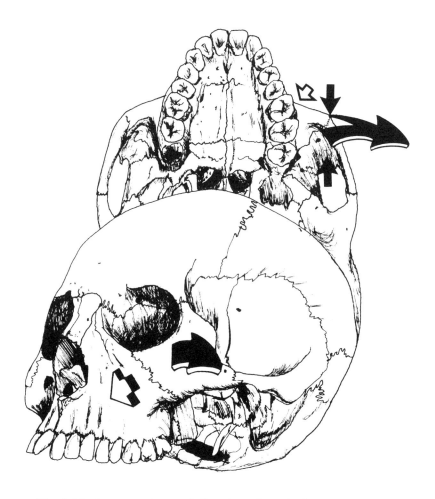

Fig. 6-14 Contact points and direction of manipulation (arrows) for releasing the left zygomaticomaxillary suture

Articular Reengagement

CONTACTS

The optimal zygomatic contact point to close this suture is located on the anterior external surface of the zygomatic bone, superolateral to the zygomaticomaxillary suture. The maxillary contact is located inside the mouth in the osseous depression of the hard palate, on the same side as the suture (Fig. 6-15).

MANIPULATION

At the zygomatic contact, W¼R-level pressure is directed inferomedially toward the suture. Concurrently, at the hard palate contact point, W-level pressure is applied superolaterally to stabilize the maxilla against the stress of the zygomatic contact (Fig. 6-15).

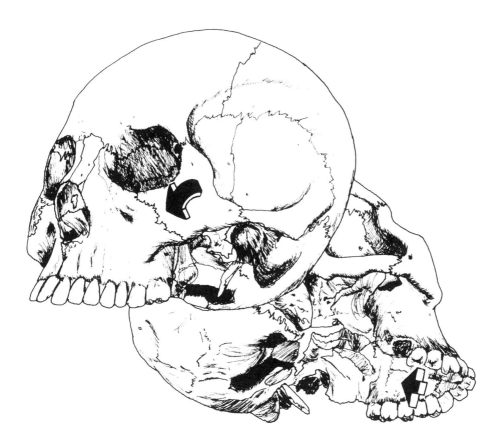

Fig. 6-15 Contact points and direction of manipulation (arrows) for closing the left zygomaticomaxillary suture

Intermaxillary Suture (Singular)

MORPHOLOGY

Located along the sagittal midline of the hard palate, the intermaxillary suture divides the right and left maxillary horizontal palatal plates. The suture originates along the anterior facial surface (between the nasal floor and the two superior incisor teeth) and courses posteriorly to terminate at the intersection of the interpalatine suture and the traversing palatine-maxillary suture (Fig. 6-16A).

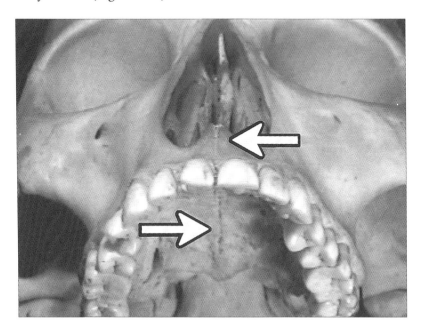

Fig. 6-16A Anteroinferior view exposing the topographic location of the intermaxillary suture

During the first three decades of life, the articular surface anterior to the incisive fossa is predominately plane-like and covered with uneven smooth shaped lumps. As this surface approaches the anterior wall of the incisive fossa, the surface changes into a series of vertical ridges and grooves. Upon closer inspection, the ridge-and-groove formations are found to traverse in an anteroinferior to posterosuperior direction along a path that runs parallel to the incisive fossa (Fig. 6-16B). By the middle of the third decade, the suture's anterior surface takes on a more weathered appearance, including irregular shaped grooves and branching ridges. During this stage of morphologic change, a large irregular shaped cavernous configuration is often noted around the center of the right or left articular surface (Fig. 6-16C).

Adjacent to the side with the central cavernous groove is a corresponding irregular prominence. Even though the surface undergoes this noticeable change in texture, the long articular posterosuperior ridges and grooves that parallel the incisive fossa's anterior marginal edge do not change, suggesting that their presence may play a significant role in the suture's mobility.

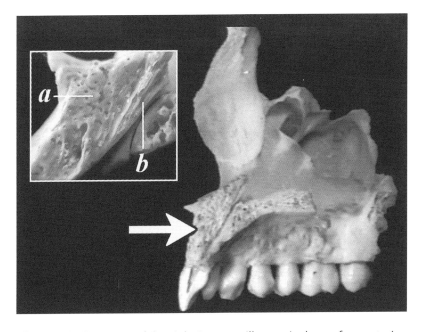

Fig. 6-16B Exposure of the right intermaxillary articular surface anterior to the incisive fossa revealing a typical surface topography found within the first three decades of life

a. Anterior bumpy plane surface
b. Posterior ridge-and-groove formations

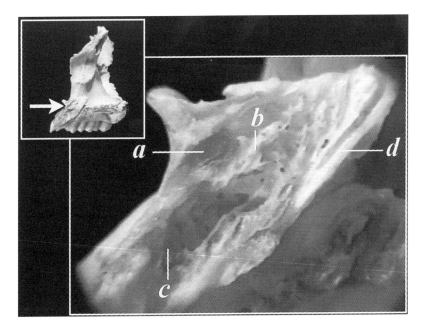

Fig. 6-16C Exposed right anterior intermaxillary articular surface revealing a typical surface topography as seen in the third decade or above

a. Typical irregular shaped groove
b. Branching irregular shaped ridge
c. Central cavernous groove
d. Posterior vertical ridge-and-groove formations

Posterior to the incisive fossa the articular surface narrows, and the surface transforms to rostral-caudal grooves inundated with shallow traversing serrated projections (Figs. 6-16D and E).

Fig. 6-16D Exposure of the right intermaxillary articular surface posterior to the incisive fossa

a. Socket for adjacent intermaxillary serration
b. Large groove-shaped socket posterior to a typical ridge formation

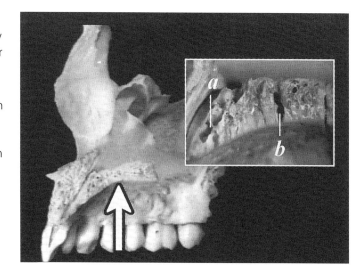

Fig. 6-16E Superior view. The suture has been disengaged to expose the articulation's traversing serrations, posterior to the incisive fossa.

a. Exposed traversing serrated projection

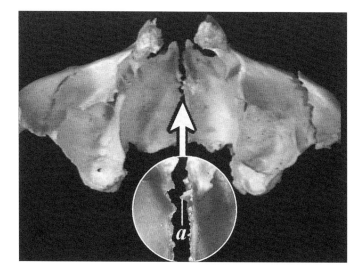

MOTION

Due to the combined configurations of grooves and serrations throughout this suture, the articular margins appear to encourage lateral expansion to medial compression and rostral flexion to caudal extension (Figs. 6-17 and 6-18).

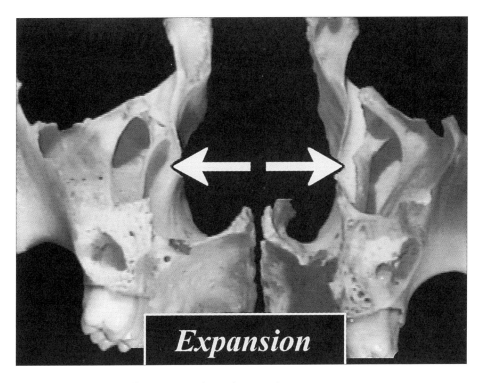

Fig. 6-17A Intermaxillary motion: lateral expansion

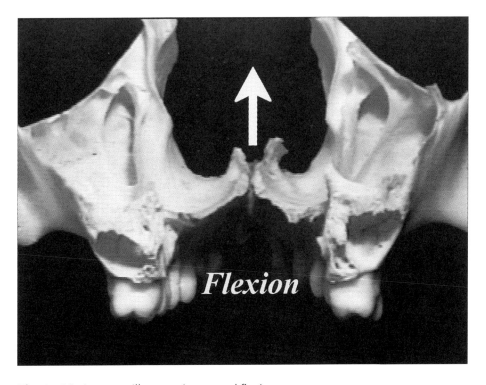

Fig. 6-18A Intermaxillary motion: rostral flexion

Compare with next photos →

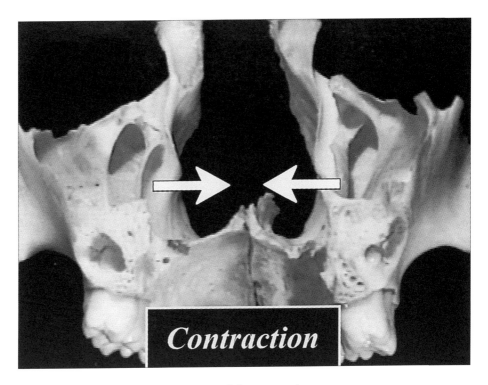

Fig. 6-17B Intermaxillary motion: medial compression

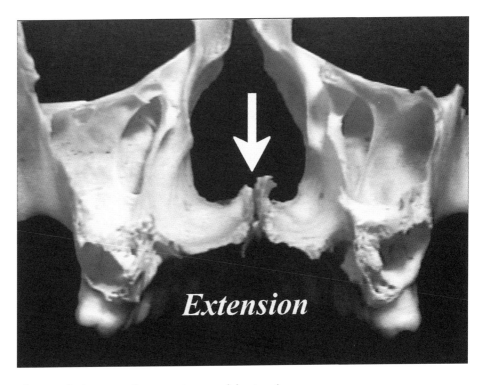

Fig. 6-18b Intermaxillary motion: caudal extension

Articular Disengagement

CONTACTS

The optimal contact points for disengaging the intermaxillary suture are located bilateral to the suture, inside the mouth and on the underbelly of the maxillary hard palate.

MANIPULATION

W¼R-level pressure is directed laterally away from the suture at a 90° angle (Fig. 6-19).

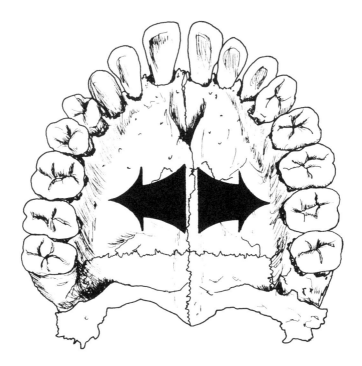

Fig. 6-19 Inferior view of the maxillary hard palate depicting the contacts and direction of manipulation (arrows) to separate the intermaxillary suture

Articular Reengagement

CONTACTS

Contact points used to reengage the intermaxillary suture are located on the external lateral surface of the right and left maxillary bones. *Note:* The contacts should be posterior to the zygomatic bones and level with the inferior border of the opening to the zygomatic fossa.

MANIPULATION

W⅓R-level force is directed toward the suture along the midsagittal plane of the face (Fig. 6-20).

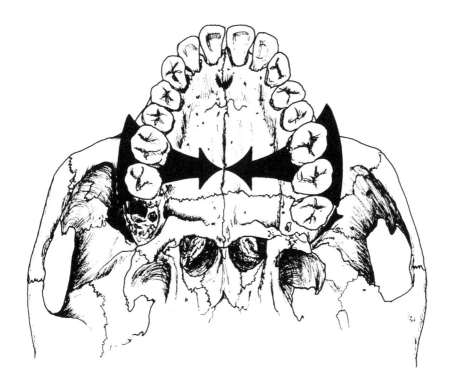

Fig. 6-20 Inferior view of the maxillary hard palate depicting the contacts and direction of manipulation (arrows) to close the intermaxillary suture

Interpalatine Suture (Singular)

MORPHOLOGY

Located along the sagittal midline posterior to the intermaxillary suture, the interpalatine suture originates at the terminal of the intermaxillary suture. The area of transition from the intermaxillary suture to the inter-palatine suture often coronally aligns with the maxilla's second and third intermolar space (Fig. 6-21).

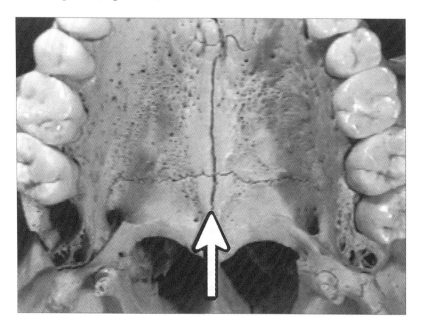

Fig. 6-21 Inferior view depicting the topographic location of the interpalatine suture

Unlike the ridge-and-trench surface of the intermaxillary suture, the inter-palatine sutural articular surface is packed with serrated teeth. The teeth pro-ject perpendicular to the opposing articular surface and insert into uneven sockets that are embedded within the opposing surface's wall (Fig. 6-22).

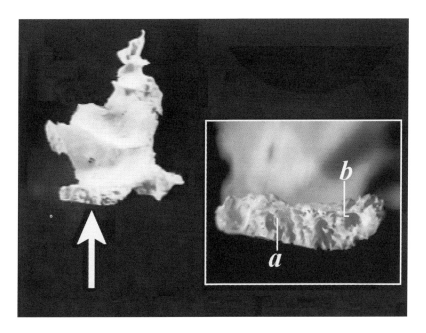

Fig. 6-22A Sagittal plane exposure of the interpalatine's articular surface

a. Serrated projection
b. Socket for an adjacent serration

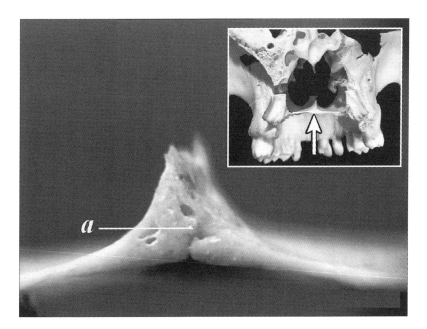

Fig. 6-22B Coronal exposure of the interpalatine suture

a. Typical serrated projection

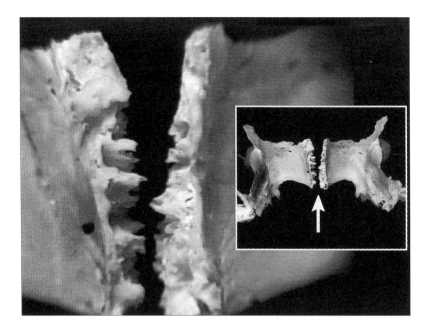

Fig. 6-22C Viewed from its superior aspect, the suture is separated to expose its serrated surface. Note that the serrations traverse the suture at right angles to the opposing articular surface.

MOTION

Because of the suture's articular interlocking serrations, this articulation (like the intermaxillary suture) allows lateral expansion to medial contraction as well as rostral flexion to caudal extension (Figs. 6-23 and 6-24).

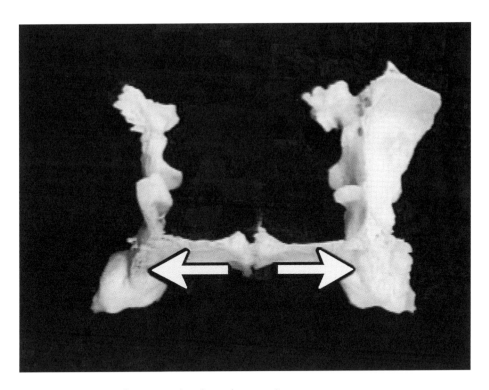

Fig. 6-23A Interpalatine motion: lateral expansion

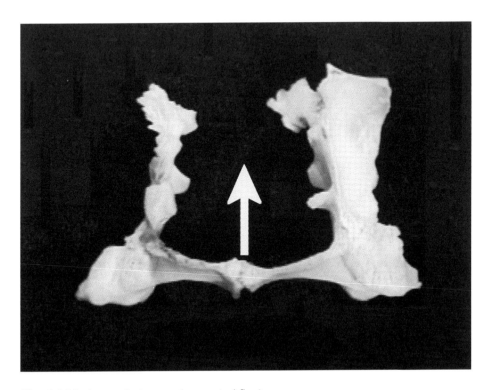

Fig. 6-24A Interpalatine motion: rostral flexion

Compare with next photos →

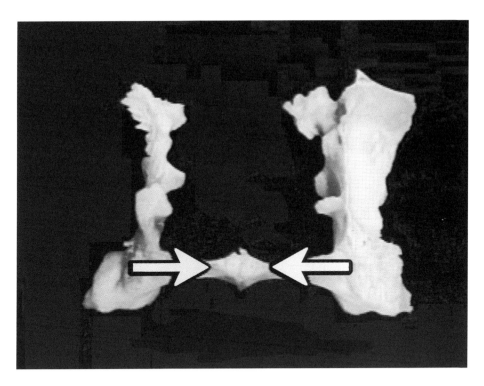

Fig. 6-23B Interpalatine motion: medial compression

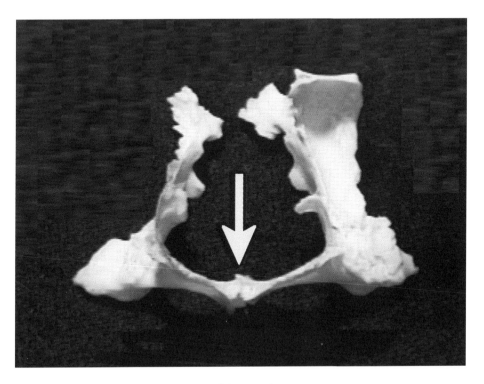

Fig. 6-24B Interpalatine motion: caudal extension

Articular Disengagement

CONTACTS

The optimal contact points for releasing this suture are located lateral to the suture on the palatine's horizontal plates.

MANIPULATION

W⅛R-level pressure is directed laterally, perpendicular to the sutures articular surface. *Note:* Care must be taken not to apply excessive pressure in a cephalad direction during this procedure, or the practitioner runs the risk of locking the serrated edge along its corresponding articular socket wall (Fig. 6-25).

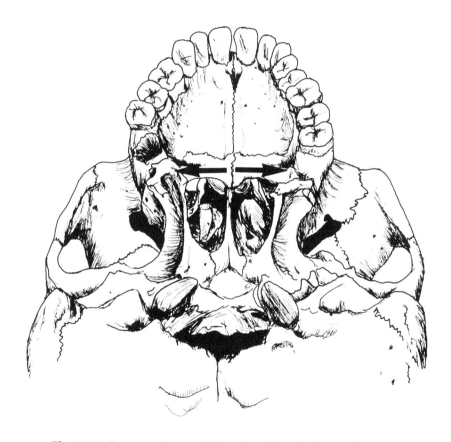

Fig. 6-25 Contact points and direction of manipulation (arrows) to release the interpalatine articular surface

Articular Reengagement

CONTACTS

The contact points used to release the interpalatine suture also serve to close the suture.

MANIPULATION

W⅛R-level pressure is applied medially toward the suture's articular surface (Fig. 6-26).

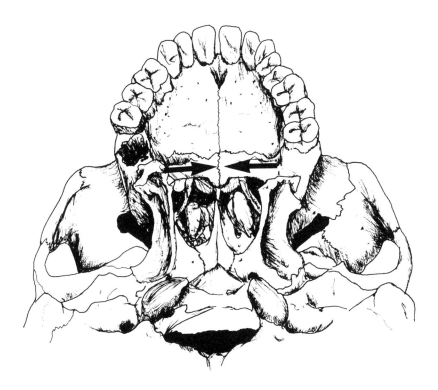

Fig. 6-26 Contact points and direction of manipulation (arrows) to close the interpalatine articular surface

Palatomaxillary Suture (Paired)

MORPHOLOGY

To efficiently study the morphology of the palatomaxillary suture, the suture has been divided into four primary subdivisions: the (1) horizontal, (2) rostral-vertical, (3) rostral-orbital, and (4) caudal-posterolateral. Each skull has two sets of divisions (right and left). This text will only address one and asks the reader to think of the other as its mirrored structure.

1. The *horizontal division* is located along the posterior border of the maxillary hard palate. As the palatomaxillary suture laterally extends from the palate's midsagittal plane, it traverses the maxilla's posterior horizontal margin to inferiorly terminate adjacent to the second molar (Fig. 6-27). When viewed from its superior nasal aspect, the palatine's horizontal margin laterally terminates in a convex curve as the suture shifts rostrally to enter its vertical division along the maxilla's posterolateral nasal wall. The majority of the maxillary articular surface is beveled along its superior nasal surface to allow for its superior overlapping by the palatine's articular surface. However, the maxilla reverses its articular beveled surface around the palate's sagittal midline to project over the palatine's anterior nasal crest. Upon initial inspection, the articular veneer appears to be primarily plane-like. However, when observed macroscopically, the presence of anteroposterior serrations are seen embedded throughout the articulation's surface (Fig. 6-28).

2. The *rostral-vertical division* originates from the superolateral terminal aspect of the horizontal division. As the palatine's horizontal articular surface approaches the maxilla's posterolateral nasal wall, it rostrally curves to form an external convex seal against the maxilla's internally concave surface (Fig. 6-29A). Once the suture has passed through its rostrally directed curve, the articulation's surface appears almost squamosal, with the exception of an anteroinferior to posterosuperior vertical ridge that traverses the maxilla's posterior internal articular surface (Fig. 6-29B).

Fig. 6-27 Topographic location of the maxillo-palatine's horizontal sutural division, as viewed from the inferior

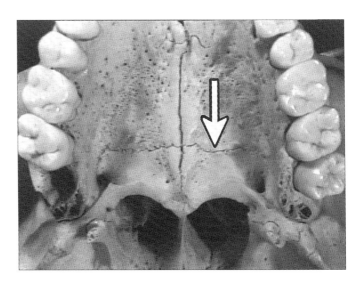

Fig. 6-28A Sagittal section through the right palatomaxillary suture exposing the suture's internal antero-posterior serrations as they zig-zag the suture's articular seam. Note the palatine's general rostral overlapping of the max-illa's articular surface.

a. Maxilla
b. Palatine

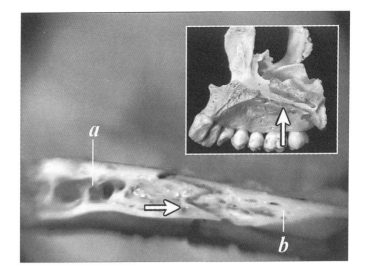

Fig. 6-28B Midsagittal view of the horizontal division, exposing the maxilla's general rostral overlapping of the pala-tine's articular surface

a. Maxilla
b. Palatine

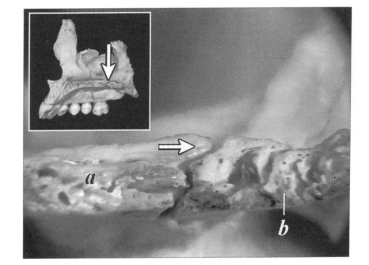

Fig. 6-28C Anterosuperior view exposing the horizontal division's overlapping arrangements. Note the small serrations hidden along the maxilla's inter-nal surface.

a. Palatine's horizontal plate
b. Maxilla's tangent horizontal plate

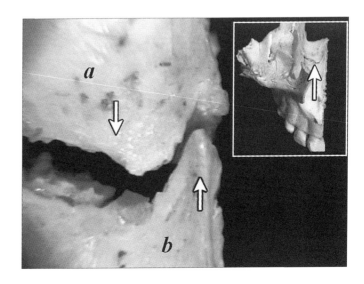

Fig. 6-29A
Anteromedial exposure
of the rostral vertical
suture. Note the pala-
tine's lateral convexity as
its horizontal division
curves rostrally to
become the rostral verti-
cal division.

a. Maxilla
b. Palatine's vertical
   division

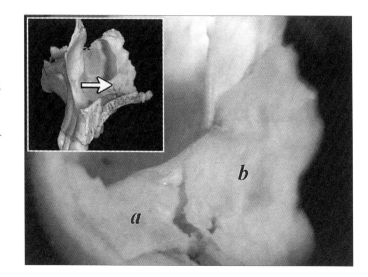

Fig. 6-29B Anteromedial
exposure of the disen-
gaged rostral vertical
articular surface. The
arrow depicts the suture's
internal maxillary ridge.
Note the ridge's vertical
posture which suggests a
possible anteroinferior to
posterosuperior glide
path for the palatine's
articular surface.

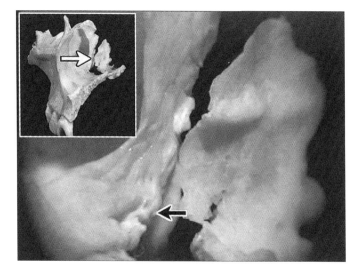

3. The *rostral-orbital division* is posteriorly located along the inferomedial wall of the eye socket (Fig. 6-30A). Projecting in a superior direction from
the top of the vertical division, the suture obliquely angles to traverse anterolaterally over the posterior medial corner of the maxilla's horizontal orbital
plate. When disarticulated and inspected through macroscopic enlargement,
the maxilla's articular surface often appears sparsely covered with uneven
ridges and indentations. However, in spite of its uneven veneer, the surface
consistently appears to maintain an overall smooth texture (Fig. 6-30B).

4. The *caudal-posterolateral division* originates from the inferior lateral
aspect of the horizontal division and descends along the maxilla's posteromedial wall to terminate in a medial-posterosuperior direction to the alveolar
process of the maxilla's third molar. Upon external inspection, the perimeter of
this articulation appears smooth and plane-like in nature (Fig. 6-31A).

Fig. 6-30A
Posterolateral exposure
of the palatomaxillary's
orbital margins

a. Rostral orbital suture
b. Superior vertical
   suture

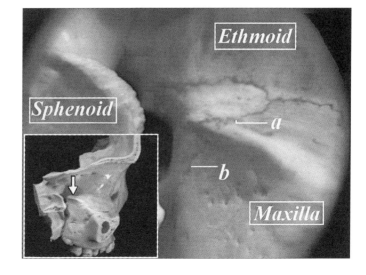

Fig. 6-30B Posterior
view. The suture has
been disarticulated to
expose the maxilla's
anterolateral articular
surface.

a. Horizontal orbital
   plate
b. Posterior ascending
   maxillary wall
c. Typical ridge
   formation
d. Palatine's orbital
   process

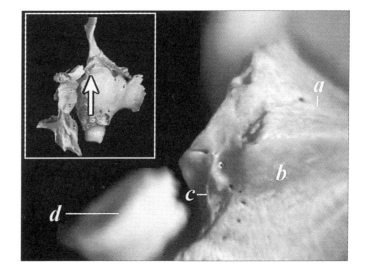

Fig. 6-31A
Posteroinferior exposure
of the caudal postero-
lateral maxillopalatine
division. Note the smooth
plane-like appearance of
the articulation's peri-
meter.

a. Palatine
b. Maxilla

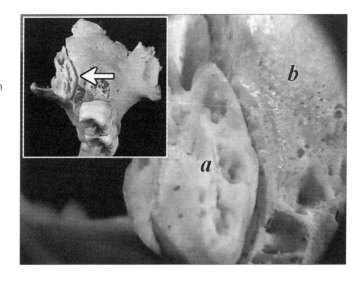

However, when the articular surfaces are separated and exposed, the maxilla's internal surface appears as a spooned-out oviform shape containing small posteromedial serrations. The palatine's adjacent surface bulges to conform with the maxilla's oval indentation and projects anterolateral serrations to interlock the suture's seam (Figs. 6-31B and C).

Fig. 6-31B
Perpendicular view of the maxilla's concave oval formation when exposed from a posteromedial perspective

a. Oviform's floor covered with shallow posteromedial projecting serrations
b. Elevated articular border to encase the palatine's adjacent articular surface

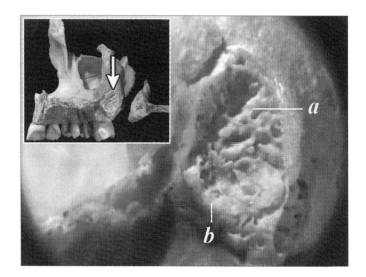

Fig. 6-31C Lateral-oblique view of the oval articular formation when exposed from a postero-inferior prospective. Note the oviform's concave appearance as its articular perimeter projects posteromedially.

a. Articular perimeter
b. Serrated articular floor
c. Palatine

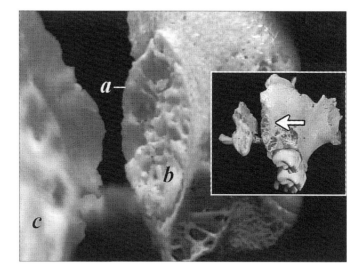

MOTION

The horizontal plate's articular surface has the appearance of a plane-like surface (to allow for gliding). However, superficial serrations extending anteroposteriorly along the articular margins appear to rule out medial to lateral motion, while the planar surface appears to allow for independent anteroposterior gliding (Fig. 6-32).

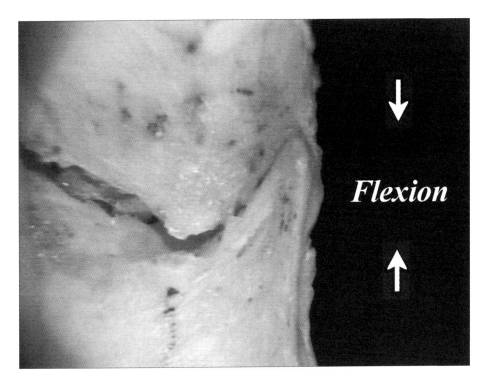

Fig. 6-32A Palatomaxillary motion: gliding flexion

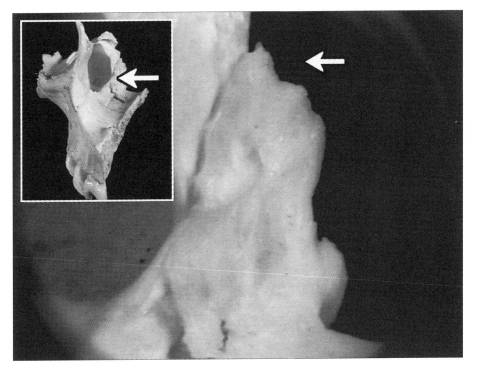

Fig. 6-33A Palatomaxillary motion: lateral

Compare with next photos →

The rostral-vertical division's squamous-like surface appears to support articular gliding, but the presence of the articulation's internal ridge suggests the addition of anteroinferior to posterosuperior tracking. Indeed, all four divisions would appear to prefer some form of anterior to posterior gliding. However, because the rostral-vertical division lacks interlocking serrated projections, this portion of the articulation appears to be somewhat capable of medial to lateral movement and may allow such motion within the confines of the maxilla's outer nasal wall (Fig. 6-33).

The smooth anterolateral surface of the rostral-orbital division permits superior-anterolateral to inferior-posteromedial gliding.

The caudal-posterolateral division's anterolateral encasement of the palatine's bulging surface into the maxilla's serrated oval articular formation appears to encourage posteromedial to anterolateral mobility and would support the medial to lateral motion dynamics of the rostral-vertical and rostral-orbital divisions.

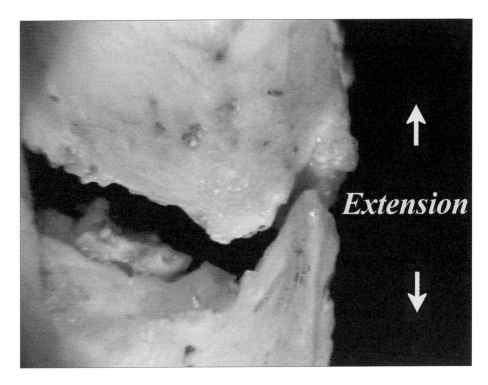

Fig. 6-32B Palatomaxillary motion: gliding extension

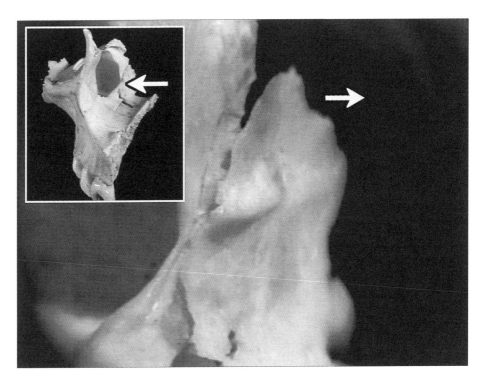

Fig. 6-33B Palatomaxillary motion: medial

Articular Disengagement

CONTACTS

The optimal contact points for releasing the palatomaxillary suture are located on the maxillary hard palate (restricted side) anterior to the suture, and on the posterior lateral aspect of the palatine's involved horizontal plate.

MANIPULATION

W¼R-level pressure in a superior direction to the maxillary contact disengages the maxilla's superior beveled surface. When a release has been accomplished, the force then shifts in an anterior direction to separate the maxillary's serrated, plane-like surface from the palatine's. The palatine contact is counter-applied posteriorly with W-level pressure to stabilize the palatine's articular surface against the anterior pull of the maxilla (Fig. 6-34).

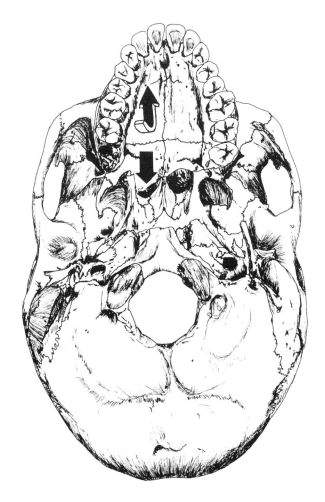

Fig. 6-34 Inferior view of the contact points and direction of manipulation (arrows) to release the right palatomaxillary

Articular Reengagement

CONTACTS

The optimal maxillary contact points to close the palatomaxillary suture are located on the maxillary hard palate anterior to the separated suture and on the anterior external surface of the maxilla superior to the front incisor teeth. The palatine contact is on the palatine's horizontal plate, immediately posterior to the separated suture (Fig. 6-35).

MANIPULATION

W¼R-level pressure to the maxillary contacts are directed posteriorly to close the serrated, plane-like articular surface. As the maxilla contact is being directed posteriorly, the anterior incisor region is drawn caudally to rock the posterior maxillary surface superiorly. This secondary maneuver aids in the engagement of the inferior beveled surface of the maxilla against the superior beveled surface of the palatine. A W-level counterforce to the maxillary maneuvers is applied to the palatine contact and draws the palatine contact in an anterior-cephalad direction against the invasive motion of the maxilla (Fig. 6-35).

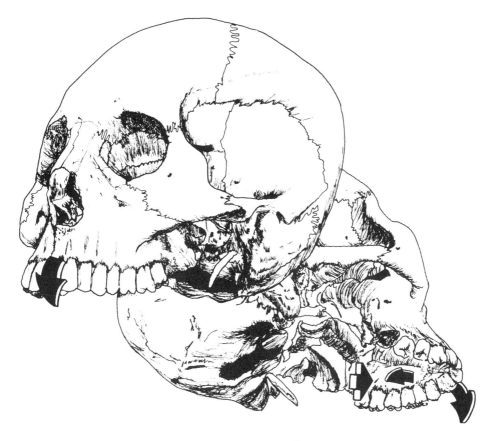

Fig. 6-35 Contact points and direction of manipulation (arrows) to reengage the left palatomaxillary suture

Frontozygomatic Suture (Paired)

MORPHOLOGY

Anteriorly joining the frontal bone's zygomatic process with the zygomatic's frontal process, the frontozygomatic suture originates on the anterolateral margin of the orbital rim and extends posteromedially to terminate with the anterosuperior corner of the sphenoid's greater wing (Fig. 6-36). The suture's thickest articular surface is found around the orbital rim in its anterior one-third (Fig. 6-37A). Beveled along its internal plane, the zygomatic's articular surface is inundated with many anterosuperior serrations, ridges, and trenches (Figs 6-37B and 6-38A). The adjacent overlapped frontal bone's border is externally beveled and articulates with the zygomatic through a series of trenches, ridges, and posteroinferior interlocking serrations (Fig. 6-38).

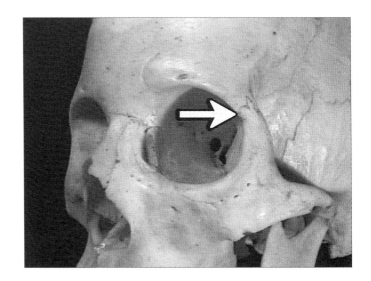

Fig. 6-36A Anterior view of the anterior topographic location of the left frontozygomatic suture

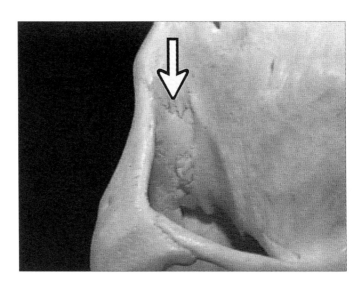

Fig. 6-36B Left posterior oblique view of the posterior topographic location of the frontozygomatic suture

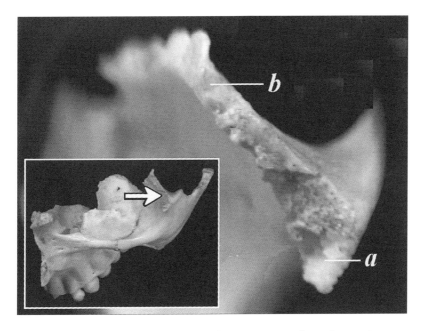

Fig. 6-37A Superior view exposing the zygomatic's frontal articular surface

a. Anterolateral marginal surface
b. Narrowing posteromedial margin

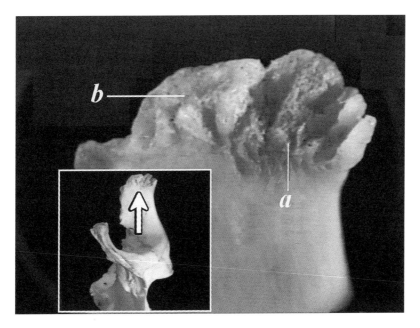

Fig. 6-37B Anteromedial oblique view exposing the left zygomatic's beveled internal articular surface

a. Anterolateral surface covered with serrations, ridges, and trenches
b. Narrowed posteromedial surface appearing somewhat smoother and less serrated

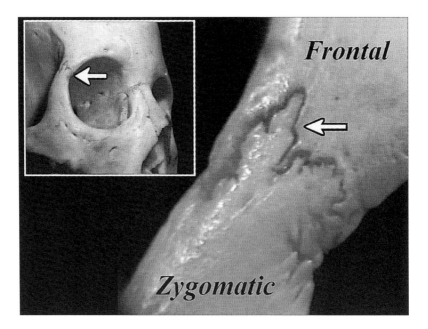

Fig. 6-38A Macroscopic exposure of the right frontozygomatic suture's external anterolateral margin. Note the anterosuperior growth pattern of the zygomatic's serrations.

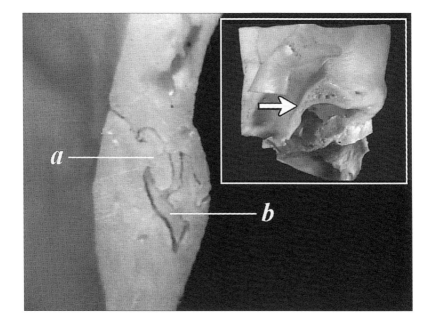

Fig. 6-38B Cross-sectional slice through the suture's narrowed posteromedial articular surface. Note the hidden internal interlocking hammer-shaped denticulate projections that often form after the second decade of life.

a. Zygomatic projection
b. Frontal bone projection

As the suture enters the posterior two-thirds of its articular sector, the osseous structure narrows considerably and the suture's marginal surface appears to take on a smoother characteristic (Figs. 6-37A and B). This, however, is not always the case, as noted in the cross-sectional view (Fig. 6-38B). Here we see, hidden deep within the narrow posteromedial articular seam, interlocking hammer-shaped denticulate projections extending from both the zygomatic and frontal margins. *Note:* The zygomatic's articular borders initially overlap the frontal bone's both anteriorly and posteriorly.

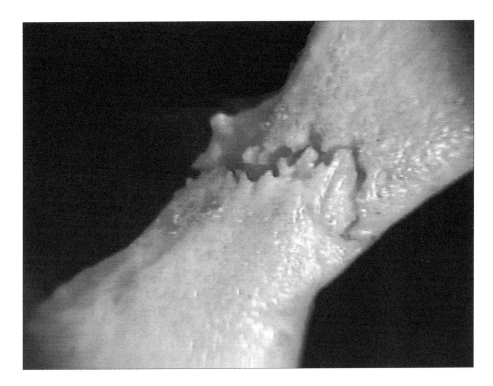

Fig. 6-39A Frontozygomatic motion: anterosuperior rocking

Compare with next photo ➜

MOTION

Although the suture's serrations appear to allow for complete disarticulation through a posteroinferiorly directed lateral traction of the zygomatic bone, the procedure is discouraged beyond the second decade of life by the development of hidden interlocking projections deep within the suture's articular margin. While existence of these interlocking denticulate formations prevents the suture's disarticulation, a rocking motion from superior-anteromedial to inferior-posterolateral is still possible (Fig. 6-39). Consequently, with the application of proper directional manipulation, it is still possible to disengage fixations along the suture's articular junction and return marginal pliability.

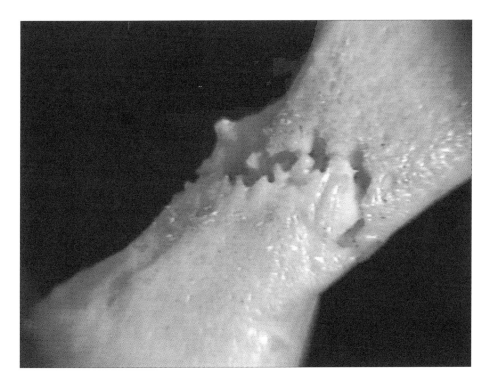

Fig. 6-39B Frontozygomatic motion: posteroinferior rocking

Articular Disengagement

CONTACTS

The optimal zygomatic contact points to release the frontozygomatic suture are located inferior to the suture along the anterior (inner) border of the zygomatic's frontal process, and along the zygomatic's inferior lateral edge (Fig. 6-40). The frontal bone's contact points are located superiorly to the suture along the anterior and posterior orbital borders of the frontal bone's zygomatic process.

MANIPULATION

Using W-level pressure, the zygomatic's superior contact compresses in a posterocaudal direction to disengage the suture's serrated articular margin. Synchronous W⅓R-level compression to the inferior zygomatic contact generates rocking of the zygomatic bone, which in turn externally flares the zygomatic's frontal process. Simultaneous to the zygomatic's manipulative procedure, W⅓R-level counterforce to the frontal bone's contacts directs the frontal bone in an anterior-rostral direction and thus completes the suture's release (Fig. 6-40).

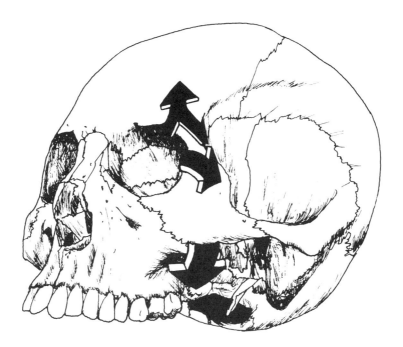

Fig. 6-40 Left anterior oblique view of the contact points and direction of manipulation (arrows) used in releasing the fronto-zygomatic suture

Articular Reengagement

CONTACTS

The optimal contact points to reengage the frontozygomatic suture are along the lateral external orbital rim of the zygomatic's frontal process below the suture's articular junction, and above the suture on the frontal bone's zygomatic process.

MANIPULATION

Using medial compression, W⅛R-level force is directed in an anterosuperior direction at the zygomatic's contact, while W-level caudal-posterior pressure is applied to the frontal bone's contact (Fig. 6-41).

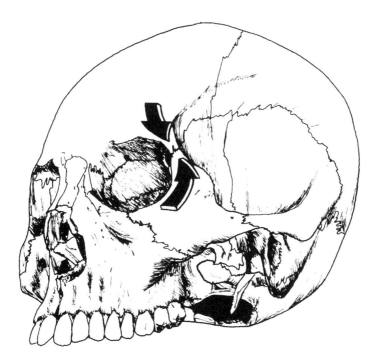

Fig. 6-41 Left anterior oblique view of the contact points and direction of manipulation (arrows) used in closing the fronto-zygomatic suture

Nasomaxillary Suture (Paired)

MORPHOLOGY

The nasomaxillary suture emanates from the lateral aspects of the nasion and descends along the superior medial margins of the maxillary frontal processes (Fig. 6-42). The superior one-quarter of this suture's articular surface runs deep into the anteroinferior underbelly of the glabella. As the suture descends, the remaining three-quarters of its articular surface often narrows to the thickness of approximately 1 to 2mm. Eighty-five percent of the maxilla's articular surface houses a trench-like formation created by the internal beveling of its anterior and posterior margins. The adjacent nasal surface appears shaved to form a shallow longitudinal wedge for the maxilla's articular trench, and tends to suggest that the two surface areas may permit interarticular gliding (Fig. 6-43). However, when the sutures are viewed from an anterior direction, a distinct bottleneck formation is created by the combined shapes of the two nasal bones. This bottleneck shape is located between the first and second superior quarters of the two bones and creates an interlocking surface that does not permit independent superior-to-inferior gliding (Fig. 6-42).

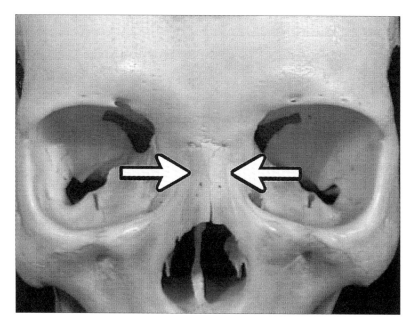

Fig. 6-42 Arrows depict the topographical location of the nasomaxillary sutures and the superior bottleneck shape created by the nasal bones

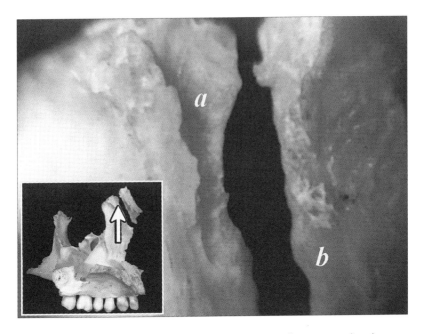

Fig. 6-43A Posteromedial view. The left nasomaxillary suture has been opened to expose its articular surface.

a. Maxillary articular trench
b. Nasal articular wedge

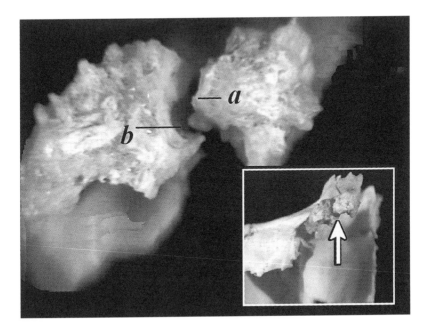

Fig. 6-43B Left nasomaxillary articulation, exposed from its superior aspect

a. Nasal wedge
b. Maxillary trench

MOTION

Because of the combined structural makeup of the nasomaxillary articular surfaces and the interlocking bottleneck shape of the upper nasal bones, independent gliding of the nasal bones along the articular surface of the maxillary frontal processes appears to be limited. However, limited antero-inferior to posterosuperior gliding seems to be possible considering the overall associated movements of the nasal bones within the maxillary articular margins (Fig. 6-44).

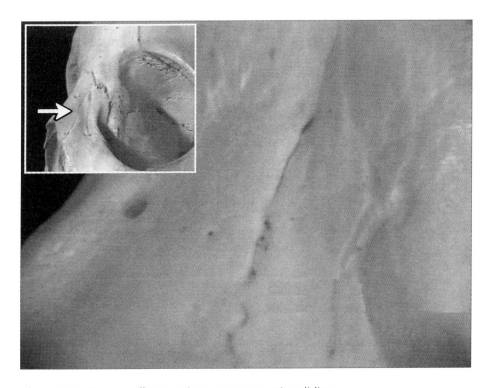

Fig. 6-44A Nasomaxillary motion: posterosuperior gliding

Compare with next photo ➡

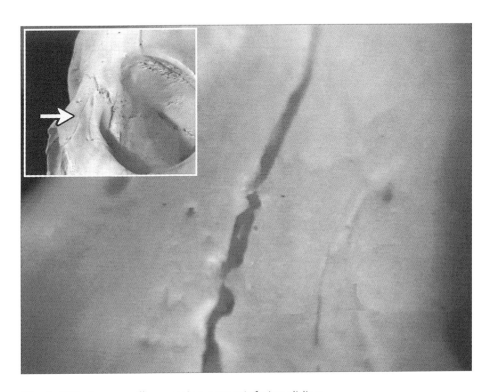

Fig. 6-44B Nasomaxillary motion: anteroinferior gliding

Articular Disengagement

CONTACTS

To disengage this suture, the practitioner must keep in mind the bottleneck shape of the superior nasal bones. Since this shape serves to discourage caudal release, attention is directed toward disengaging the maxillary surface from the nasal bone rather than the nasal bone from the maxilla. There are three optimal contact points to achieve this suture's release. Two are located on the maxilla of the involved articular side: inside the mouth on the anterolateral aspect of the hard palate, and on the external anterior surface medial to the infraorbital foramen. The third contact is located on the anterosuperior aspect of the involved nasal bone immediately below the nasion (Fig. 6-45).

MANIPULATION

W-level pressure applied to the maxillary contacts compresses into the contact surface, thus clamping onto the structure. With the maxilla firmly engaged by the clamp-like grip, the line of force is directed in an anterolateral-caudal direction using W⅓R-level force to draw the maxilla away from the nasal bone. Counterpressure is simultaneously applied using W⅓R-level pressure to the nasal bone contact, stabilizing the bone in a medial-caudal direction. The overall process thus causes the specific release of the nasomaxillary suture (Fig. 6-45).

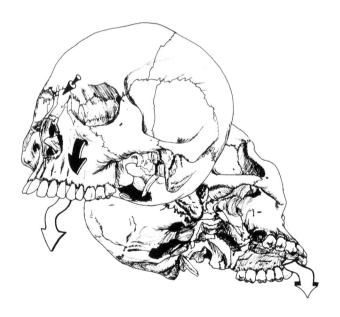

Fig. 6-45 Contact points and direction of manipulation (arrows) for releasing the nasomaxillary suture

Articular Reengagement

CONTACTS

Contact points used to reengage the nasomaxillary suture are located on the anterior surface of the nasal bone, medial to the involved suture, and on the involved external maxillary frontal process, medial to the eye socket.

MANIPULATION

W⅛R-level pressure is directed superolaterally to the nasal contact while W-level pressure to the maxillary contact directs the force superomedially (Fig. 6-46). The superior manipulative force aligns the gliding surfaces between the wedge and trench while the lateral and medial forces compress the wedge into the trench to secure the suture's articular surface.

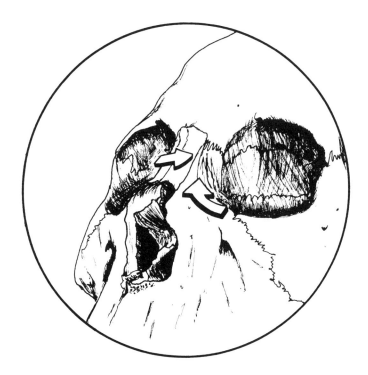

Fig. 6-46 Contact points and direction of manipulation (arrows) for closing the nasomaxillary suture

Internasal Suture (Singular)

MORPHOLOGY

The internasal suture is located between the two nasal bones on the mid-sagittal plane of the nasal bridge (Fig. 6-47). Characteristically zig-zagged in its upper-third articular seam, the suture appears to articulate as two flat surfaces butting together. However, upon separation, the articular borders reveal a series of superficial, alternating, beveled undercuts that line the suture's upper articular borders and prevent anteroposterior slippage. The first overlapping bony flap is located along the superior one-sixth of the suture and usually crosses from right to left. The second overlapping osseous flap usually crosses the suture within the second superior one-sixth from left to right (Fig. 6-48A). As the articular margins descend into the suture's inferior two-thirds, the borders take on a more linear surface devoid of overlapping edges and alternating bevels (Fig. 6-48B). Just as with the lateral articular margin, the nasal bone's sagittal surface appears thicker superiorly and thins to approximately 1mm as it descends toward the opening of the nasal passage.

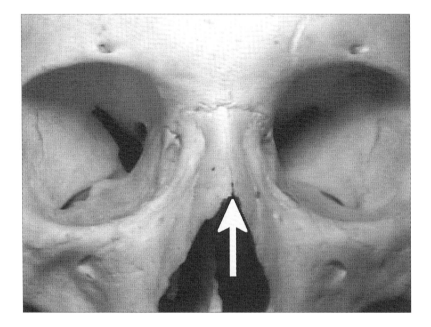

Fig. 6-47 Topographic location of the internasal suture

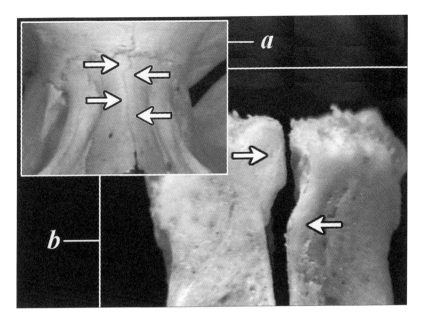

Fig. 6-48A Internasal suture

a. Zig-zag articular seam that interlocks the suture and inhibits gliding

b. Macroscopic view: the internasal suture has been opened to expose its superior alternating articular formation

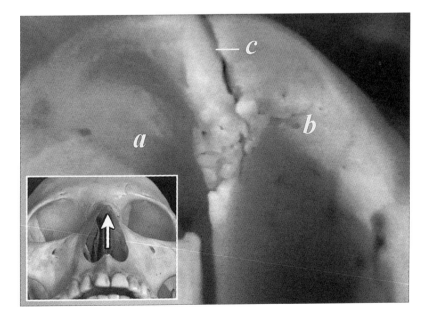

Fig. 6-48B Inferior exposure depicting the edge-to-edge articular seam of the suture's lower region. *Note:* Although the suture terminates close to the sagittal midline, it is not uncommon for it to deviate slightly during its ascent.

a. Right nasal bone

b. Left nasal bone

c. Internasal suture

MOTION

Because of the structural characteristics of its articulations, the suture appears to be capable of anteroposterior hinge-like activity. The suture's morphology suggests lateral separation along its longitudinal seam. However, the practitioner should keep in mind that the nasal bones articulate superiorly with the frontal bone, and articulate laterally between the two maxillary frontal processes. It is this enveloped association that dictates hinge-like motion as opposed to lateral expansion (Figs. 6-49 and 6-50).

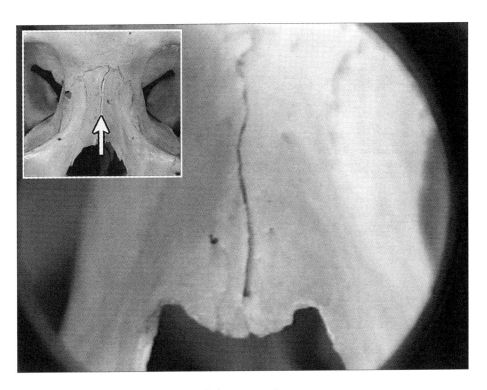

Fig. 6-49A Internasal motion: medial compression

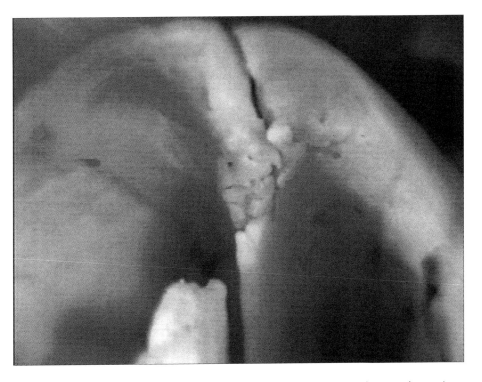

Fig. 6-50A Internasal motion (inferior view): lateral expansion with central anterior shift

Compare with next photos →

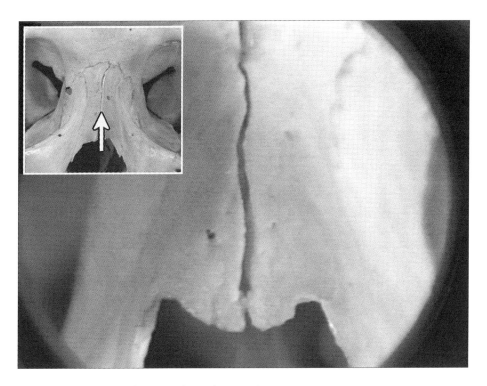

Fig. 6-49B Internasal motion: lateral separation

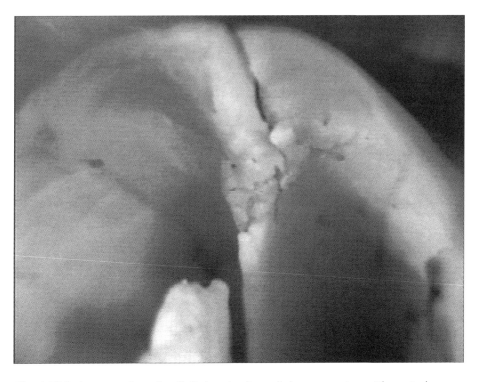

Fig. 6-50B Internasal motion (inferior view): medial compression with central posterior shift

Articular Disengagement

CONTACTS

The optimal contacts for releasing the internasal suture are located along the anterior surface of the nasal bones. Since the overlapping beveled articular surfaces tend to act as an interlocking device, contacts should be approached with this in mind. The contact on the left nasal bone is located immediately inferior to the nasion or nasal frontal suture. The contact on the right nasal bone should be on the second one-sixth superior aspect of the nasal bone inferior to the level of the left contact (Fig. 6-51).

MANIPULATION

W⅛R-level pressure is initially directed posteriorly at the two contact points to release the overlapping beveled articular surfaces. The pressure is then altered to draw the nasal bones apart by maintaining the posterior compression, but shifting the force laterally away from the suture (Fig. 6-51). *Note:* Release of this suture is limited by the surrounding structures that envelop the nasal bones. Consequently, disengagement will be perceived as a softening rather than a separation.

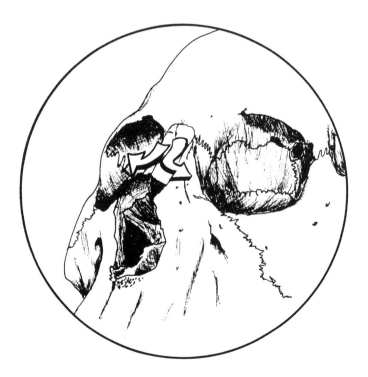

Fig. 6-51 Contact points and direction of manipulation (arrows) to release the internasal suture

Articular Reengagement

CONTACTS

The optimal contacts for reengaging the internasal suture are located within the superior one-third of the two nasal bones. As a rule, the left nasal contact is on the anterior surface of the bone, half a finger width inferior to the nasal-frontal suture. The right nasal bone is contacted along its anterior surface immediately inferior to the nasion (Fig. 6-52). *Note:* The contact points are dictated by the suture's overlaying sagittal zig-zag formation.

MANIPULATION

W⅛R-level pressure is directed posteromedially through both contact points. This action serves to compress the two overlapping beveled surfaces of the suture and close or tighten the interlocking articular surface of the two nasal bones below the points of contact (Fig. 6-52).

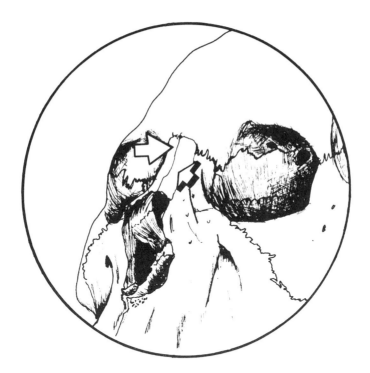

Fig. 6-52 Contact points and direction of manipulation (arrows) to close the internasal suture

Frontonasomaxillary Suture (Interconnected Pair)

The frontonasomaxillary suture consists of the paired frontomaxillary and frontonasal sutures; in this text, the four sutures have been grouped under one common name. The discussion that follows is based upon the structural similarity of the four sutures' articular surfaces and their interlocking articular associations, which renders them incapable of independent manipulation. Consequently, the articular contours that will be depicted here are those found along the entire articular surface, and manipulative strategies address the relationship of the frontal bone to the entire nasomaxillary articular surface.

MORPHOLOGY

Inferiorly bordered by the superior articular surfaces of the two nasal bones and the frontal processes of the paired maxillary bones, the suture is unified superiorly by the single articular surface of the frontal bone below the region of the glabella (Fig. 6-53). Located superior to the nasal bridge in a region known as the nasion, this suture is invested with serrated teeth that anchor the four inferior bones to the frontal bone's socket-and-trench articular surface. The teeth emerge posterosuperiorly from the nasal and maxillary processes to enter the frontal bone's adjacent articular surface. Once inside their respective sockets, the teeth slightly alter their course to an anterosuperior direction. This creates a small sickle-shaped serration that serves to anchor the articular surfaces together (Figs. 6-54 and 6-55).

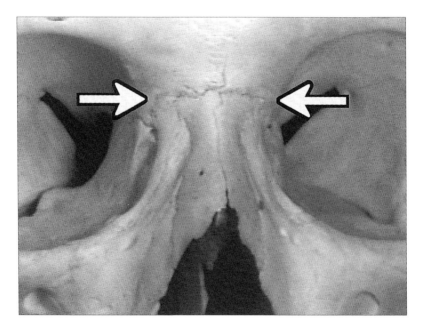

Fig. 6-53 Topographic location of the frontonasomaxillary suture

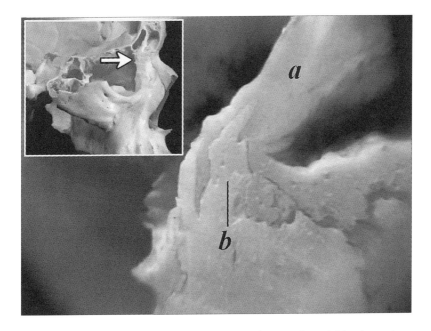

Fig. 6-54 Sagittal section exposing a typical ascending sickle-shaped projection from the maxilla's frontal process

a. Frontal bone
b. Maxillary's serrated projection

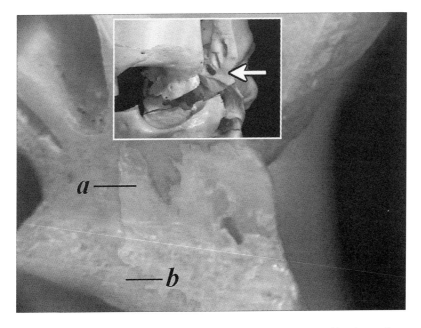

Fig. 6-55 Sagittal section exposing a typical ascending sickle-shaped projection from the nasal bone's articular surface into its adjacent frontal bone's socket

a. Projecting nasal serration
b. Anteroinferior projecting surface of the frontal bone

MOTION

Because of the unusual sickle shape of the articular serrations in this suture, it appears that direct caudal descent of the inferior osseous structures is impossible. However, the serrations do allow for caudal descent if it is accompanied with an anterior shift at the end (Fig. 6-56).

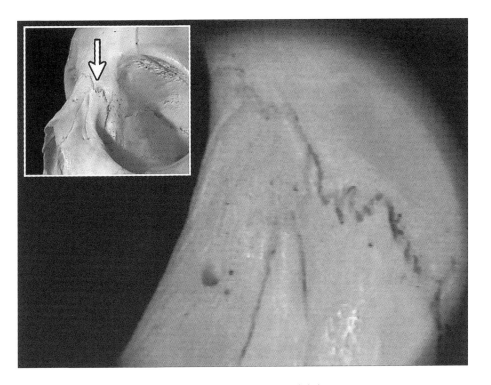

Fig. 6-56A Frontonasomaxillary motion: anterocaudal descent

Compare with next photo ➔

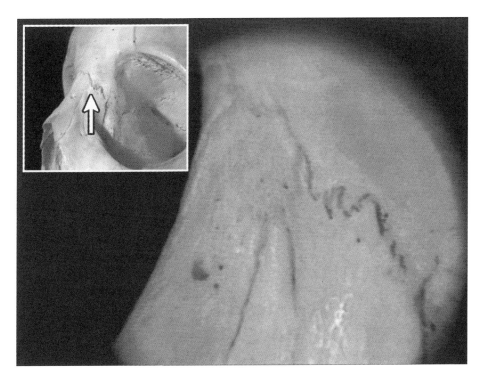

Fig. 6-56B Frontonasomaxillary motion: posterocephalad ascent

Articular Disengagement

CONTACTS

Optimal contact points for disengaging this suture are located on the frontal bone, overlapping the two nasomaxillary sutures, and inside the mouth on the anterior hard palate. The frontal bone's contacts are placed on the superomedial rims of the eye-sockets, inferior to the medial margins of the superciliary aches. The nasomaxillary contacts overlap the nasomaxillary sutures, and the hard palate's contact is located along the anterior sagittal midline, posterior to the front incisor teeth (Fig. 6-57).

MANIPULATION

Posterosuperior W-level pressure on the frontal bone's contacts secure its position against the tug generated by the following maneuvers. The contacts over the nasomaxillary regions are directed caudally with W⅓R-level force, while the hard palate's contact utilizes W⅛R-level force to draw the inferior maxillary surface in an anteroinferior direction (Fig. 6-57).

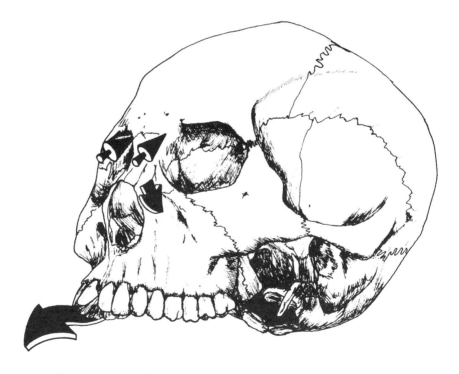

Fig. 6-57 Optimal contact points and direction of manipulation (arrows) used to release the frontonasomaxillary suture

Articular Reengagement

CONTACTS

The optimal maxillary contacts for reengaging this suture are the same as those used in releasing the suture. However, the frontal bone's contacts are positioned over the medial aspects of the superciliary arches, adjacent to the frontal bone's sagittal squamous and superior to the level of the frontal eminences (Fig. 6-58).

MANIPULATION

W⅛R-level pressure is employed on the frontal bone's contacts in an anterior-caudal direction toward the suture's articular surface. W-level force is applied to the nasomaxillary contacts in a rostral direction toward the suture as the maxillary palate contact swings posterosuperiorly (Fig. 6-58).

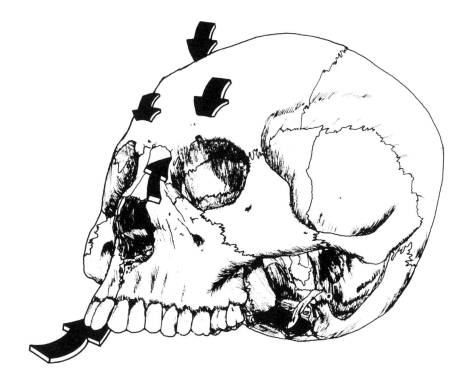

Fig. 6-58 Optimal contact points and direction of manipulation (arrows) to close the left frontonasomaxillary suture

CHAPTER SEVEN

Inaccessible Sutures

IN THIS CHAPTER, inaccessible facial sutures are studied first. This is followed by a study of inaccessible base and vault sutures. As in Chapters 5 and 6, the morphological attributes, description of motion, and manipulative strategies are given for each suture. To aid the practitioner, one or more paired images are found within each section on motion.

Facial Sutures

Frontolacrimal Suture (Paired)

MORPHOLOGY

The frontolacrimal suture is located inside the anteromedial aspect of the eye socket. This small suture originates anteriorly at the lateral border of the frontomaxillary suture and posteriorly terminates at the frontoeth-moidal suture (Fig. 7-1A). Because of the suture's position under the medial fat pad of the eyeball, the suture is considered inaccessible.

Viewed externally, the suture's articular margins appear to be lined with bevels or overlapping serrations. The serrated formations projecting rostrally from the lacrimal's articular border and caudally from the frontal bone's articular border appear to consistently overlap their adjacent surfaces (Fig.

7-1B). However, when observed from a coronal slice, the alternating serrations are definitely superficial, and the deeper articular configuration is characterized by the frontal bone's shaved internal edge, which mostly descends to externally overlap the lacrimal's articular border (Fig. 7-2).

Fig. 7-1A Topographical location of the fronto-lacrimal suture

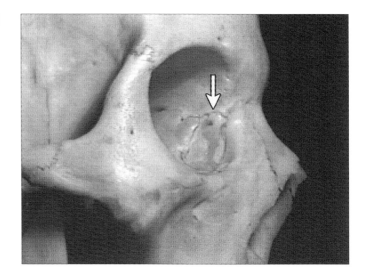

Fig. 7-1B Magnified external view of the frontolacrimal suture. Arrows depict the direction of alternating articular overlaps.

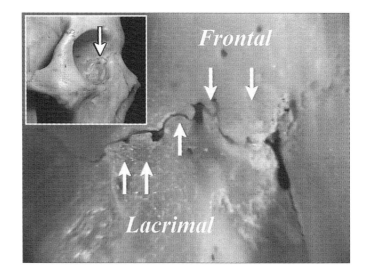

MOTION

The superomedial to inferolateral angular configuration of the overlapping frontal bone's articular margin appears to allow inferolateral to superomedial gliding along the lacrimal's superior articular surface. Because the frontal bone's articular border appears to be slightly concave while the lacrimal's adjacent margin is convex, this curved articular junction is also capable of medial to lateral rocking (Fig. 7-3).

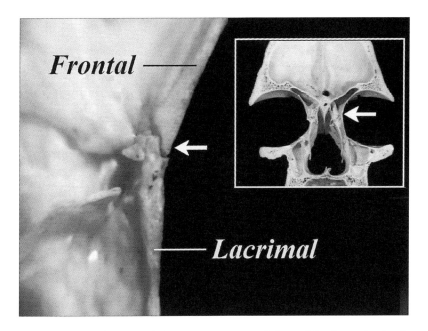

Fig. 7-2 Magnification of the posterior coronal slice of the frontolacrimal suture. Arrow depicts the frontal bone's internally beveled overlapping border.

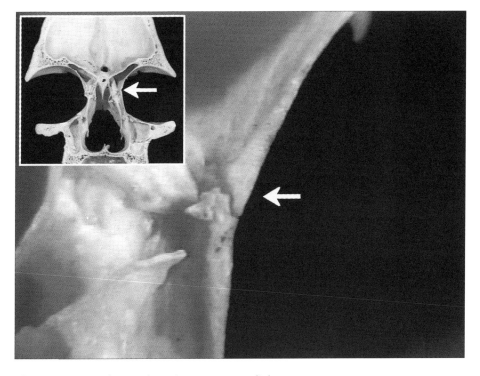

Fig. 7-3A Frontolacrimal motion: superomedial

Compare with next photo ➡

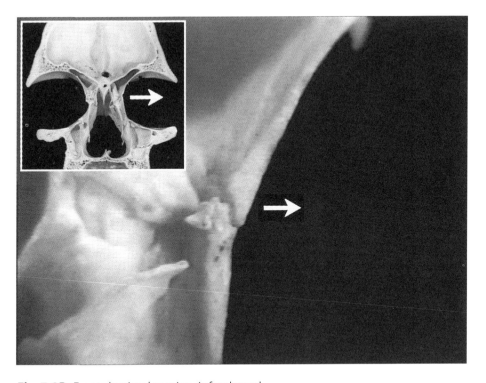

Fig. 7-3B Frontolacrimal motion: inferolateral

Articular Disengagement

CONTACTS

Although this suture cannot be palpated, the practitioner may use associated landmarks to access the necessary releasing points. To locate the
frontal contact, an imaginary horizontal line is followed from the top of
the frontomaxillary suture to a location inside the superomedial orbital
rim of the eye socket (Fig. 7-4A). This should place the contact on the
frontal bone, rostral to the suture. The maxillary contacts that are used
in conjunction with the frontal bone contact are located on the external
maxillary surface, lateral to the floor of the nasal cavity and posterior to
the last molar on the side of sutural fixation (Fig. 7-4B).

Fig. 7-4A Location of
the frontal bone's con-
tact. Arrow delineates
the imaginary horizontal
line as it courses over the
frontomaxillary suture to
end inside the supero-
medial orbital rim.

a. Frontal contact
b. Frontomaxillary suture

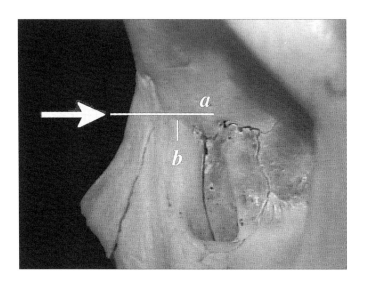

MANIPULATION

W¼R-level pressure is applied rostrally to the frontal bone's contact as
W¼R-level pressure is applied to the maxilla's contacts, drawing the maxilla in a caudal-anterior direction (Fig. 7-4B).

Articular Reengagement

CONTACTS

The frontal bone's contact used to reengage the suture is located over the
medial supraorbital arch. The maxillary contacts are identical to those used
to disengage the suture (Fig 7-5).

MANIPULATION

W¼R-level pressure is applied to the frontal bone's contact in a medial-
caudal direction toward the suture as the maxillary contacts are drawn
rostrally and posterior using W-level pressure to counter the pressure of
the frontal bone's maneuver (Fig. 7-5).

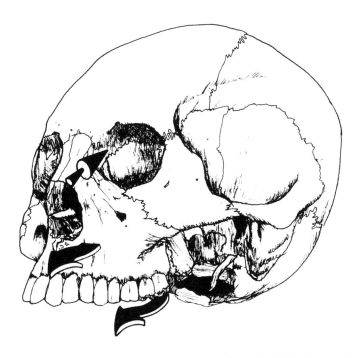

Fig. 7-4B Contact points and direction of manipulation (arrows) for releasing the left frontolacrimal suture

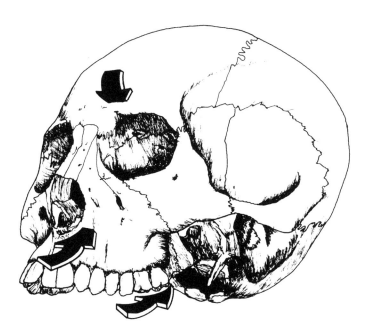

Fig. 7-5 Contact points and direction of manipulation (arrows) for closing the left frontolacrimal suture

Anterior Lacrimomaxillary Suture (Paired)

MORPHOLOGY

This suture is located along the posterolateral border of the frontomaxillary process (Fig. 7-6). Upon initial observation, the osseous borders appear to align edge to edge (Fig. 7-7A). However, when examined from its posterior aspect, the superior one-fourth of the articular surface displays a hidden internal lacrimal ledge that appears to be sparsely serrated on its anterior edge (Fig. 7-7B). As the articular margin descends into its remaining inferior border, the lacrimal's beveled surface changes to externally overlap its adjacent maxillary articular border. Although the suture's overall articular contour supplies medial-lateral stability, very little posteroanterior support seems to be furnished. Therefore, it appears that the suture's posteroanterior articular integrity is based upon the lacrimal's remaining articular associations.

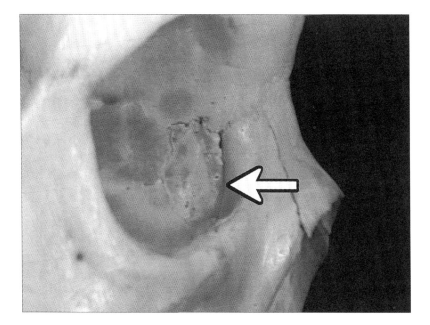

Fig. 7-6 Topographical location of the anterior lacrimomaxillary suture

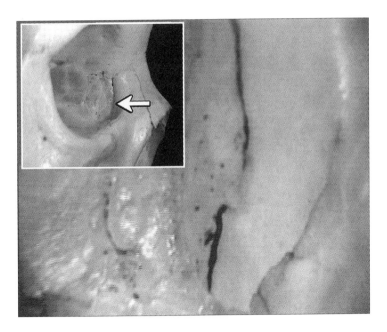

Fig. 7-7A External topographic exposure depicting the suture's illusionary edge-to-edge articular junction. Note the external overlapping flap from the middle of the lacrimal's articular border.

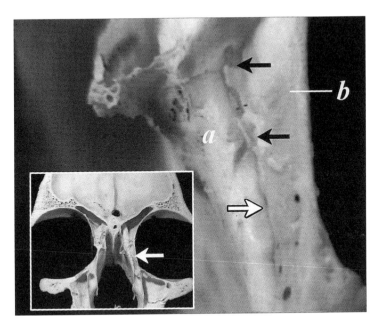

Fig. 7-7B Posterior view exposing the lacrimal's anterior articular junction with the frontomaxillary process. Arrows depict the internal areas of articular overlapping along the suture's superior articular margin.

a. Maxilla
b. Lacrimal bone

MOTION

Dictated by the suture's articular configurations and the lacrimal's associated structures, two primary movements along this articular junction are possible. The first primary motion is posterosuperior-lateral flaring, which disengages the lacrimal's anterior articular border from its adjacent maxillary margin. The second primary motion reengages the suture's articular seam when the lacrimal's anterior border is drawn in an anteroinferior-medial direction (Figs. 7-8 and 7-9).

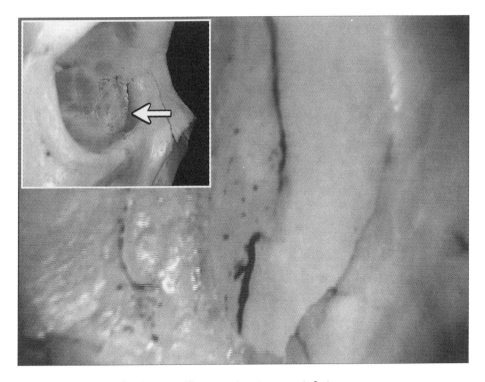

Fig. 7-8A Anterior lacrimomaxillary motion 1: anteroinferior

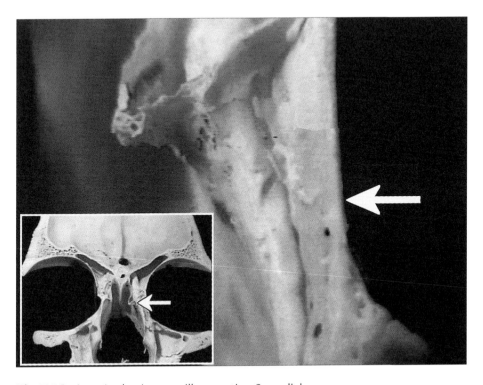

Fig. 7-9A Anterior lacrimomaxillary motion 2: medial

Compare with next photos →

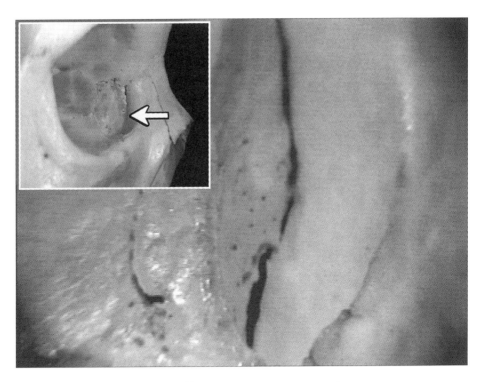

Fig. 7-8B Anterior lacrimomaxillary motion 1: posterosuperior

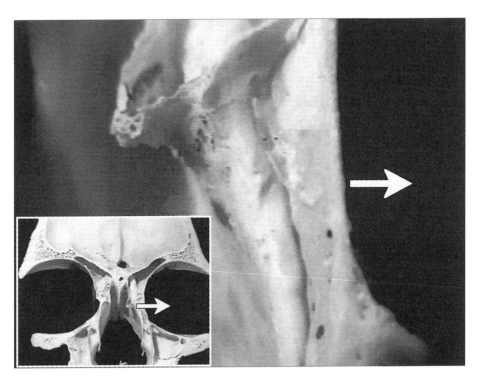

Fig. 7-9B Anterior lacrimomaxillary motion 2: lateral

Articular Disengagement

Because of the unusual nature and location of this suture, direct attempts to independently disengage it are highly unlikely. However, the release of sutural fixations may be accomplished using the following strategic manipulation.

CONTACTS

The following contacts are applied to the side of the involved lacrimal fixation and can be regarded as a combined direct-indirect manipulative protocol. Located on the maxilla's lateral frontomaxillary process, the direct contact is inside the medial rim of the eye socket while the indirect contact is inside the mouth along the crown surfaces of the first and second maxillary molars (Fig. 7-10).

MANIPULATION

The lateral maxillary process's contact is coerced in a caudal-anterior direction with W-level force to disengage the process's serrating junction to the frontal bone's articular margin. The process is then drawn medially toward the opposite facial side with W⅓R-level pressure to separate the maxilla's process from the lacrimal's anterior articular margin. Synchronous W⅓R-level force on the molar contacts in a medial-rostral direction indirectly secures the lacrimal between the maxilla's inferior orbital articular junction and the superior frontal bone's articular margin (Fig. 7-10).

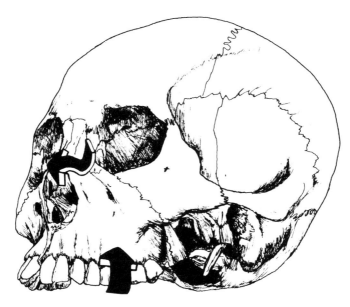

Fig. 7-10 Contact points and direction of manipulation (arrows) for releasing the anterior lacrimomaxillary suture

Articular Reengagement

CONTACTS

The same contacts are used to close and release the anterior lacrimomaxillary articular surface.

MANIPULATION

W⅓R-level pressure guides the maxillary process's contact posteriorly into the suture while simultaneous superomedial W-level tension on the molar contact secures the articular binding between the medial orbital floor and the frontal bone's articular margin (Fig. 7-11).

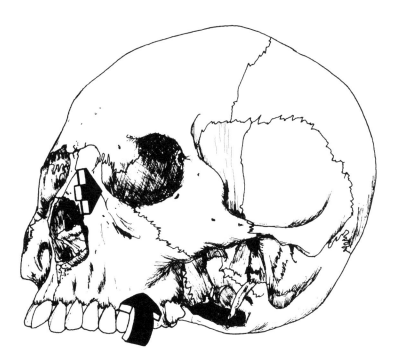

Fig. 7-11 Contact points and direction of manipulation (arrows) for closing the anterior lacrimomaxillary suture

Inferior Lacrimomaxillary Suture (Paired)

MORPHOLOGY

Bordered posteriorly by the ethmoid and anteriorly by the maxilla's lacrimal groove, the inferior lacrimomaxillary suture is located superomedially to the anterior maxillary orbital surface along the anteromedial inferior wall of the eye socket (Fig. 7-12A). When observed laterally from inside the eye socket, the border between the lacrimal's articulation and the adjacent maxillary surface appears to have an edge-to-edge bond. However, a posterior coronal slice exposure of the suture's anterior one-fifth articular seam reveals that the lacrimal's inferior articular surface is noticeably bifurcated to straddle its adjacent articular borders. Squamosal in configuration, the lacrimal's internal surface extends caudally along the inner wall of the maxilla's lacrimal groove, and its external surface projects inferolaterally to externally overlap its adjacent maxillary orbital surface (Fig. 7-12B). As the suture extends posteriorly, the lacrimal's remaining articular border alters its configuration, and its internal descending surface disappears. No longer straddled over the maxilla, the lacrimal's articular edge hovers superiorly over its juxtaposed articular surface formed by the union of the inferior nasal concha and the maxilla's medial orbital margin (Fig. 7-12C). *Note:* It has been observed in some specimens that lacrimal overlapping occurs along the anterior one-fifth and posterior two-fifths of the suture's articular surface, while the region in between articulates marginally end to end.

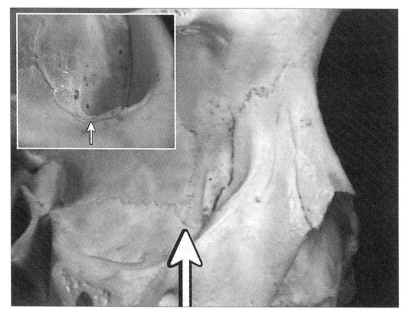

Fig. 7-12A Viewed laterally from inside the eye socket, the arrow depicts the topographic location of the inferior lacrimomaxillary suture

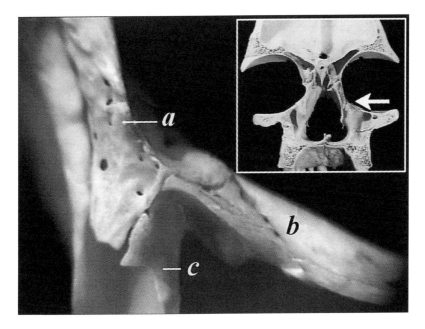

Fig. 7-12B Posterior coronal section exposing the inferior lacrimomaxillary suture's anterior one-fifth articular seam

a. Lacrimal bone
b. Maxilla's orbital plate
c. Maxilla's caudal projection to the inferior nasal concha

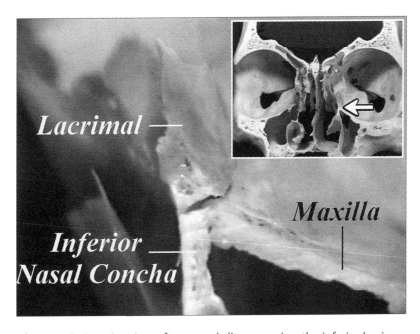

Fig. 7-12C Anterior view of a coronal slice exposing the inferior lacrimomaxillary suture's posterior four-fifths articular seam. *Note:* The lacrimal's inferior juxtaposed articular border runs in a superolateral to inferomedial direction and maintains a persistent rostral overlap of the maxilla's border throughout the suture.

MOTION

The lacrimal's anterior bifurcation and posterosuperior angular overlay suggests the possibility of internal-to-external rocking over the maxilla's adjacent articular border. To fully understand the dynamics that govern this suture's release or engagement, the practitioner should keep in mind the difference between the lacrimal's anterior and posterior articular contours. The bifurcated anterior aspect of the lacrimal's orbital articular seam tends to release or open as its outer articular ledge lifts and externally flares into the orbital socket (Fig. 7-13). However, as the external margin lifts from its adjacent maxillary border, the lacrimal's internal caudal projecting surface tends to compress against its juxtaposed articular surface. Thus, from a lateral orbital view, the suture may appear to be releasing when in fact it is engaging along its anterointernal junction. Unlike the anterior articular junction, the suture's posterior four-fifths is less restricted because of the absence of an internal articular ledge. Therefore, upon external orbital surface flaring, this portion truly releases as its articular surface lifts and courses laterally over the maxilla's adjacent rim (Fig. 7-14). Although the suture's profile does permit rostral elevation of the lacrimal from its seat along the maxilla's adjacent border, this motion is somewhat limited by the lacrimal's superior articular association with the frontal bone.

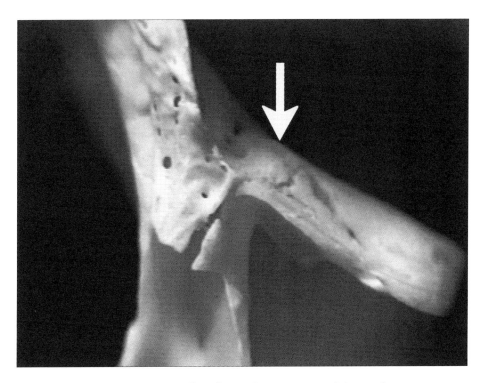

Fig. 7-13A Inferior lacrimomaxillary flaring (anterior aspect): internal

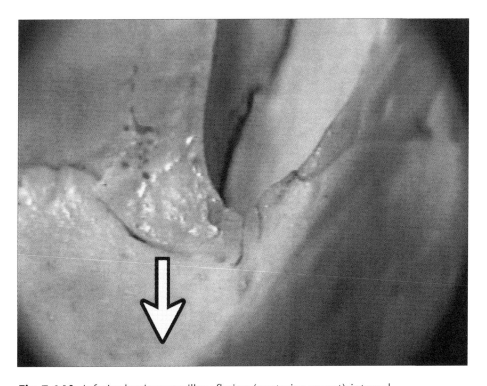

Fig. 7-14A Inferior lacrimomaxillary flaring (posterior aspect): internal

Compare with next photos →

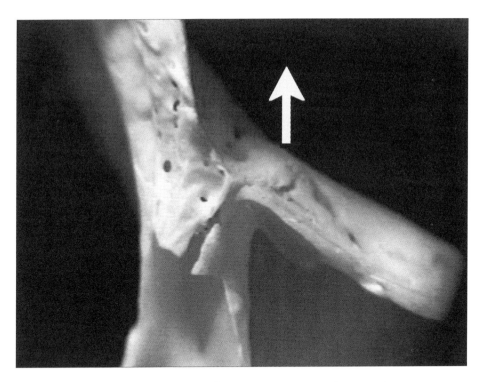

Fig. 7-13B Inferior lacrimomaxillary flaring (anterior aspect): external

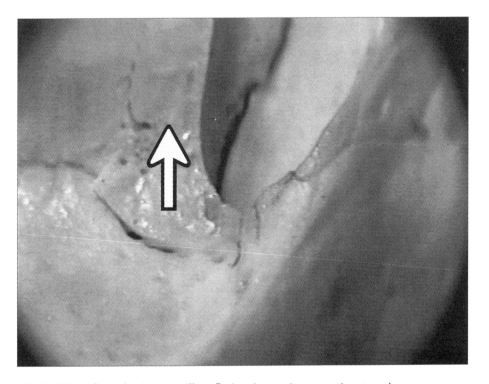

Fig. 7-14B Inferior lacrimomaxillary flaring (posterior aspect): external

Articular Disengagement

CONTACTS

The optimal contact points for releasing this suture are located on the superior frontomaxillary process below the frontomaxillary suture, and inside the mouth along the lateral aspect of the last three maxillary molars. This greater contact surface aids in disengaging (Fig. 7-15).

MANIPULATION

The application of posterior W⅓R-level pressure through the maxillary process secures the lacrimal bone. Simultaneous W-level force on the lateral molars' contact separates the inferior lacrimomaxillary suture by drawing the molars' contact in a caudal-medial direction (Fig. 7-15).

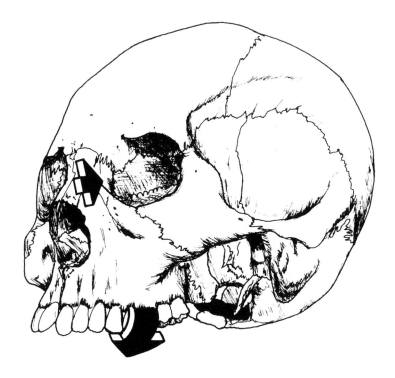

Fig. 7-15 Contact points and direction of manipulation (arrows) for releasing the inferior lacrimomaxillary suture

Articular Reengagement

CONTACTS

The optimal contact points for closing the inferior lacrimomaxillary suture's articular surface are located on the superior frontomaxillary process, inferior to the frontomaxillary suture, and along the inferior crown surfaces of the maxilla's first and second molars (Fig. 7-16).

MANIPULATION

W-level pressure is applied posterosuperiorly to the frontomaxillary process to compress the superior lacrimomaxillary suture and stabilize the lacrimal bone. To engage the suture, W⅓R-level pressure is applied rostrally to the molar's contact toward the inferior lacrimomaxillary margins (Fig. 7-16).

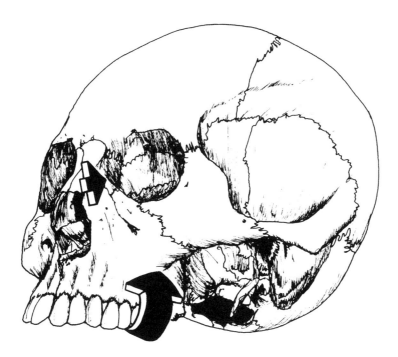

Fig. 7-16 Contact points and direction of manipulation (arrows) for closing the inferior lacrimomaxillary suture

Ethmoidolacrimal Suture (Paired)

MORPHOLOGY

Located approximately 1.5cm posterior to the anteromedial orbital rim, the ethmoidolacrimal suture resides along the medial wall of the eye socket and runs in a rostral to caudal direction along the anterior articular surface of the ethmoid bone (Fig. 7-17). The lacrimal's posterior internal articular edge is frequently shaved to overlap the ethmoid's anterior articular border. The ethmoid's externally overlapped anterior articular margin is often sparsely lined with miniature anteroposterior serrated teeth, suggesting a moderate interlocking of the suture's articular border (Fig. 7-18).

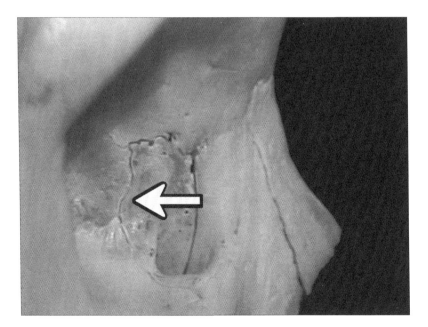

Fig. 7-17A Topographic location of the ethmoidolacrimal suture

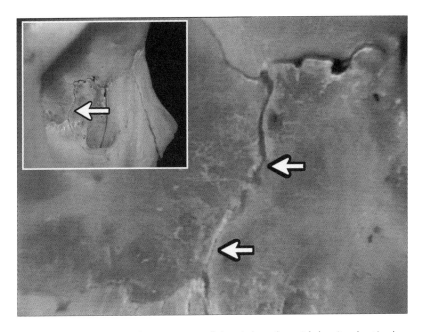

Fig. 7-17B Macroscopic exposure of the right ethmoidolacrimal articular seam. Arrows depict the direction of sutural overlap.

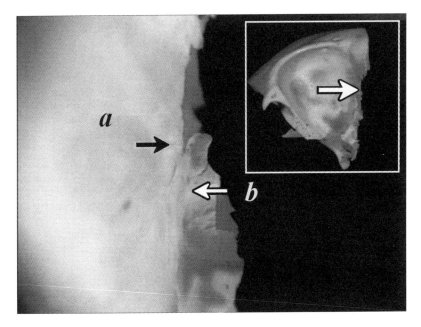

Fig. 7-18 Inferior axial exposure through the articular surface of the right ethmoidolacrimal suture. The majority of the ethmoid has been cut away to enhance the exposure of the suture's articulation.

a. Lacrimal bone
b. Ethmoid bone

MOTION

The suture's general articular configuration appears to permit anteroposterior gliding (Figs. 7-19 and 7-20).

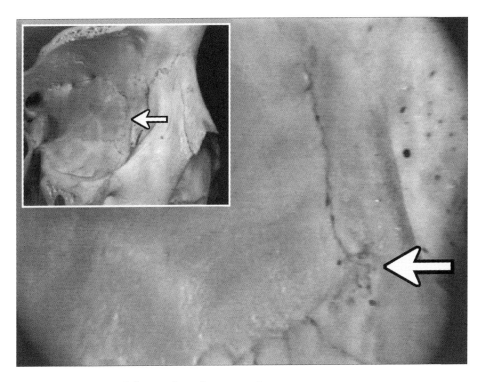

Fig. 7-19A Ethmoidolacrimal motion: posterior engagement

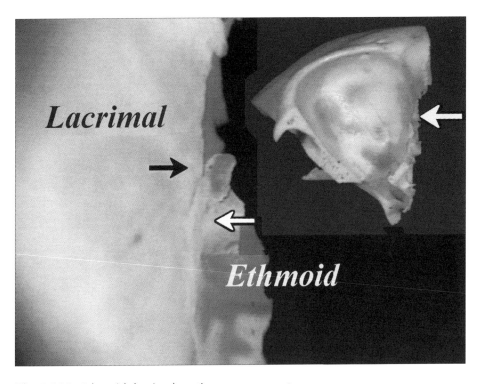

Fig. 7-20A Ethmoidolacrimal motion: engagement

Compare with next photos ➡

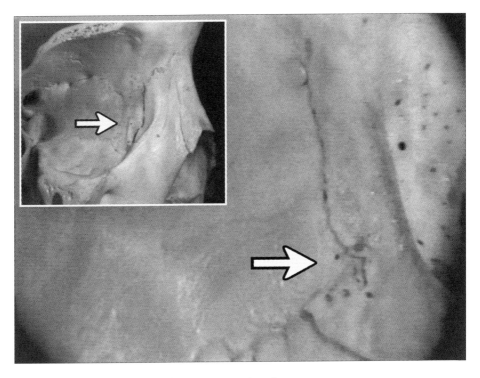

Fig. 7-19B Ethmoidolacrimal motion: anterior disengagement

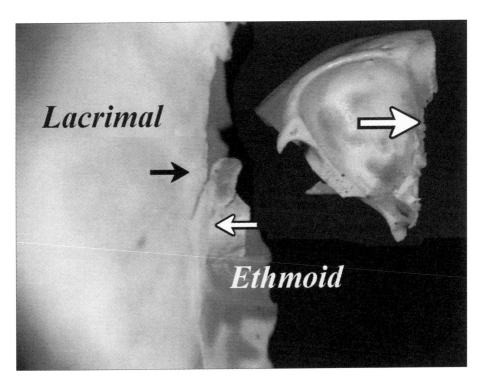

Fig. 7-20B Ethmoidolacrimal motion: disengagement

Articular Disengagement

CONTACTS

The optimal contacts for releasing this articulation are located along the external maxillary alveolar margins, inferior to the zygomaticomaxillary processes and bilaterally posterior to the frontozygomatic processes in the anterior rostral indentation over the sphenofrontal suture (Fig. 7-21).

MANIPULATION

To coercively draw the maxilla away from the side of sutural fixation, apply W¼R-level anteromedial rotational force to the maxillary contacts. This rotational force causes the maxilla's medial orbital border to elevate and secure the lacrimal's inferior articular seam while separating the lacrimal from its articular association with the ethmoid. W¼R-level counterpressure on the frontal contacts compresses the frontal bone toward the side of sutural fixation. This maneuver creates a counterstrain to the ethmoid's rostral articular surface and torques the ethmoid's superior surface laterally. Maintaining the lateral rotational pressure on the frontal bone's contacts, the contacts are then compressed with W⅓R-level force toward the sagittal midline of the ethmoid notch. This creates a secondary bilateral internal rotation of the frontal bone and shifts the glabella anteriorly. As the glabella moves anteriorly, the superior frontolacrimal suture locks along its posterior portion and draws the lacrimal bone away from its ethmoid articular surface (Fig. 7-21).

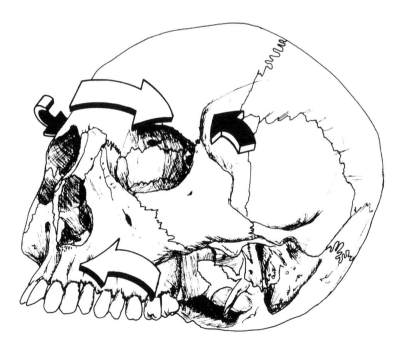

Fig. 7-21 Contact points and direction of manipulation (arrows) for releasing the left ethmoidolacrimal suture

Articular Reengagement

CONTACTS

The same contacts are used to reengage and disengage the ethmoido-lacrimal suture. However, the manipulation is altered to produce reengagement of the suture rather than disengagement (Fig. 7-22).

MANIPULATION

To close the suture, W⅓R-level rotational force is applied to the maxillary contact toward the side of sutural involvement. The rotation is directed across the anterior external surface of the two maxillary bones and guides the structure in a lateral-posterior direction on the involved side. Counter W-level pressure applied to the frontal bone's contacts draws the frontal bone (on the side of the involved suture) medially or toward the opposite side (Fig. 7-22). This generates a counterstrain to the invasive motion of the maxillary contacts and secures the ethmoidolacrimal suture.

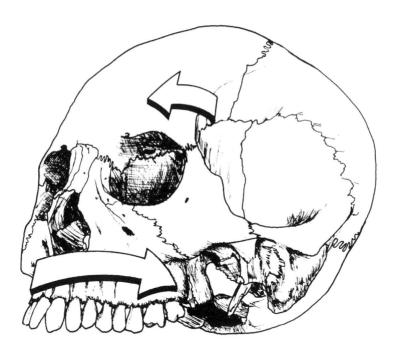

Fig. 7-22 Contact points and direction of manipulation (arrows) for closing the left ethmoidolacrimal suture

Frontoethmoidal Suture (Singular)

MORPHOLOGY

Topographically located along the superomedial wall inside the right and left eye sockets, the frontoethmoidal suture is often thought of as paired (Fig. 7-23). However, when disarticulated, the surface reveals that it is uninterrupted around the ethmoid's anterior border, creating a unique single horseshoe-like articular formation (Fig. 7-24A). For this reason, this text will combine the two sides and treat them as one suture with right and left halves.

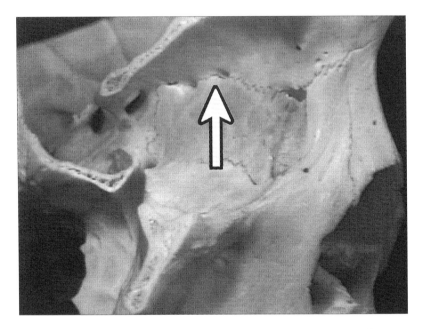

Fig. 7-23 Topographic exposure depicting the location of the right lateral portion of the frontoethmoidal suture

The frontal bone's posterior one-third articular surface is covered with shallow serrations that project posteroinferiorly into the ethmoid's adjacent facet (Figs. 7-24A and B). As the articular surface travels anteriorly toward the glabella, the serrated veneer disappears, and the surface divides to form an internal and external articular edge that is segmentally divided by traversing osseous plates. These plates create a series of interosseous pockets (Fig. 7-24A).

The ethmoid's corresponding superior articular surface consists of a thin convex osseous plate that bulges into the frontal bone's pockets and adheres to their enclosed walls. This results in the general encapsulation of the ethmoid's articular surface between its internal and external articular edges by the frontal bone (Fig. 7-24C).

The anterior traversing pole where the suture crosses the sagittal midline is posterior to the frontonasomaxillary suture. This is the region that

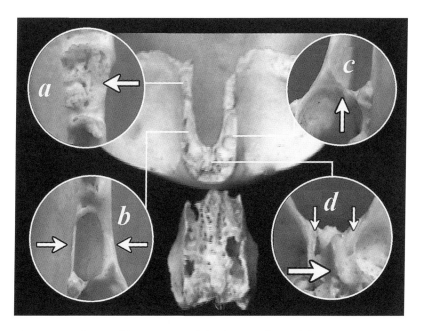

Fig. 7-24A Opened hinge view of the frontoethmoidal suture exposing the inferior frontal bone and superior ethmoid articular surfaces

a. Posterior serrated surface
b. External and internal articular borders with interosseous pocket
c. Traversing osseous partition
d. Inferior anterior serrated surface. Arrows depict anteroposterior sockets for the ethmoid's superior projecting serrations.

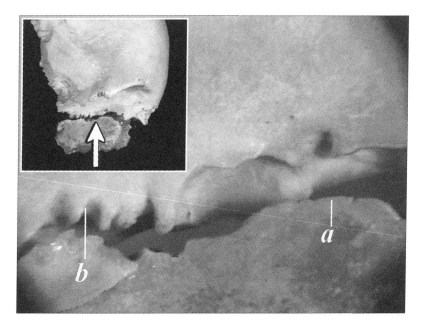

Fig. 7-24B Lateral exposure depicting the sutures transitional morphogenesis from posteriorly serrated to anteriorly planed

a. Anterior plane-type border
b. Posterior serrated border

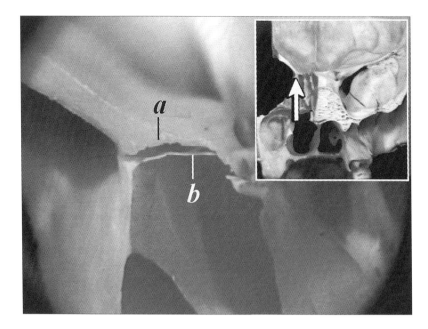

Fig. 7-24C Posterior coronal section exposing the frontal bone's superior interosseous pocket and the ethmoid's superior convex articular plate

a. Frontal bone's articular pocket
b. Ethmoid's superior articular plate

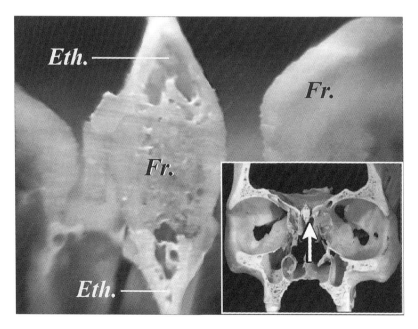

Fig. 7-24D Anterior coronal slice exposing the ethmoid's superior and inferior envelopment of the frontal bone's anterior sagittal articular region

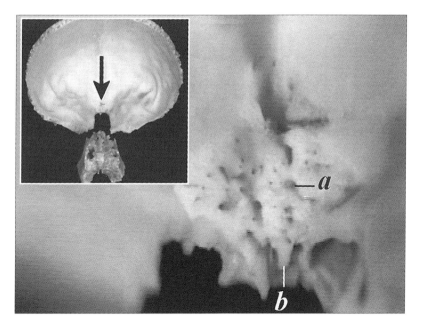

Fig. 7-24E Posterior exposure of the frontal bone's internal superior overlapped oval articular surface

a. Socket formation for one of the ethmoid's anterior projecting serration
b. Typical posterior serration commonly found projecting from the frontal bone's articular surface

connects the right and left lateral articular segments and affirms their status as one continuous suture. Until this region, there is superior overlapping by the frontal bone of the ethmoid's right and left lateral articular associations.

Once the ethmoid enters into this articular segment, its configuration undergoes a superior and inferior overlapping dominance as its articular surface splits to "sandwich" the frontal bone (Fig. 7-24D). Somewhat ovoid in shape, the frontal bone's superior internal articular surface is laced with serrated sockets to receive the anteroinferiorly projecting teeth that protrude from the anterior underbelly of the ethmoid's crista galli (Fig. 7-24E). The ethmoid's inferior articular projections that complete the frontal bone's encasement consists primarily of anterior projecting serrations that extend from the ethmoid's anterior articular surface and insert along the inferior frontal surface near its nasal spine (Fig. 7-24A).

MOTION

The direction of sutural mobility is dictated by the location of the suture and the configuration of its articular margins. To assist in deciphering the motions, the suture has been divided into the following three primary divisions:

1. Division one consists of the anteromedial (nasion) region. The serrations, sockets, and grooves found within this division permit anteroinferior to posterosuperior rocking.
2. Divisions two and three consist of the frontal bone's right and left lateral articular association with the ethmoid's superior air-cell plates. The ostensible motion within both lateral divisions consists of drawing the frontal bone's articular margins in an inferomedial to superolateral direction over the ethmoid's adjacent articular borders (Figs. 7-25 and 7-26).

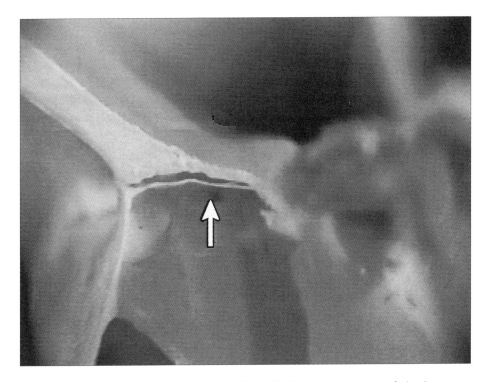

Fig. 7-25A Frontoethmoidal motion (divisions 2 & 3, posterior coronal view): ethmoid superolateral

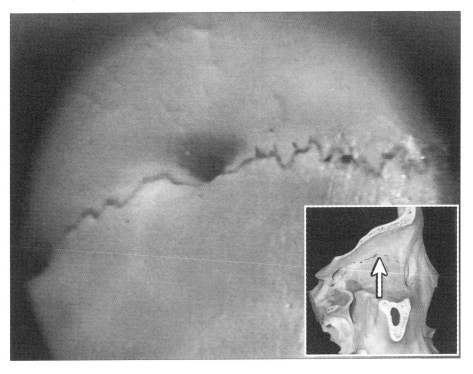

Fig. 7-26A Frontoethmoidal motion (divisions 2 & 3): frontal inferomedial

Compare with next photos ➡

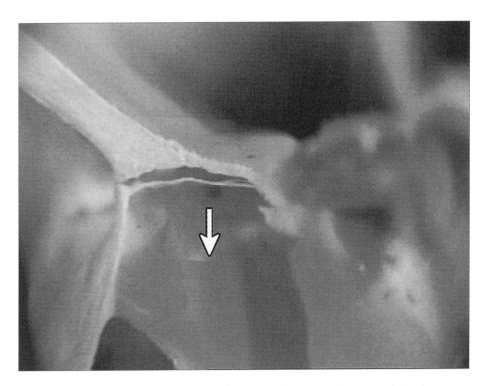

Fig. 7-25B Frontoethmoidal motion (divisions 2 & 3, posterior coronal view):
ethmoid inferomedial

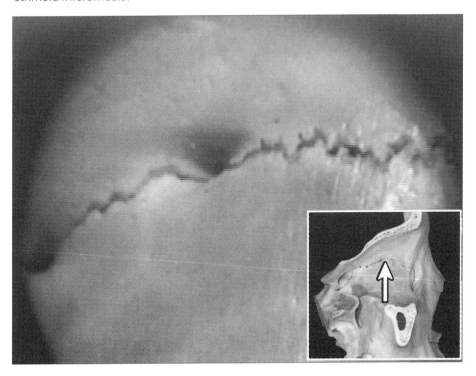

Fig. 7-26b Frontoethmoidal motion (divisions 2 & 3): frontal superolateral

Articular Disengagement and Reengagement

Because of the unusual nature of this suture, the practitioner must first determine which aspect of the suture needs to be disengaged. This will in turn determine which contact points to use. Because this suture is continuous from both sides of the ethmoid notch, the practitioner will often find it necessary to close one portion of the suture to open the other. An example of this can be seen when releasing the suture's anterior portion. To achieve anterior release, the frontal bone's lateral surface is compressed into internal rotation, thus drawing the metopic region anteriorly and releasing it from the ethmoid. However, this maneuver also compresses the lateral frontoethmoidal suture, resulting in the closure of its lateral articular surfaces. It is for this reason that disengaging and reengaging manipulations are combined in this section. The contacts and manipulations described below are used for:

1. Releasing the anterior frontoethmoidal suture around the crista galli or closing the lateral frontoethmoidal suture along the superomedial orbital wall
2. Releasing the lateral articular surfaces or closing the anterior articular surface of the frontoethmoidal suture.

CONTACTS

To release the anterior frontoethmoidal suture around the crista galli or close the lateral frontoethmoidal suture along the superomedial orbital wall, the optimal contact points are located bilaterally superior to the sphenofrontal suture and along the lateral aspects of the hard palate inside the mouth (Fig. 7-27).

MANIPULATION

W⅓R-level force through the frontal bone's contacts is directed medially toward the central sagittal midline of the posterior ethmoid notch. This maneuver will compress the frontal bone into internal rotation and secure the lateral frontoethmoidal articular surfaces while shifting its anteriorly serrated articular surface forward. The anterior shift of the frontal bone's metopic surface unlocks the serrated articulations and releases the frontal bone from the ethmoid. Simultaneous W⅓R-level pressure to the maxillary hard palate compliments the frontal bone's maneuver by directing its force laterally to secure the articular surface of the ethmoidomaxillary suture. As the maxillary contacts expand the hard palate and rotate the ethmoidomaxillary articular borders internally against the ethmoid, the maxilla is pulled in an anterior direction to enhance the ethmoid's separation from the frontal bone's metopic surface. The caudal tugging of the vomer and the sphenoid draws the ethmoid in a posterior direction (Fig. 7-27).

CONTACTS

To release the lateral articular surfaces or close the anterior articular surface of the frontoethmoidal suture, the optimal contact points are located along the frontal metopic region, extending laterally over the superciliary

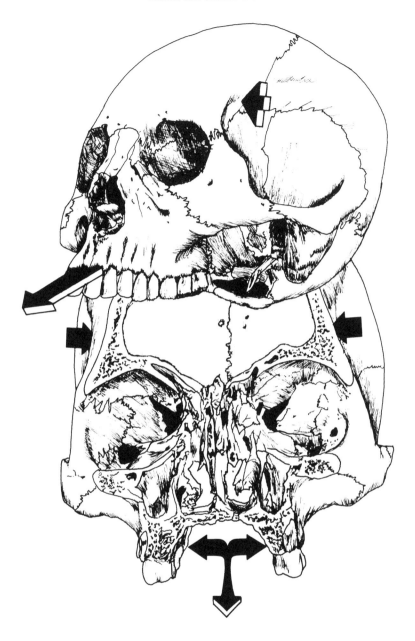

Fig. 7-27 Optimal contact points and direction of manipulation (arrows) for releasing the anterior frontoethmoidal articular surface and closing the lateral frontoethmoidal articular surfaces

aches and caudally over the anterolateral surfaces of the maxillary bones. The point for counterpressure is located across the squamous portion of the occiput, level with the external occipital protuberance (Fig. 7-28).

MANIPULATION

W⅓R-level pressure is directed posteriorly at the frontal bone's contact toward the external occipital protuberance, as the maxillary contacts are compressed toward the sphenobasilar junction using W⅓R-level pressure. This maneuver releases the frontal bone's medial orbital plate articulation with the lateral frontoethmoidal suture as the frontal bone rotates externally. Simultaneously, W/R-level pressure on the occiput's contact in an anterior direction toward the glabella (1) generates anterior-directing force on the ethmoid's posterior wall through the sphenoid bone while it also (2) reacts to the manipulation at the frontal bone's contact to close the anterior portion of the frontoethmoidal suture (Fig. 7-28).

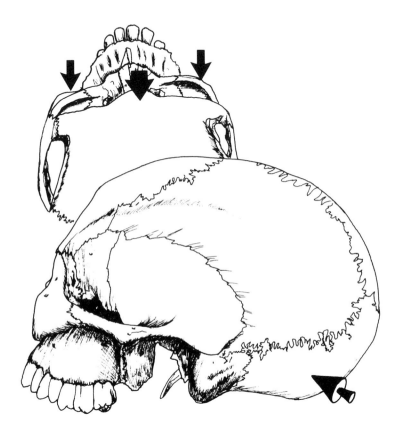

Fig. 7-28 Optimal contact points and direction of manipulation for closing the anterior frontoethmoidal articular surface and releasing the lateral frontoethmoidal articular surfaces

Ethmoidomaxillary Suture (Paired)

MORPHOLOGY

Located along the inferior medial wall of the eye socket, the ethmoido-maxillary suture runs posteriorly from the lacrimal bone to the medial aspect of the inferior orbital fissure (Fig. 7-29). Because of the presence of alternating caudal and rostral serrations in the suture's outer edge, the initial impression is that this is a serrated suture. However, the serrations are only located along the outer marginal seam, while the internal configuration is smooth and absent of pin or socket formations (Fig. 7-30). When coronally sliced and viewed posteriorly, the maxilla's articular surface appears to widen rostrally to externally overlap the ethmoid's inferior lateral border, and to project a small inferomedial ledge to support the ethmoid's adjacent inferior articular border (Fig. 7-30B).

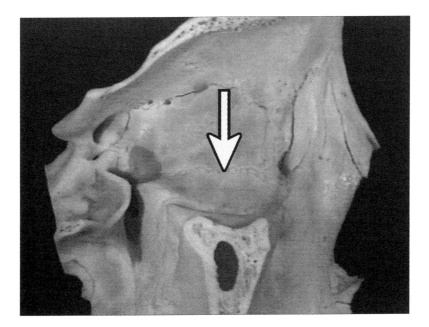

Fig. 7-29 Topographic location of the ethmoidomaxillary suture

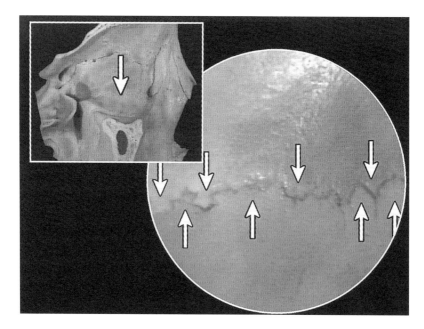

Fig. 7-30A Lateral view exposing the articulation's serrated projections. Arrows in the macroscopic enlargement delineate the characteristic alternating serrations.

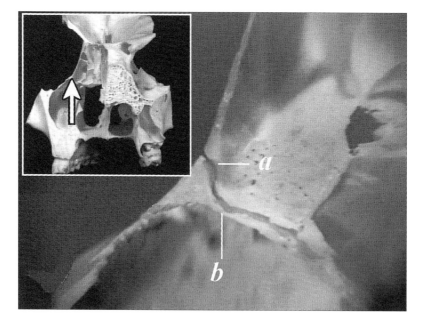

Fig. 7-30B Macroscopic coronal section exposing the ethmoidomaxillary articular junction posteriorly. Note the maxilla's external elevation and how it externally overlaps the ethmoid's inferolateral articular edge.

a. Ethmoid's overlapped inferolateral articular border
b. Maxilla's inferior supporting ledge

MOTION

The miniature serrations aligning the suture's external articular border appear to allow rostral to caudal mobility but not anteroposterior gliding. However, when sliced coronally and observed from a posterior direction, the sanctioned motion appears to be in a superomedial to inferolateral direction (Fig. 7-31).

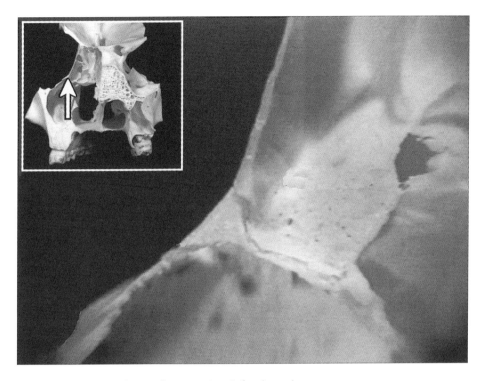

Fig. 7-31A Ethmoidomaxillary motion: inferolateral

Compare with next photo ⇨

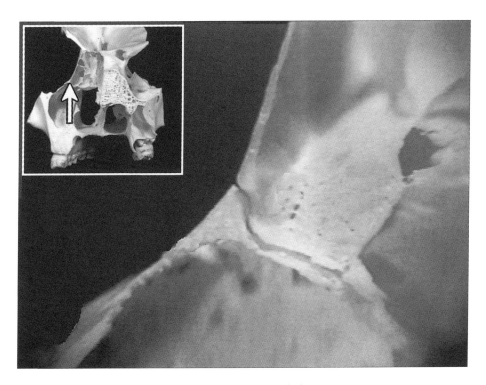

Fig. 7-31B Ethmoidomaxillary motion: superomedial

Articular Disengagement

CONTACTS

The optimal contact points for releasing the ethmoidomaxillary suture are located bilaterally superior to the anterior borders of the sphenofrontal suture and bilaterally on the external maxillary surface, inferior to the maxilla's zygomatic processes (Fig. 7-32).

MANIPULATION

W⅓R-level medial pressure to the frontal bone's contacts grips the frontal bone's surface and stabilizes the ethmoid against the maxilla's counter-pressure. W⅓R-level medial pressure on the maxillary contacts directs the molar surface below the hard palate toward the sagittal midline of the mouth. This, in turn, rotates the articular surface of the maxilla supero-laterally away from the ethmoid's articular surface (Fig. 7-32).

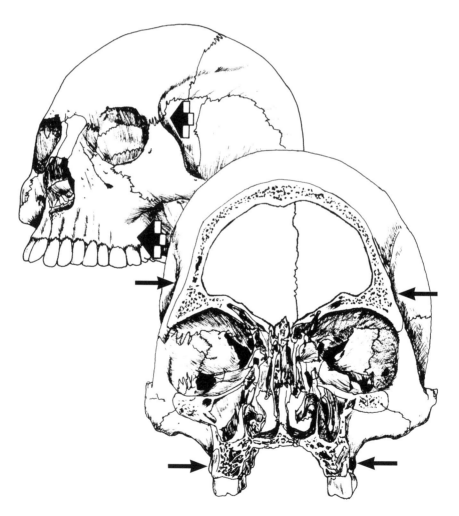

Fig. 7-32 Contact points and direction of manipulation for releasing the ethmoidomaxillary suture

Articular Reengagement

CONTACTS

The optimal contact points for reengaging the ethmoidomaxillary suture are located bilaterally superior to the frontal bone's zygomatic process and on the hard palate medial to the maxilla's first molar alveolar processes (Fig. 7-33).

MANIPULATION

W⅓R-level force is applied to the frontal bone's contacts in an anterocaudal direction. This maneuver locks the frontoethmoid suture and stabilizes the ethmoid bone against the countering lateral-superior W-level pressure of the maxillary contacts. The maxillary maneuver is designed to expand the lateral surface area below the hard palate, and to compress the maxillary articular surface medially against the ethmoid's articular surface (Fig. 7-33).

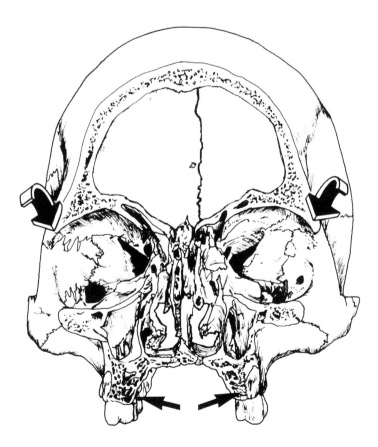

Fig. 7-33 Contact points and direction of manipulation (arrows) for closing the ethmoidomaxillary suture

Ethmoidonasal Suture (Paired)

MORPHOLOGY

The ethmoidonasal suture is located on the anterosuperior aspect of the nasal cavity. Enveloping the posterior crest of the nasal bones, the suture superiorly extends bilaterally to partially cross the superior posterior surfaces of the nasal bones (Fig. 7-34).

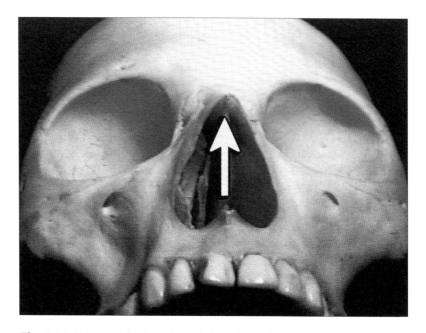

Fig. 7-34 Topographic location of the ethmoid-nasomaxillary suture

Although variations have been observed, the following description depicts the suture's most common structural configuration. Upon initial observation, the ethmoid's perpendicular plate in the suture's inferior superficial articular border appears to form an edge-to-edge articulation with the nasal crest. However, macroscopic inspection of twenty-five human skulls revealed that the ethmoid's perpendicular plate often articulated with the nasal crest of the right nasal bone and was only minimally associated with the left (Fig. 7-35A). It is unknown at this time if this finding is an aberration or is a result of genetic programming.

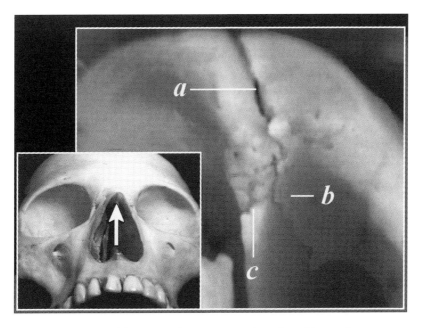

Fig. 7-35A Viewed from its inferior aspect, the ethmoidonasal suture has been magnified to expose its inferior articular characteristics.

a. Internasal suture
b. Left nasal bone
c. Ethmoid perpendicular plate's plane-type articular junction with the nasal crest

Hidden deep within the suture's superior articular formation, the ethmoid's perpendicular plate bifurcates to envelop the posterior projecting surface of the nasal crest. The internasal suture is often found coursing posteriorly toward the perpendicular plate's bifurcated surface but appears to fall short of actually entering the bifurcation zone. This is because the right ethmoidonasal suture frequently deflects laterally, preventing the right nasal bone from entering the bifurcated region. Meanwhile, the left nasal crest enters the bifurcated zone and posteromedially projects its serrations deep into the V-shaped formation (Fig. 7-35B). As the suture expands bilaterally over the posterosuperior surfaces of the nasal bones, its margins form a convex irregular appearance that would appear to discourage lateral mobility.

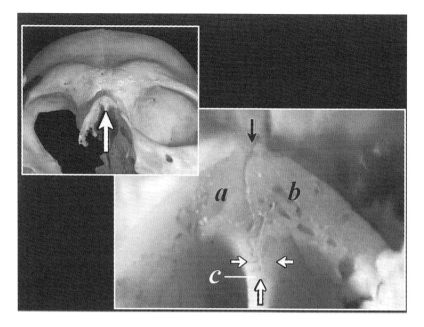

Fig. 7-35B Anteroinferior view depicting the ethmoidonasal suture's superior articulating characteristics. An axial slice through the nasal bone's and ethmoid's perpendicular plate exposes the rostral portion of the suture from its inferior aspect.

a. Right nasal bone

b. Left nasal bone

c. Perpendicular plate. White arrows delineate the bifurcation formation. Black arrow depicts the internasal suture.

MOTION

The internasal suture's anteroposterior hinge-like structure apparently permits anterior disengagement and posterior reengagement along the ethmoid's anteromedial perpendicular border. Although this might be construed as the suture's sanctioned mobility, this motion actually serves to release or stabilize the suture's articular osseous components. However, the angular contour of the ethmoid's lateral articular surface on its adjacent posterior nasal walls seems to permit posterosuperior to anteroinferior gliding (Fig. 7-36).

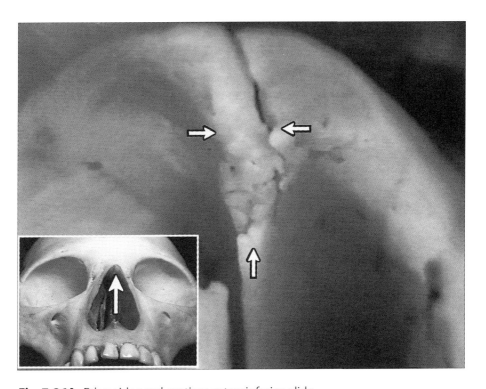

Fig. 7-36A Ethmoidonasal motion: anteroinferior glide

Compare with next photo ➡

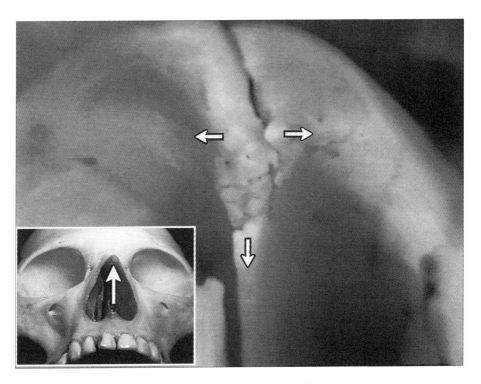

Fig. 7-36B Ethmoidonasal motion: posterosuperior glide

Articular Disengagement

Because of the pattern of the suture's deep internal serrations, substantial anterior or caudal disengagement is apparently discouraged. Although consummate disengagement is unlikely, pliable stress release may be achieved through caudal gliding of the nasal and frontomaxillary process while the frontal bone's ethmoidal notch margins secure the ethmoid.

CONTACTS

The primary contacts for releasing the ethmoid-nasomaxillary suture are located bilaterally over the nasion region of the nasal bones and the maxillary processes. The ancillary contacts employed to stabilize the ethmoid against maneuvers of the primary contacts are bilaterally located immediately posterior to the frontal bone's temporal line above the frontal bone's zygomatic processes (Fig. 7-37).

MANIPULATION

W⅓R-level pressure on the primary nasion contacts draws the nasal bones and maxillary processes in a caudal-anterior direction. This maneuver slides the nasal and maxillary articular surfaces caudally, loosening the sutural margins to the ethmoid's bifurcated surfaces. Concurrent W-level medial pressure on the ancillary contacts compresses and rostrally elevates the frontal bone. This maneuver secures the ethmoid's cribriform margins within the frontal bone's ethmoid notch and stabilizes the ethmoid to the drawing action at the primary contacts (Fig. 7-37).

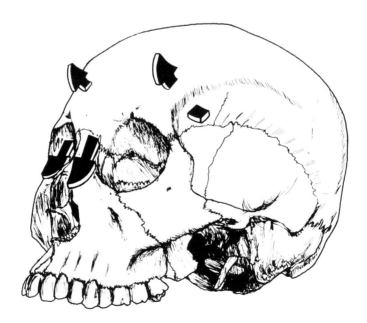

Fig. 7-37 Contact points and direction of manipulation (arrows) for releasing the ethmoid-nasomaxillary suture

Articular Reengagement

CONTACTS

The primary contacts for reengaging the ethmoid-nasomaxillary suture are located bilaterally over the nasion region of the nasal bones and the frontomaxillary processes. The ancillary contacts are bilaterally located immediately posterior to the frontal bone's temporal line above the frontal bone's zygomatic processes (Fig. 7-38).

MANIPULATION

Rostral-posterior W-level pressure to the primary nasion contacts compresses the maxilla's frontal process and nasal articular margins against the ethmoid's anterior perpendicular articular surface. Synchronous $W\frac{1}{3}R$-level medial pressure to the ancillary contacts secures the ethmoid in the frontal bone's ethmoid notch. Once the ethmoid is secured, the direction of force is altered anteriorly using W-level force to secure the ethmoid's anterior perpendicular articular surface to the nasal and maxillary counter surfaces (Fig. 7-38).

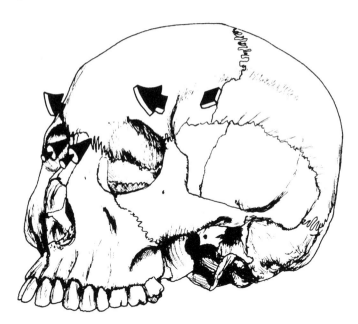

Fig. 7-38 Contact points and direction of manipulation (arrows) for reengaging the ethmoid-nasomaxillary suture

Sphenoethmoidal Suture (Paired)

MORPHOLOGY

Topographically located along the eye socket's posterior-medial wall, the sphenoethmoidal suture runs in a superior to inferior direction and joins the ethmoid bone to the anterior surface of the sphenoid's body (Fig. 7-39). Superiorly divided into right and left parts by a central perpendicular septum, the ethmoid's kidney-shaped posterior walls are slightly concave and often function as the sphenoid body's anterior wall (Fig. 7-40A). The external borders around the ethmoid's posterior articular surfaces are externally beveled and divided into upper serrated and lower squamosal margins to accommodate the overlapping internally beveled edges of the sphenoid's anterior margins (Figs. 7-40B and C). Sagittally, the ethmoid's medial articular border is smooth and elevated to superficially join the sphenoid's anterior body superolateral to the sphenoidal sinus opening. As previously noted, the ethmoid's perpendicular septum posteriorly divides the superior articular surface into right and left parts. Posteriorly bifurcating, the perpendicular septum straddles the sphenoid's anterior central septum, thereby securing the suture's position against lateral instability (Fig. 7-40D).

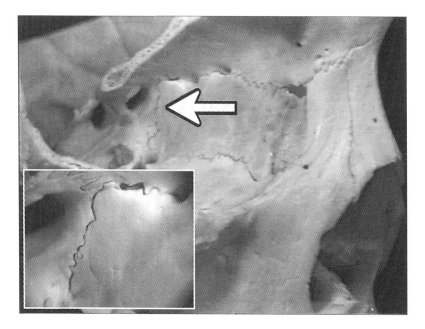

Fig. 7-39 Topographic location of the sphenoethmoidal suture

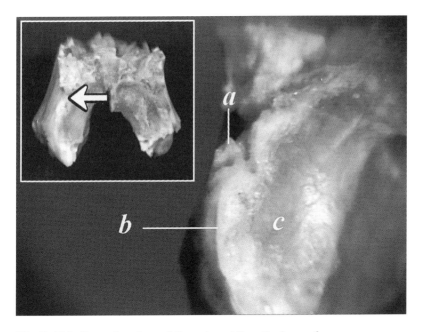

Fig. 7-40A Posterior view of the ethmoid's articular surface

a. Externally beveled superolateral serrated borders
b. Inferolateral squamous edge
c. Concave kidney-shaped condylar surface

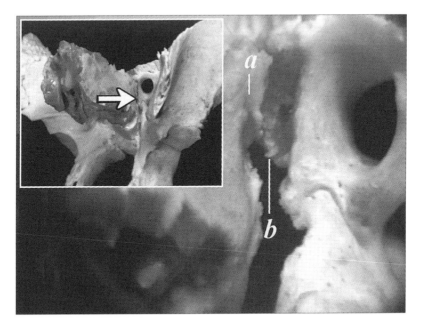

Fig. 7-40B Anterolateral exposure of the sphenoethmoidal suture. The articulation has been disengaged to expose the laterally affiliated articular surfaces.

a. Ethmoid's overlapped articular groove
b. Sphenoid's superior serrated surface

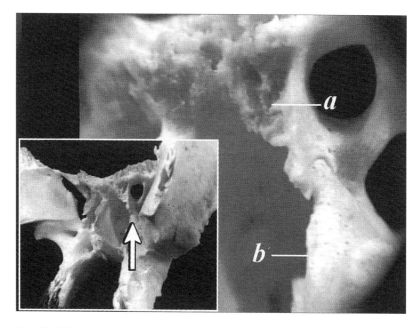

Fig. 7-40C Exposure of the sphenoid body's anterolateral articular surface

a. Lateral internally beveled serrated socket
b. Squamous articular surface area

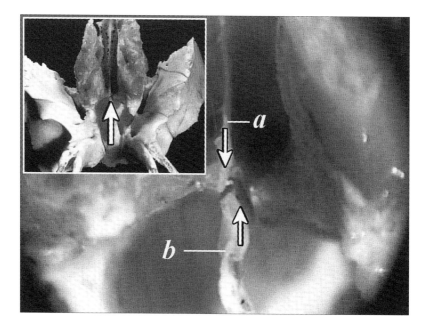

Fig. 7-40D Inferior view exposing the ethmoid's perpendicular plate articulation with the sphenoid's anterior central septum. Note that the sphenoid's septum is anteriorly wedged within the posterior bifurcated margins of the ethmoid's perpendicular plate.

a. Ethmoid's perpendicular plate
b. Sphenoid's central septum

MOTION

The combination of anteroposterior serrations and inferior squamosal margins suggests that anterior to posterior gliding along the articulation's perimeter is allowed. However, the enveloping overlap of the ethmoid's boundary by the sphenoid also suggests that disengagement may be obstructed during the ethmoid's expansion phase of both primary and pulmonary respiration (Fig. 7-41).

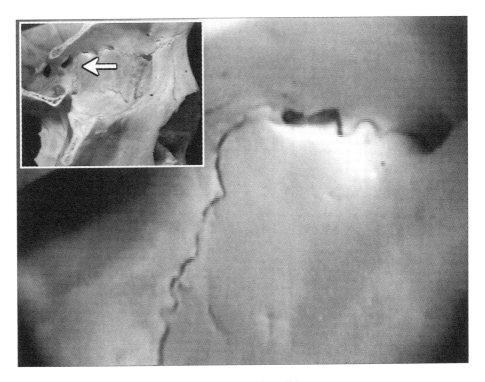

Fig. 7-41A Sphenoethmoidal motion: posterior glide

Compare with next photo ➡

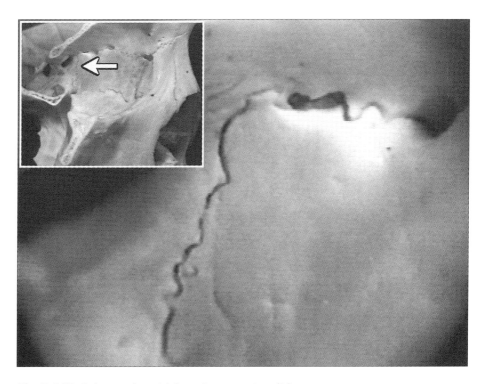

Fig. 7-41B Sphenoethmoidal motion: anterior glide

Articular Disengagement

CONTACTS

The optimal contact points for releasing the sphenoethmoidal suture are located on the frontal bone, bilaterally superior to the sphenofrontal sutures and inferior to the sphenoid's pterygoid process on the affected side (Fig. 7-42).

MANIPULATION

At the frontal bone's contacts, W/R-level pressure is applied into the vault toward the midsagittal line of the ethmoid notch. This pressure compresses the frontal bone's articular surface against its corresponding ethmoid surface and serves to confine the ethmoid between the frontal bone's supraorbital plates. The frontal bone's contacts then shift their course and draw the inferior frontal surface in a caudal-anterior direction, swinging the ethmoid from the sphenoid body. Simultaneous posterosuperior W-level force to the pterygoid contact serves to push the sphenoid away from the ethmoid (Fig. 7-42).

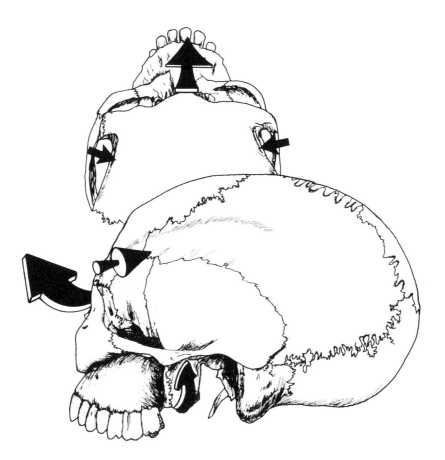

Fig. 7-42 Contact points and direction of manipulation (arrows) for releasing the left sphenoethmoidal suture

Articular Reengagement

CONTACTS

The optimal contact points for reengaging the sphenoethmoidal suture are located on the glabella, extending bilaterally across both superciliary arches and posteriorly to the tip of the pterygoid process on the side of fixation (Fig. 7-43).

MANIPULATION

At the frontal bone's contacts, W⅓R-level force toward the external occipital protuberance engages and secures the ethmoid against the counterforce generated during the pterygoid's manipulation. Synchronous W¼R-level pressure to the pterygoid contact draws the pterygoid in an anteroinferior direction to secure the sphenoid's body against the posterior bulging articular surface of the ethmoid (Fig. 7-43).

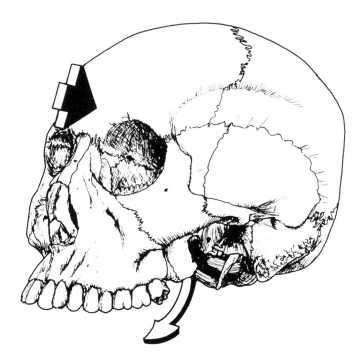

Fig. 7-43 Contact points and direction of manipulation (arrows) for reengaging the left sphenoethmoidal suture

Palatoethmoidal Suture (Paired)

MORPHOLOGY

Located in the posteromedial-inferior wall of the orbital socket, the palato-ethmoidal suture laterally wraps around the posteroinferior corner of the ethmoid and extends anteriorly to join with the maxillopalatine's superior orbital suture and the posterior border of the ethmoidomaxillary suture (Fig. 7-44A). Unique in its formation, the palatine's articular surface takes on the appearance of a reclining chair with a high backrest (Fig. 7-44B). With its seat extending medially under the ethmoid's posterior articular surface, the high backrest superolaterally extends along the ethmoid's posterolateral marginal border. Closer observation of the backrest formation shows that its veneer appears smooth and scooped out to form a cup-shaped configuration for the envelopment of the ethmoid's posterolateral corner (Fig. 7-44B). Although this suture's overall surface is smooth, its orbital margin is superficially jagged, discouraging anteroposterior slippage along the ethmoid's outer articular seam (Fig. 7-44A).

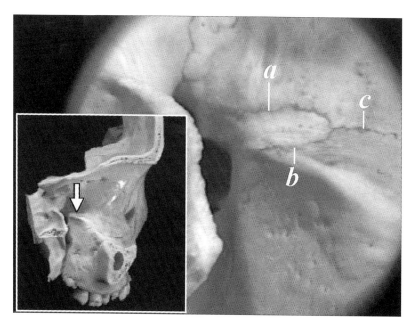

Fig. 7-44A Posterior-oblique exposure delineating the topographic location of the palatoethmoidal suture

   a. Palatoethmoidal suture
   b. Superior palatine-maxillary orbital suture
   c. Ethmoidomaxillary suture

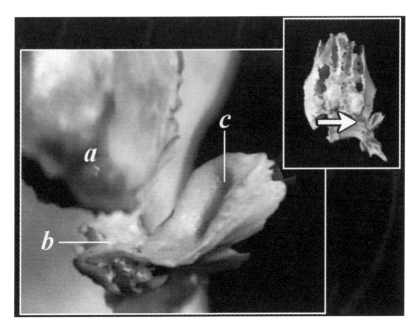

Fig. 7-44B Posterosuperior view exposing the palatine's superior ethmoidal articular surface. Note the reclining chair formation.

a. Ethmoid's posterolateral articular corner as seen from above
b. Palatine's medial projecting seat formation that supports the ethmoid from below. Note the concave anteroposterior surface combines with a medial-lateral convexity, suggesting that the articular surface can tolerate either anterior-to-posterior or medial-to-lateral rocking.
c. Characteristic spoon-shaped backrest that envelops the ethmoid's posterolateral corner. Note the articular surface's smooth superior-anterolateral incline.

MOTION

An initial investigation of the suture's jagged superficial orbital margin would appear to rule out independent anterior or posterior gliding. However, its unique cup-like encasement of the ethmoid's posterolateral corner combined with its inclined angulation and smooth articular veneer would appear to sanction posteromedial to anterolateral rocking (Figs. 7-45).

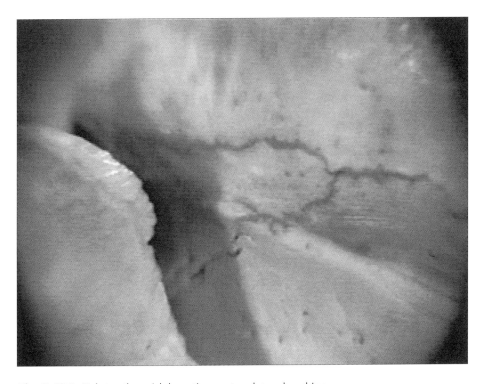

Fig. 7-45A Palatoethmoidal motion: anterolateral rocking

Compare with next photo ➔

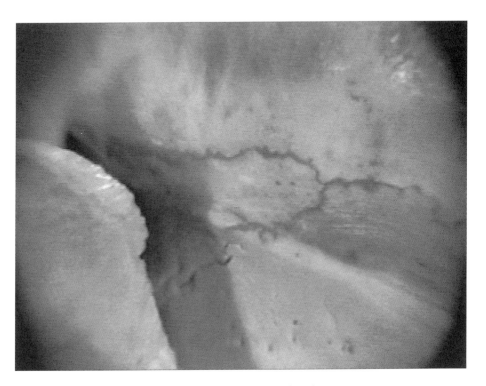

Fig. 7-45B Palatoethmoidal motion: posteromedial rocking

Articular Disengagement

CONTACTS

To achieve maximum sutural release, a trisurface contact of the frontal bone, sphenoid, and maxilla is suggested. The frontal bone is contacted at the anterior-inferolateral border of the coronal suture. The sphenoid is contacted over the external surface of its greater wing. The maxilla is approached from inside the mouth, along its posterolateral wall, and anterior to the pterygomaxillary fissure (Fig. 7-46).

MANIPULATION

The frontal and sphenoid contacts may be manipulated separately or simultaneously as one continuous contact overlaying the sphenofrontal suture. Using W⅓R-level pressure, the contacts are directed toward the midsagittal plane of the vault to secure the ethmoid's posterosuperior articular seam with the frontal bone. Once engaged, the frontal bone is then directed superiorly to elevate the ethmoid from its palatine surface. As the ethmoid is elevated, the maxilla is simultaneously drawn anteriorly with W⅓R-level force to interlock its orbital palatine affiliation and secure the palatine from the ethmoid's elevating tug (Fig. 7-46).

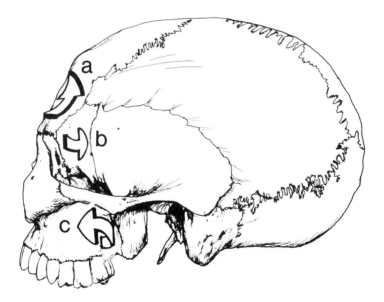

Fig. 7-46 Left posterolateral-oblique view of the contact points and direction of manipulation (arrows) used in disengaging the palatoethmoidal suture

a. Frontal bone's contact superior to the sphenofrontal suture and anterior to the coronal suture
b. External contact overlapping the sphenoid's greater wing
c. Maxilla's posterolateral wall contact

Articular Reengagement

CONTACTS

The identical vault contacts are recommended for reengaging the suture. However, the maxillary contact should be repositioned to the posteroinferior border of the pterygoid process. *Note:* Optimally, the contacts should be administered on the side of sutural instability. The frontal bone's contact is then located along its inferolateral border, anterior to the coronal suture and superior to the sphenofrontal articular seam. The second and third contacts are administered to the sphenoid's central external greater wing surface and the posteroinferior edge of its pterygoid process (Fig. 7-47).

MANIPULATION

The frontal bone's contact is guided in a caudal to medial direction with W⅓R-level pressure as the sphenoid's greater wing is maneuvered anteromedially with equal force. The combined application secures the ethmoid's superior and posterior surfaces. Simultaneous W⅓R-level force maneuvers the pterygoid contact superiorly to coerce the reengagement of the palatine's orbital margin with the ethmoid (Fig. 7-47).

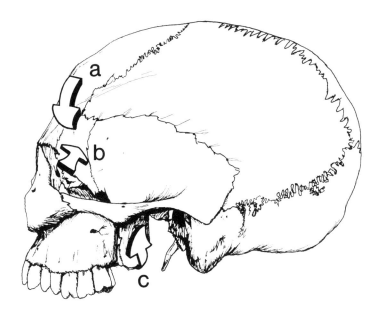

Fig. 7-47 Left posterolateral-oblique view of the contact points and direction of manipulation (arrows) used in reengaging the palatoethmoidal suture

a. Frontal contact anterior to the coronal suture and superior to the sphenofrontal suture

b. External contact overlaying the center of the sphenoid's greater wing

c. Pterygoid's posteroinferior contact

Vomeronasal Crest Articulation (Singular)

MORPHOLOGY

The vomeronasal crest articulation is located along the nasal floor, superior to the nasal crest of the intermaxillary and interpalatine sutures (Fig. 7-48). Classified as a schindylesis articulation, the vomer's thin wedged articular border lodges between the nasal crests of the two maxillary and palatine bones (Fig. 7-49A and C). *Note:* Although the majority of the vomer's articular surface is encased between the intermaxillary and interpalatine nasal crests, it is not uncommon to find a reversal of its articular formation along the suture's midarticular region. When this occurs, the vomer's fragile border bifurcates to overlap the posterior maxillary crest; this may occur to stabilize the suture's interlocking structures (Fig. 7-49B).

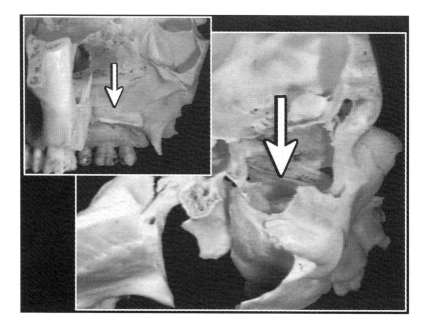

Fig. 7-48 Vomeronasal crest topographic location

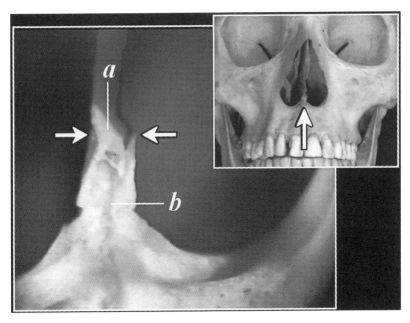

Fig. 7-49A Anterior view exposing the articular junction of the vomer between the maxillary nasal crests. Arrows delineate the maxillary crest's bifurcated margins.

  a. Vomer   b. Intermaxillary suture

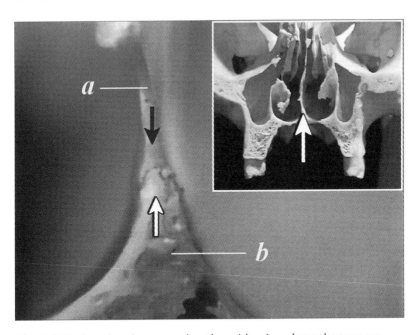

Fig. 7-49B Anterior view exposing the midregion along the vomeronasal crest articulation. Note that the articular formation reverses in this region, and the vomer's articular margin bifurcates to envelop the maxillary crest.

  a. Vomer with its bifurcated border (black arrow)
  b. Intermaxillary suture and the nasal crest as it enters the vomer's bifurcation zone (white arrow)

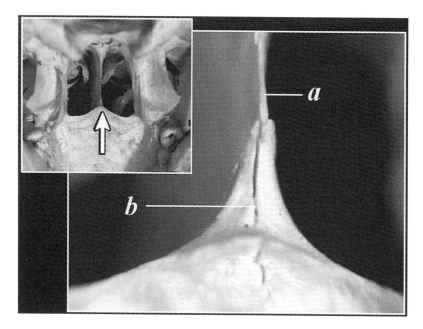

Fig. 7-49C Posterior view revealing the posterior articular junction of the vomer to the interpalatine suture. Note that the articular surface has reverted back to the vomer's wedge-shaped insertion between the nasal crest's interpalatine suture.

a. Posterior vomer surface
b. Interpalatine suture as it ascends through the elevated nasal crest

MOTION

Dissection of the suture reveals that the vomer's articular position is either locked or unlocked by the coordinated movements of the intermaxillary and interpalatine sutures. When the suture is unlocked, the vomer is further coerced into anteroposterior sagittal rocking by associated motions of the sphenoid. Consequently, the articular configurations of the suture and its neighbors determine this suture's movements (Fig. 7-50).

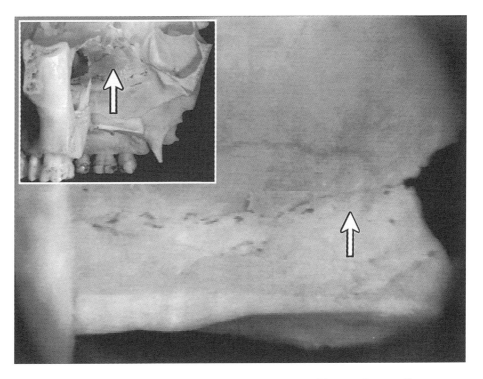

Fig. 7-50A Vomeronasal crest motion: anterior vomer with superior maxilla

Compare with next photo ⇨

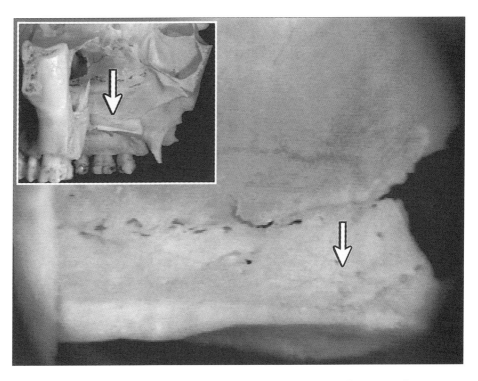

Fig. 7-50B Vomeronasal crest motion: posterior vomer with inferior maxilla

Articular Disengagement

CONTACTS

The optimal contacts for releasing this suture are located bilaterally on the superior external surfaces of the sphenoid's greater wings, and inside the mouth, along the lateral margins of the hard palate (Fig. 7-51).

MANIPULATION

At the sphenoidal contact, W-level pressure is directed toward the sagittal midline of the vault. The sphenoid is then rotated in an anterosuperior direction to create a posterior shift of its body. The shift draws the vomer in a posterosuperior direction relative to the sphenoid's body and lifts the vomer from between the nasal crests. At the intraoral hard palate contacts, W⅓R-level lateral pressure opens the intermaxillary and interpalatine sutures. This releases the wedged compression of the hard palate's nasal crest from the vomer and allows the manipulation of the sphenoid to elevate the vomer from its seat between the nasal crests (Fig. 7-51).

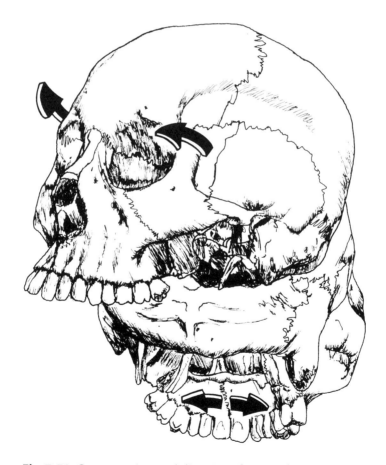

Fig. 7-51 Contact points and direction of manipulation (arrows) for releasing the vomeronasal crest articulation

Articular Reengagement

CONTACTS

The optimal contact points for closing this suture are found bilaterally on the external surface of the sphenoid's greater wings and along the external surface of the maxillary bones. To reach the maxillary contact, the practitioner's fingers are placed inside the mouth inferior to the maxillary zygomatic processes and superior to the lateral alveolar borders (Fig. 7-52).

MANIPULATION

At the sphenoid's contacts, W-level pressure is directed toward the sagittal midline of the vault. The sphenoid is then rotated in a posteroinferior direction to create an anterior shift of its body. The sphenoid body's countershift compresses the vomer in an anteroinferior direction and wedges the vomer between the nasal crests of the maxillopalatine bones. Simultaneously, W/R-level pressure is applied on the lateral maxillary contacts toward the sagittal midline of the hard palate. This pressure forces the intermaxillary and interpalatine sutures to tighten the furrow around the vomer's articular surface (Fig. 7-52).

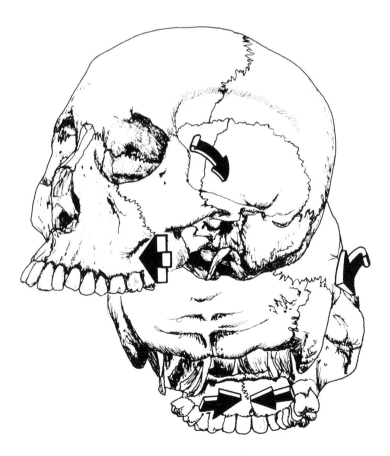

Fig. 7-52 Contact points and direction of manipulation (arrows) for reengaging the vomer-palatomaxillary suture

Vomeroethmoidal Suture (Singular)

MORPHOLOGY

Located along the posteroinferior marginal half of the ethmoid's perpendicular plate, the vomeroethmoidal suture joins the vomer to the ethmoid and constitutes the posterior osseous portion of the nasal septum (Fig. 7-53). Often absent of bevels or serrations, the articular margins connect edge to edge along the suture's anterior articular surface (Fig. 7-54A). Magnification of the suture's anterior articular seam reveals that the vomer's transverse articular surface appears to randomly evolve into either a concave or convex shape. Occasionally, the ethmoid's perpendicular plate is found to be deviated with the vomer often supplying the plate with an articular ledge (Fig. 7-54B). This "accommodation" may be a result of genetic programming, trauma, arthritis, or the introduction of articular stress generated by cranial distortions.

As the suture approaches its posterior quadrant, the vomer's marginal edge often bifurcates, and the perpendicular plate takes on a knife-edge formation as it inserts into the bifurcated furrow. This altered contour apparently secures the suture along its articular seam and guarantees its position against lateral deviations. This can be seen in the illustration of the sphenovomerine suture (Fig. 7-59B).

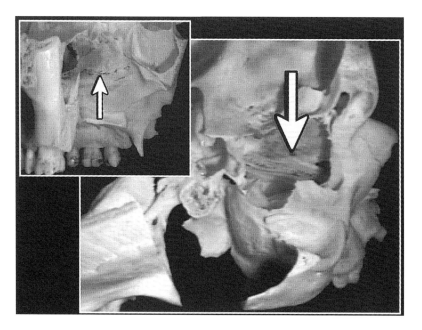

Fig. 7-53 Vomeroethmoidal suture's topographic location

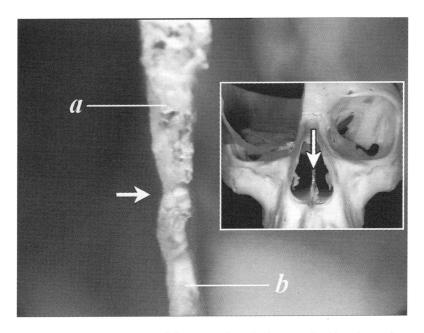

Fig. 7-54A Anterior view of the vomer's articular marginal border with the ethmoid's nasal septum. Arrow depicts articular union.

a. Ethmoid's perpendicular plate
b. Vomer

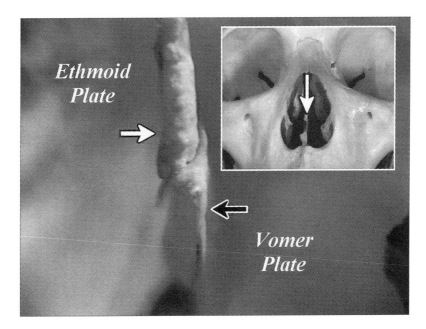

Fig. 7-54B A common lateral articular deformity that is often referred to as a partially deviated septum

MOTION

Whether the vomer's articular border is convex or concave, the suture's articular configuration apparently permits anteroposterior gliding, sagittal separation or compression, and transverse lateral rocking (Fig. 7-55).

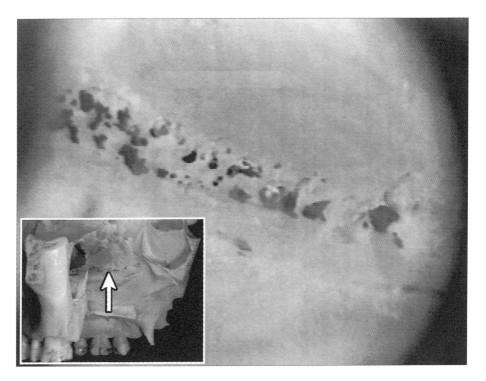

Fig. 7-55A Vomeroethmoidal motion: sagittal separation

Compare with next photo ➡

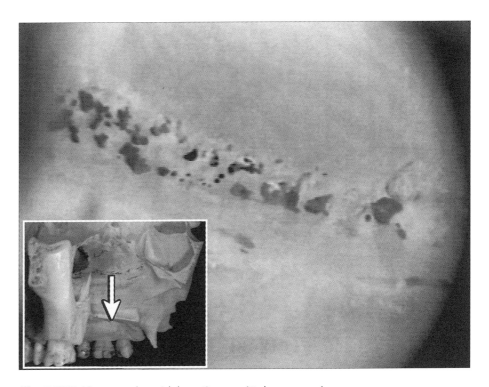

Fig. 7-55B Vomeroethmoidal motion: sagittal compression

Articular Disengagement

CONTACTS

To release the vomeroethmoidal suture, the optimal contact points are located bilaterally on the external maxillary surfaces, inferior to the zygomatic processes of the maxillae, and on the anteroinferior tips of the pterygoid processes (Fig. 7-56).

MANIPULATION

W⅔R-level pressure is applied to the maxillary contacts toward the sagittal midline. This maneuver secures the articular surface of the nasal crest around the vomer's inferior articular margin and serves to stabilize the vomer against the elevating draw of the ethmoid. Posterosuperior W⅓R-level pressure is simultaneously applied to the pterygoid contacts, elevating the posterior sphenoid's body and shifting its anterior surface in an anteroinferior direction to interlock with the ethmoid's perpendicular plate. Upon engaging the ethmoid, the sphenoid forces the perpendicular plate to actively glide anteriorly along the vomer's articular border, releasing the suture from existing fixations (Fig. 7-56).

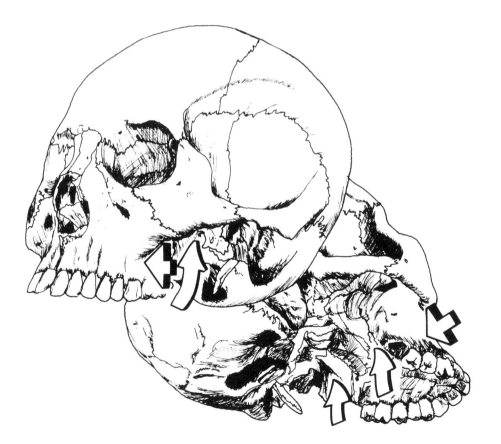

Fig. 7-56 Contact points and direction of manipulation (arrows) for releasing the vomeroethmoidal suture

Articular Reengagement

CONTACTS

The optimal contact points for closing this suture are located (1) bilaterally at the external maxillary surface inferior to the zygomatic processes of the maxillae, and (2) bilaterally posterior to the zygomatic processes of the frontal bone (Fig. 7-57).

MANIPULATION

W/R-level pressure is applied at the maxillary contacts toward the hard palate's sagittal midline. This maneuver locks the vomer's inferior surface between the intermaxillary and interpalatine nasal crests. Once the vomer is secured, the pressure on the maxillary contacts is shifted in a superior-posterior direction to elevate the vomer toward the ethmoid's perpendicular plate. W/R-level force is simultaneously applied to the frontal bone's contacts toward the midsagittal plane of the ethmoid notch. This coerces the frontal bone into internal rotation against the superior lateral margins of the ethmoid bone and drives the ethmoid in an inferior direction to secure the vomeroethmoidal suture from above (Fig. 7-57).

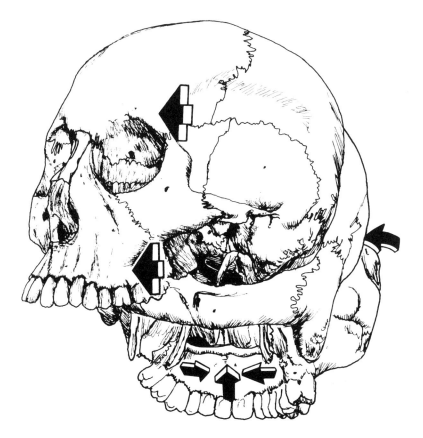

Fig. 7-57 Contact points and direction of manipulation (arrows) for closing the vomeroethmoidal suture

Sphenovomerine Suture (Singular)

MORPHOLOGY

The sphenovomerine suture is located on the posterosuperior aspect of the vomer's perpendicular plate. This unique articulation joins the vomer to the inferior belly of the sphenoid body and the pterygoid's medial vaginal processes (Fig. 7-58). The vomer's smooth articular surface is centrally gouged to envelop the sphenoid's caudally protruding V-shaped rostrum in a schindylesis-type articular union (Fig. 7-59A). As the vomer's articular surface expands bilaterally from its central groove, the vomer takes on an ala, that is, wing-like, appearance to cover the remaining underbelly of the sphenoid's body and ultimately terminates with the vaginal processes protruding from the medial pterygoid base (Figs. 7-59B~D). The alae's lateral articular margins are beveled and plane-like, and extend in an anterolateral to posteromedial direction. Articulating from one margin to the other, the pterygoid's vaginal processes caudally overlap the vomer's lateral margins posteriorly but are often caudally overlapped by the vomer anteriorly (Fig. 7-59D).

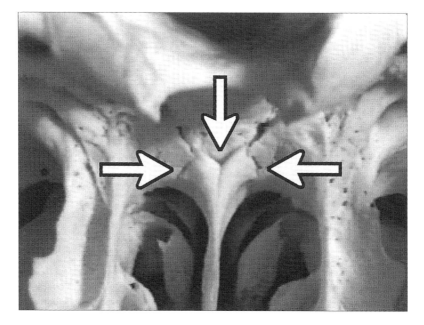

Fig. 7-58 Topographic locations of the vomer's three articular margins to the sphenoid

Fig. 7-59A Superior view exposing the rostral articular surface of the vomer

a. Vomer's articular trench that houses the sphenoid's protruding V-shaped rostrum projection

b. Vomer's lateral alae articular margins which articulate with the vaginal processes of the sphenoid's pterygoid processes

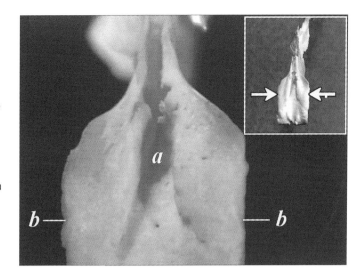

Fig. 7-59B Anterior view of the vomer's sphenoid articular surfaces

a. Vomer's articular trench that houses the sphenoid's protruding V-shaped rostrum projection

b. Vomer's lateral articular alae borders which articulate with the sphenoid's vaginal processes

c. Bifurcated groove that envelops the postero-inferior margin of the ethmoid's perpendicular plate

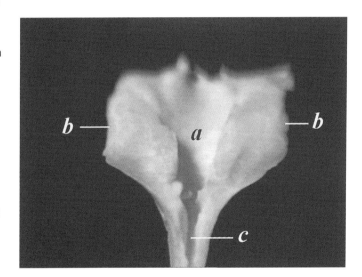

Fig. 7-59C Posteroinferior exposure depicting the sphenoid's articular surface with the vomer

a. Sphenoid's V-shaped rostrum projection

b. Pterygoid vaginal processes

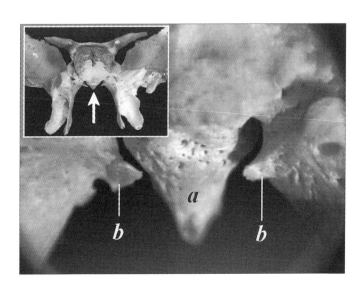

Fig. 7-59D
Posteroinferior view
exposing the vomer's
articulations with the
sphenoid's inferior body
and the pterygoid's articular vaginal processes

a. Sphenoid's body
b. Pterygoid's right
   vaginal ledge

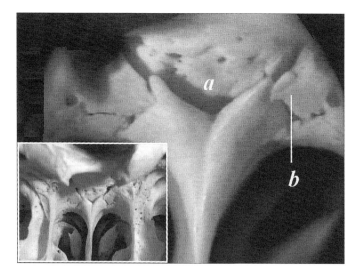

Fig. 7-59E Pterygoid's
vaginal process has been
removed to expose the
vomer's left lateral alar
articulation with the
sphenoid body. *Note:* The
vomer's hidden envelop-
ment of the sphenoid's
rostrum centrally stabi-
lizes the joint and limits
lateral deviation of the
joint. However, the joint's
anterosuperior to pos-
teroinferior articular
angulation appears to
permit anteroinferior to
posterosuperior gliding.

a. Sphenoid's body
b. Vomer bone

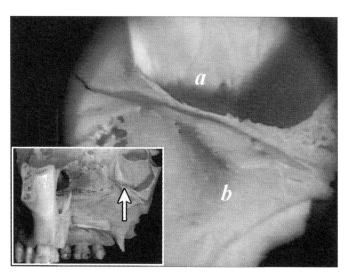

MOTION

The articulation's postural integrity is ensured, and posterior or caudal slippage of the vomer is discouraged, because of the (1) variable overlapping
of the vaginal-alar margins, (2) anteroposterior wedge configuration of the
pterygoid's vaginal ledges, (3) vomer's envelopment of the sphenoid's rostrum projection, and (4) anterior articulation with the ethmoid's perpendicular plate. Nevertheless, this articulation appears to be capable of
multidirectional movement. These movements include (1) anterocaudal to
posterorostral gliding, (2) anterosuperior to posteroinferior rocking, and
(3) lateral transverse gliding. While the sphenoid's rostrum appears to act
as a fulcrum for the vomer's multidirectional activity, its articular association with the vomer's central groove appears to predominantly support
only the anterocaudal to posterorostral gliding motion. It is the alar's
beveled articular affiliation with the pterygoid's adjacent vaginal borders
that appears to support the other two motions (Figs. 7-60 through 7-62).

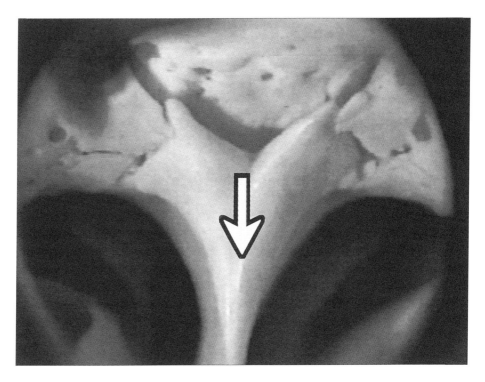

Fig. 7-60A Sphenovomerine motion: anterocaudal gliding

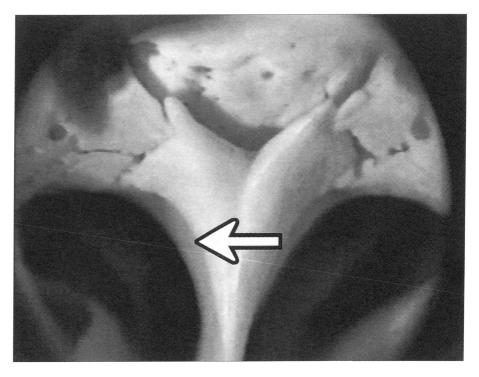

Fig. 7-61A Sphenovomerine motion: left transverse gliding

Compare with next photos →

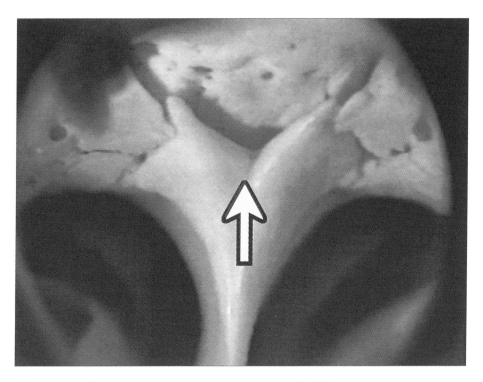

Fig. 7-60B Sphenovomerine motion: posterior-rostral gliding

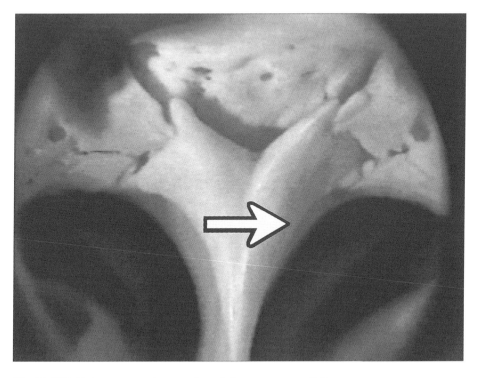

Fig. 7-61B Sphenovomerine motion: right transverse gliding

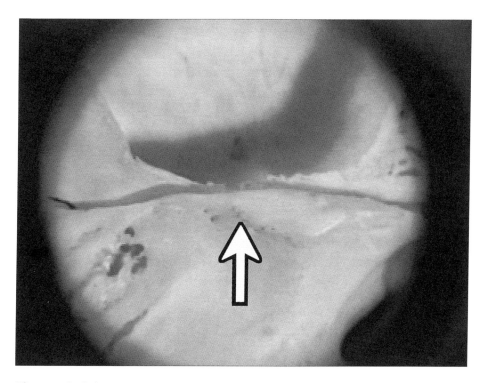

Fig. 7-62A Sphenovomerine motion: anterosuperior rocking

Compare with next photo ➡

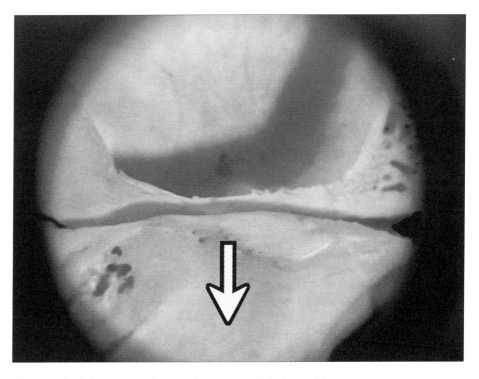

Fig. 7-62B Sphenovomerine motion: posteroinferior rocking

Articular Disengagement

Note: It is imperative for the practitioner to recognize the ethmoid's role in anteriorly securing the vomer into its anteroposterior wedged relationship with the pterygoid's medial vaginal articulations. Consequently, when attempting to disengage this articulation, attention must first be given to releasing the vomeroethmoidal suture.

CONTACTS

The optimal contacts for releasing the sphenovomerine suture are located on the hard palate along the entire surface area of the interpalatine and intermaxillary sutures. The associated sphenoid contacts are over the right and left greater wings (Fig. 7-63).

MANIPULATION

W-level pressure on the hard palate's contact compresses it into the sagittal midline. The maxillopalatine's contact is then drawn anteriorly with W¼R-level force to disengage the vomer from its seat on the sphenoid's rostrum. Concurrently, W-level force on the sphenoid's contacts is used to grip the greater wings and draw them in an anterorostral direction. This serves to complete the vomer's release as the sphenoid's body is pulled in a posterocephalad direction away from the vomer's articular surface (Fig. 7-63).

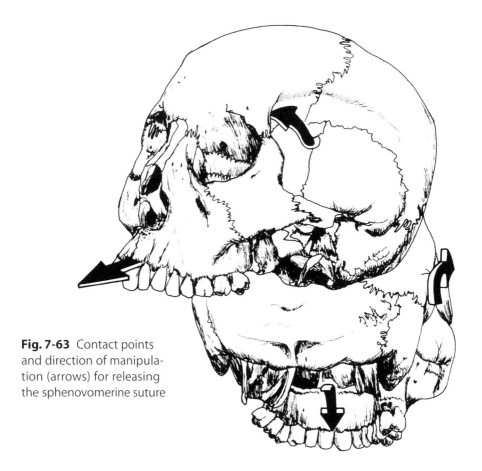

Fig. 7-63 Contact points and direction of manipulation (arrows) for releasing the sphenovomerine suture

Articular Reengagement

CONTACTS

The same contacts are used to reengage and disengage the sphenovomerine suture (Fig. 7-64).

MANIPULATION

On the hard palate's contact, W/R-level pressure is directed in a posterosuperior direction toward the sphenoid's rostrum. Concurrently, W-level compression on the sphenoidal contacts is used to grip the greater wings and draw them in a posterocaudal direction. This serves to compress the sphenoid bone to the vomer's articular margin, which is diametrically opposed to the sphenoid bone, thereby reinstating the suture's articular integrity (Fig. 7-64).

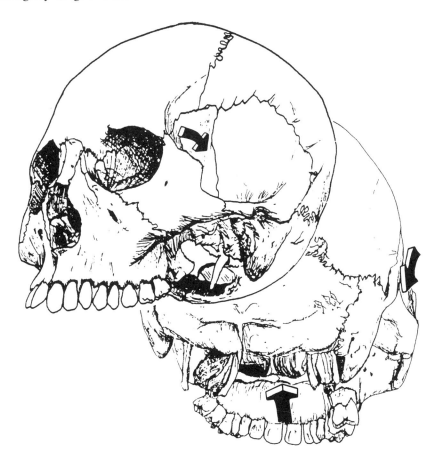

Fig. 7-64 Contact points and direction of manipulation (arrows) for closing the sphenovomerine suture

Sphenopalatine Suture (Paired)

The sphenopalatine suture is complex. Superiorly, it originates from the anteroinferior sphenoid body and extends caudally along the anterior surface of the pterygoid process (Fig. 7-65). The suture is actually composed of three primary articular divisions: superior orbital, middle perpendicular, and inferior biarticular. *Note:* Although the morphology of each articular division will be analyzed separately, the surfaces are considered to be part of the same articular suture. For this reason, the suggested manipulative protocol will combine the three divisions and address them as one.

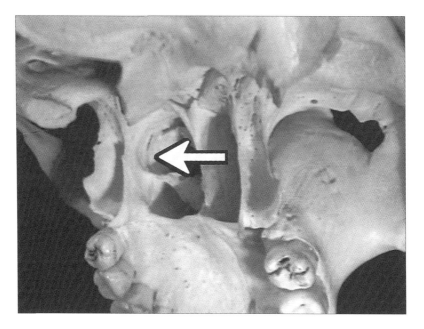

Fig. 7-65 General location of the sphenopalatine suture

MORPHOLOGY

1. *Superior orbital division.* When viewed from its sagittal midline, the superior orbital division appears as a thin strip of bone projecting postero-superiorly from the palatine's superior articular surface to the sphenoid's midsagittal anterior body (Fig. 7-66A). However, this is misleading as noted when the articular surfaces are separated and the palatine's entire surface area is revealed. The palatine's articular margin is characteristically squamosal and extends anterolaterally along the anteroinferior surface of the sphenoid body. What appears as a thin osseous strip from the midsagittal view is actually an extension of the anterosuperior palatine wall as it projects from the superior perpendicular division to become the superior orbital division.

As the osseous projection approaches the sphenoid's anteroinferior wall, it posteriorly projects a small supportive shelf under the sphenoid's anterior belly. However, upon joining with the sphenoid bone, the palatine's primary articular surface deviates rostrally to ascend the sphenoid's anteroinferior wall and stabilizes the sphenoethmoidal suture from below (Figs. 7-66B and C).

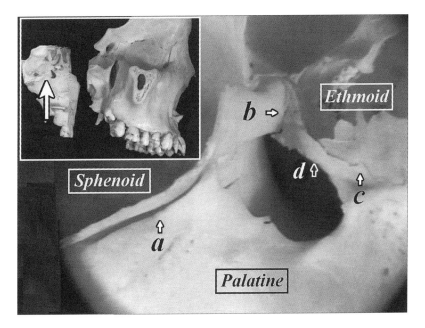

Fig. 7-66A Midsagittal slice through the posterior facial region. The left posterior portion was withdrawn to expose the palatine's upper midsagittal margins.

a. Palatine's articulation with the inferior body of the sphenoid bone
b. Palatine's superior nasal orbital articular seam
c. Midsagittal border of the palatoethmoidal suture
d. Palatine's thin osseous projection. Note that the projection courses in a posterosuperior direction to join the palatine with the sphenoid's anteroinferior border. As the two surfaces merge, the palatine projects a small shelf under the belly of the sphenoid bone before it ascends along the sphenoid's anterior wall.

Fig. 7-66B Medial view of the palatine's superior orbital division.

a. Squamosal surface for the sphenoid's anteroinferior body
b. Inferior supportive shelf
c. Superior articular border of the perpendicular division
d. Articular surface for the ethmoid

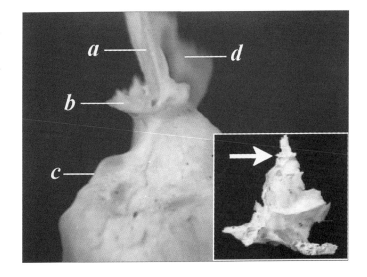

Fig. 7-66C Medial-posterior-oblique exposure of the superior orbital division

a. Palatine's sphenoidal squamosal articular surface
b. Inferior supportive shelf with rostral projecting serrations for articular stabilization
c. Superior border of the perpendicular division

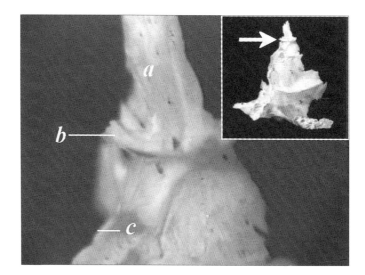

2. *Perpendicular division.* Superiorly, this division originates between the inferolateral surface of the sphenoid body adjacent to the rostrum's base and the sphenopalatine process (Figs. 7-66A and 7-67A). A coronal sectional slice reveals that the palatine's superior plane-like articular border caudally overlaps the sphenoid's adjacent surface at a 45° superolateral to inferomedial angle (Fig. 7-67A).

Looking at the articulation's longitudinal path from an inferior direction often reveals an anterolateral to posteromedial angulation fluctuating between 15° and 20° from the palatine's anterior articular border to the sphenoid's medial pterygoid base (Fig. 7-67B). When combined with its paired suture, the two articular seams create a posteriorly narrowed furrow that caudally overlaps and secures the anterolateral one-fifth of the articular margin of the vomer's ala (Fig. 7-67B). As the suture leaves its superior region, it descends in a plane-like formation articulating edge to edge with the pterygoid's anterior internal medial crest (Figs. 7-67C and D).

Fig. 7-67A Anterior-coronal exposure of the superior perpendicular palatal sphenoid articulation

a. Inferior sphenoid body
b. Superior palatine process

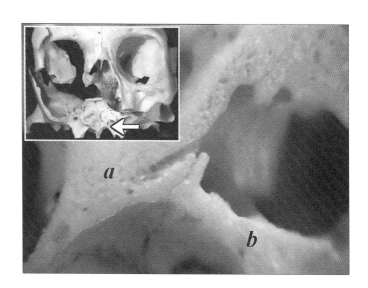

Fig. 7-67B Inferior exposure delineating the palatine's anterolateral to posteromedial longitudinal wedge-shaped articular seam

a. Palatine's superior left process
b. Left superior articular seam

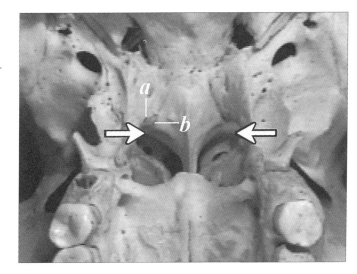

Fig. 7-67C Medial view of the palatine's left perpendicular plate. Arrows depict the palatine's superficial anteroposterior projections as they medially overlap the pterygoid's anterior-medial edge.

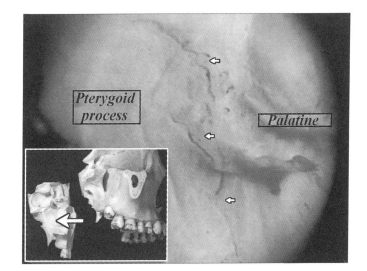

Fig. 7-67D Inferior exposure of the left perpendicular plate's articular association with the medial-anterior border of the pterygoid process. The articulation has been sliced along its axial plane and the lower half was removed to expose the suture's articular arrangement.

a. Palatine's perpendicular plate
b. Left pterygoid process

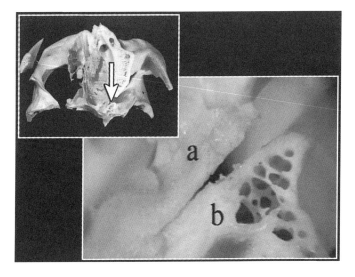

3. *Inferior biarticular division.* This division is actually a continuation of the perpendicular division as it descends into its lower terminal region. Its distinguishing characteristic is found upon entering this division: the pterygoid's anterior articular margin bifurcates to articulate with the palatine's medial and lateral articular furrows (Figs. 7-68A~C). Macroscopic enlargement of the pterygoid's bifurcated articular surfaces reveals that both articular borders appear to share a propensity toward marginal convexity (Fig. 7-68A). However, the medial articular plate's surface is smooth and the lateral articular plate is covered with anteroposterior serrated projections (Figs. 7-68B and C). Positioned between the palatine's medial and lateral pterygoid furrows is a wedge-shaped formation known as the pterygoid fossa. Although this formation is gouged and exhibits a concave surface, its marginal borders are raised and form a flush articular wedge between the pterygoid's medial and lateral plates (Figs. 7-68C and D).

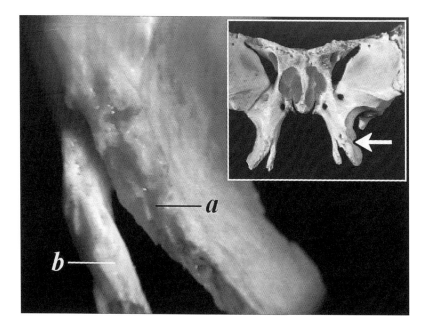

Fig. 7-68A Anterior view exposing the inferior articular division of the pterygoid's left bifurcated process

a. Serrated lateral margin
b. Smooth medial margin

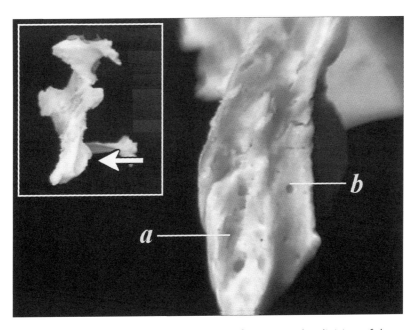

Fig. 7-68B Posterior view exposing the inferior articular division of the palatine process

a. Serrated lateral margin
b. Smooth medial margin. Note that the sphenoid's medial pterygoid process often appears smooth and plane-like, whereas the lateral process is often covered with minute serrations coursing in a postero-lateral to anteromedial direction.

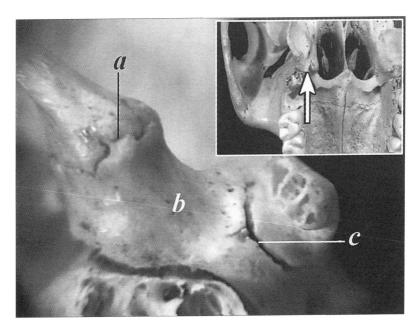

Fig. 7-68C Inferior view exposing the left sphenopalatine's inferior division and its interarticular association

a. Serrated lateral articular seam   c. Smooth medial articular seam
b. Palatine's wedge formation

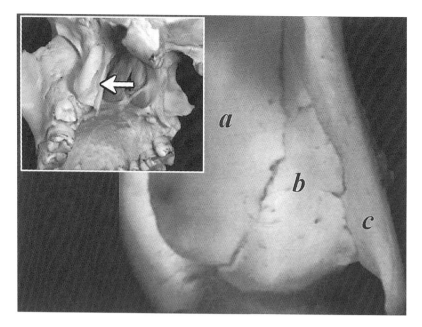

Fig. 7-68D Posteroinferior exposure delineating the wedge-and-bifurcation line within the sphenopalatine's inferior sutural division

a. Lateral pterygoid process
b. Palatine's wedge formation
c. Medial pterygoid process

MOTION

The combination of serrations, planes, and furrows appears to support superolateral to inferomedial gliding along the suture's superior articular seam and superomedial to inferolateral gliding along the suture's inferior articular margins. These diametrically opposed movements are due to a central rocking fulcrum located midway between the palatine perpendicular plate's upper and lower regions. Consequently, as the palatine's perpendicular plate glides superiorly, its superior region is coupled with the articulation's rocking motion to shift laterally, and the inferior region is coupled to rock medially. (Figs. 7-69 through 7-71).

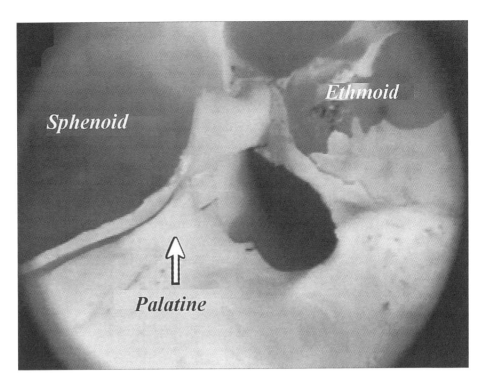

Fig. 7-69A Sphenopalatine motion: superior gliding

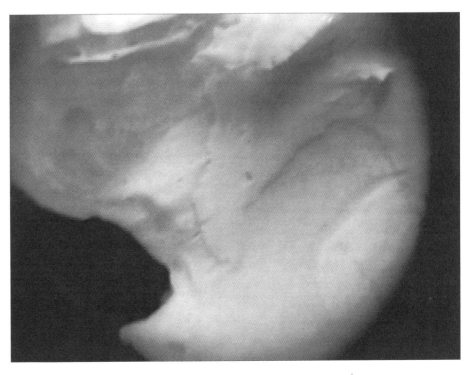

Fig. 7-70A Sphenopalatine motion: superolateral gliding

Compare with next photos →

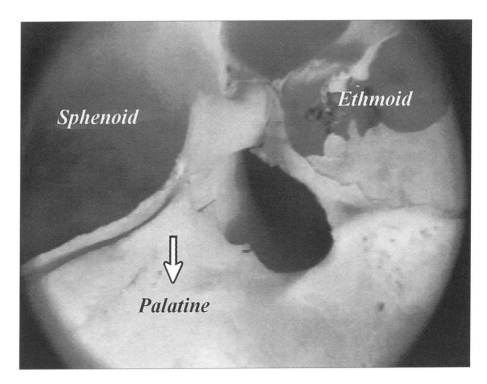

Fig. 7-69B Sphenopalatine motion: inferior gliding

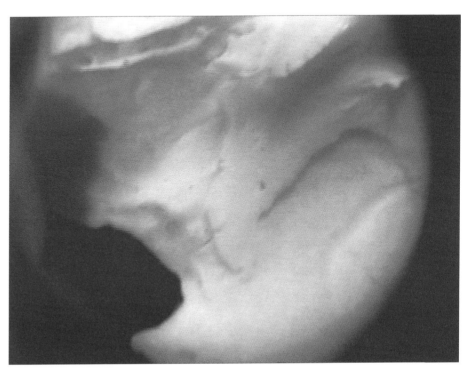

Fig. 7-70B Sphenopalatine motion: inferomedial gliding

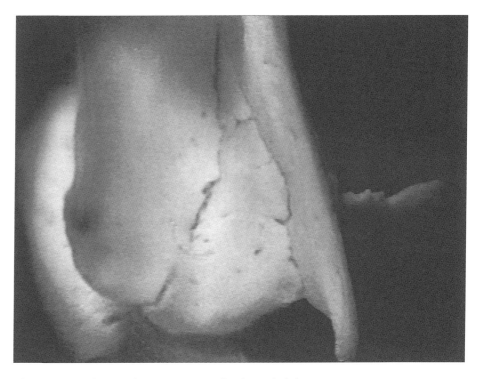

Fig. 7-71A Sphenopalatine motion: inferolateral gliding

Compare with next photo →

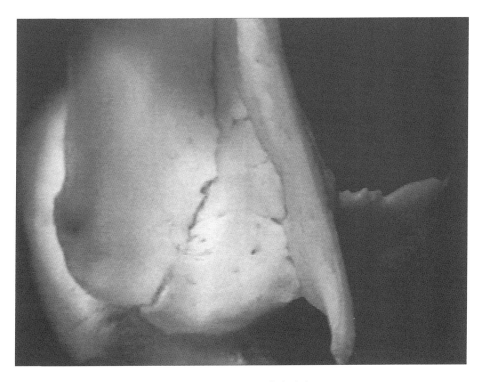

Fig. 7-71B Sphenopalatine motion: superomedial gliding

Articular Disengagement

CONTACTS

The optimal contact points for releasing the sphenopalatine suture are located inside the mouth straddling the maxilla and bilaterally contacting the posterior external surface above the last molars, and on the anterior tip of the pterygoid process (Fig. 7-72).

MANIPULATION

W-level pressure is used to grip and squeeze the maxillary contacts toward the sagittal midline of the hard palate. This maneuver compresses the two maxillary structures together and forces the palatine bones to stay with the maxilla. Once the palatines are secured, posteromedial W¼R-level pressure on the pterygoid's contact guides the pterygoid away from the palatine's articular surface (Fig. 7-72).

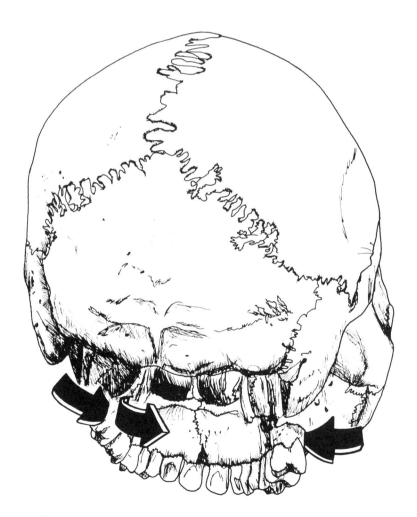

Fig. 7-72 Contact points and direction of manipulation (arrows) for releasing the left sphenopalatine suture

Articular Reengagement

CONTACTS

The optimal contacts for reengaging the sphenopalatine suture are located on the anterior external maxillary surface, in the bony depression above the alveolar processes of the incisor teeth and posterior to the lateral pterygoid process (Fig. 7-73).

MANIPULATION

W-level pressure on the maxillary contacts compress them posteriorly toward the sagittal center of the sphenobasilar junction. This manipulation secures the maxilla against the palatine's horizontal and perpendicular plates. Concurrently, anterolateral W¼R-level force on the pterygoid's contact draws the pterygoid's articular surface against the palatine's, thereby securing the suture's articular surfaces (Fig. 7-73).

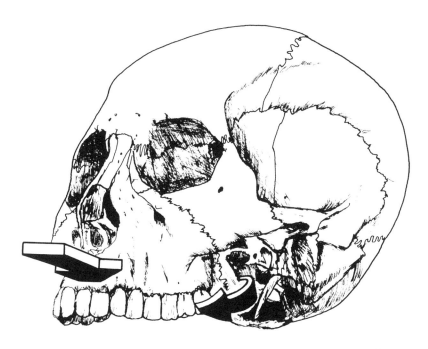

Fig. 7-73 Contact points and direction of manipulation (arrows) for reengaging the left sphenopalatine suture

Sphenozygomatic Suture (Paired)

MORPHOLOGY

Located along the internal lateral wall of the eye socket, the sphenozygomatic suture runs from the frontal bone's lateral supraorbital plate to the infraorbital fissure (Fig. 7-74A). To help clarify its morphology, the suture has been divided into three primary articular divisions. To accomplish this, the suture is first bisected into its superior and inferior halves. The inferior half is then further subdivided into its superior and inferior halves (Fig. 7-74B).

Fig. 7-74A Topographic position of the left sphenozygomatic suture when viewed from the anterior and posterior directions

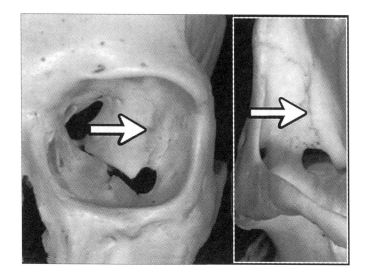

Fig. 7-74B Anterior macroscopic view of the sphenoid's left articular margin. Arrows delineate the suture's three primary articular divisions

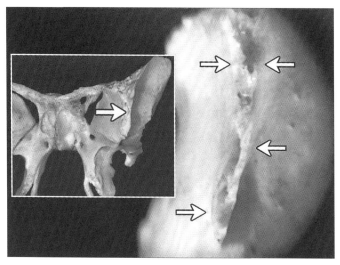

1. *Superior division.* This division of the sphenoid's articular surface is characteristically trench-like in contour and appears to be a combination of squamous and serrated formations. Macroscopic observation reveals thin, fragile, overlapping squamous ridges that project from the sphenoid's superior trench-like borders to encase the zygomatic's serrated wedge-like articular margin (Fig. 7-75A).

Fig. 7-75A Axial slice inferiorly exposing the superior articular division. Arrows in the macroscopic enlargement delineate the sphenoid's overlapping squamous ridges that envelop the zygomatic's serrated articular wedge formation

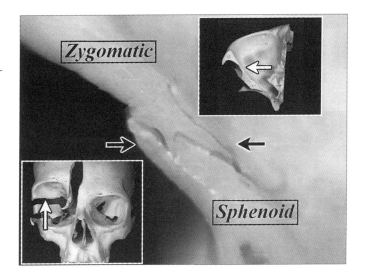

2. *Intermediate division.* Within this division, which is located in the superior portion of the suture's inferior half, the sphenoid's posterior margin extends behind the zygomatic's articular border. Macroscopic enlargement reveals anterior overlapping of the sphenoid bone by the zygomatic, which is distinctly characteristic of this division (Fig. 7-75B).

Fig. 7-75B Axial slice superiorly exposing the intermediate division

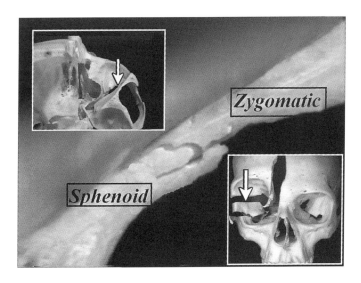

3. *Caudal division.* In this division, the sphenoid's marginal ridge reverses itself and protrudes anteriorly over the zygomatic's articular surface. In addition, the sphenoid's marginal ridge completes its interlocking hinged-like articular seam (Fig. 7-75C).

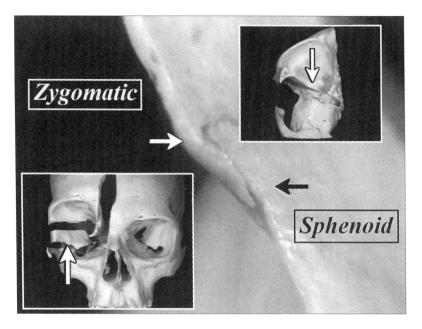

Fig. 7-75C Axial slice inferiorly exposing the caudal division. Arrows in the macroscopic enlargement delineate the anterior overlapping of the zygomatic by the sphenoid bone.

MOTION

The zygomatic's association with the frontal and temporal bones coupled with the suture's articular configuration appear to permit anteromedial to posterolateral hinging throughout the suture's articular seam (Fig. 7-76).

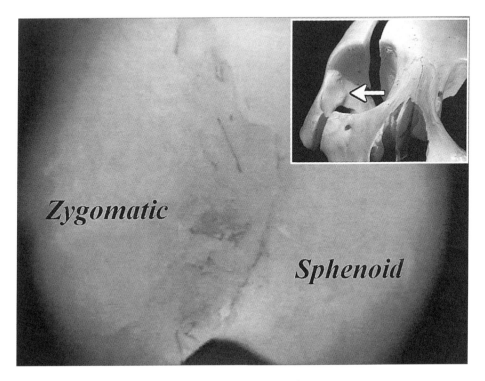

Fig. 7-76A Sphenozygomatic motion: posterolateral

Compare with next photo ⇒

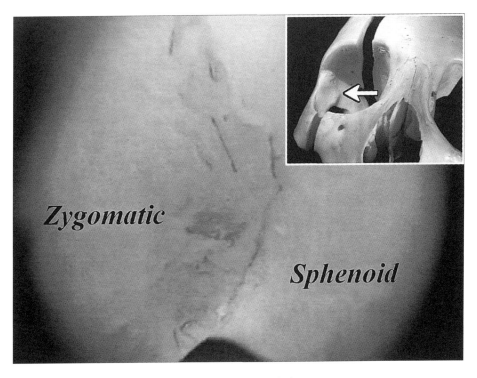

Fig. 7-76B Sphenozygomatic motion: anteromedial

Articular Disengagement

CONTACTS

The optimal contact points for releasing this suture are posterior to the lateral margin of the zygomatic frontal process and on the external surface of the sphenoid's greater wing (Fig. 7-77).

MANIPULATION

Anterior W/R-level force is applied to the zygomatic's marginal contact while W⅓R-level compressive force on the sphenoid's contact push the greater wing medially toward the sella turcica of the sphenoid body (Fig. 7-77).

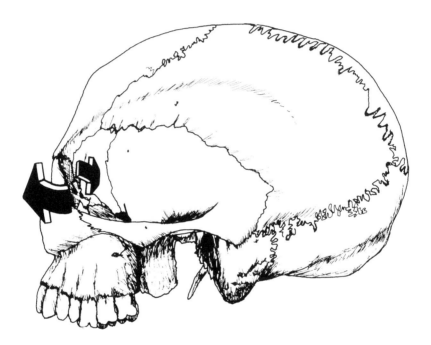

Fig. 7-77 Contact points and direction of manipulation (arrows) for releasing the sphenoid zygomatic suture

Articular Reengagement

CONTACTS

The optimal contacts for reengaging this suture are located on the anterior surface of the zygomatic's frontal process (lateral to the lower portion of the eye socket) and on the external surface of the sphenoid's greater wing (Fig. 7-78).

MANIPULATION

Manipulate the zygomatic contact posteromedially with W¼R-level pressure while W-level force on the sphenoid's contact is directed anteriorly toward the suture's articular surface (Fig. 7-78).

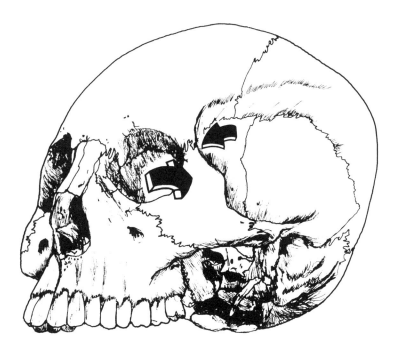

Fig. 7-78 Contact points and direction of manipulation (arrows) for closing the sphenoid zygomatic suture

Base and Vault Sutures

There are eight inaccessible articulations in the cranial vault and base. Of these, six are paired and two are singular. When addressing paired articulations, the primary characteristics of one side usually mirror its paired counterpart. Consequently, this section will address only one side unless there is a significant difference between them. *Note:* The primary characteristic that differentiates the vault sutures, both accessible and inaccessible, from facial sutures is the direct connection of the vault sutures with the intercranial meningeal membranes.

Lesser Sphenofrontal Suture (Paired)

MORPHOLOGY

The lesser sphenofrontal suture is located on the inferior surface of the vault, posterior to the supraorbital plates of the frontal bone and anterior to the lesser wings of the sphenoid bone (Fig. 7-79). In the lateral third of this suture, the lesser sphenofrontal wing's inferior articular border is smoothly beveled and acts as a superior overlapping ledge to the frontal bone's adjacent articular margin. As the suture courses medially toward the posterior midsagittal plane of the ethmoid notch, the lesser wing of the sphenoid's superior articular ledge and an inferior projecting marginal shelf "sandwich" the frontal bone's adjoining articular border (Fig. 7-80A). Serrated in nature, this portion of the suture is inundated with anteroposterior pin-to-socket formations (Fig. 7-80A).

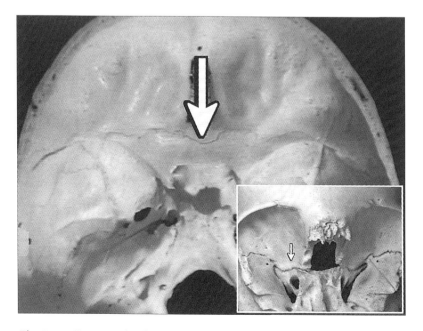

Fig. 7-79 Topographic location of the lesser sphenofrontal suture

Like the sphenoid's lateral articular margin, the frontal bone's lateral third articular edge is smoothly beveled to caudally adhere with the lesser sphenofrontal wings's inferior surface. However, the frontal bone's remaining wedged articular surface is beveled superiorly and inferiorly to form a knife-edge configuration covered with anteroposterior ridges and serrations (Fig. 7-80B).

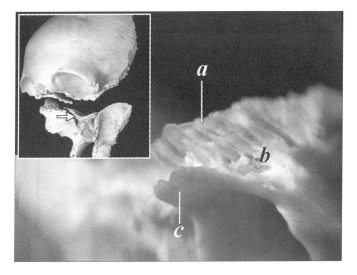

Fig. 7-80A Anterolateral-oblique view of the lesser sphenofrontal suture

   a. Lesser sphenofrontal wing's superior overlapping marginal shelf
   b. Lesser sphenofrontal wing's serrated articular trench which houses the frontal bone's articular border
   c. Sphenoid's inferior projecting shelf

Fig. 7-80B Posterior view exposing the frontal bone's serrated wedge-shaped articular surface

a. Superior marginal surface
b. Inferior marginal surface

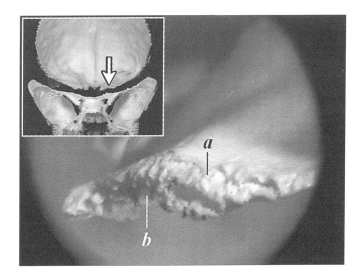

MOTION

Dictated by the suture's morphologic configurations of marginal ledges and pin-to-socket serrations, this suture's articular movements appear to be confined to anterior to posterior gliding. Rostral to caudal rocking may also be tolerated (Figs. 7-81 and 7-82).

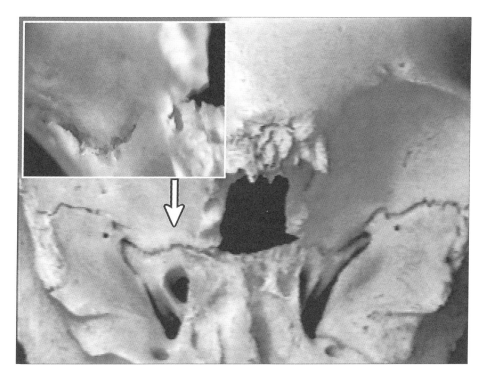

Fig. 7-81A Lesser sphenofrontal motion: posterocaudal rocking

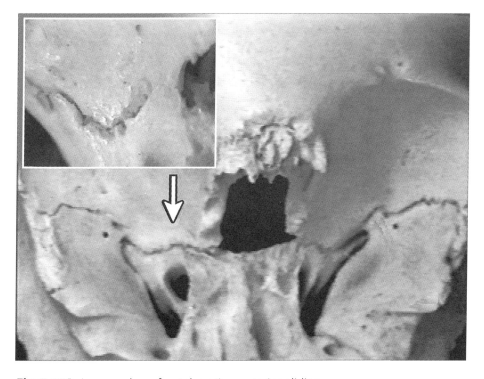

Fig. 7-82A Lesser sphenofrontal motion: anterior gliding

Compare with next photos →

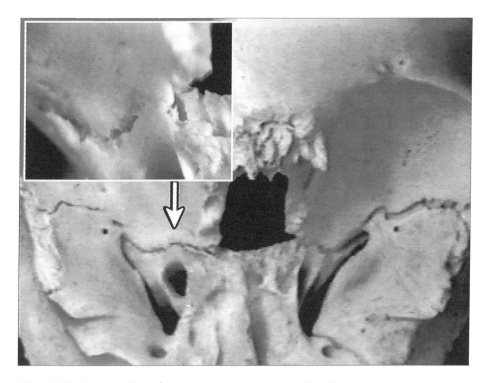

Fig. 7-81B Lesser sphenofrontal motion: anterorostral rocking

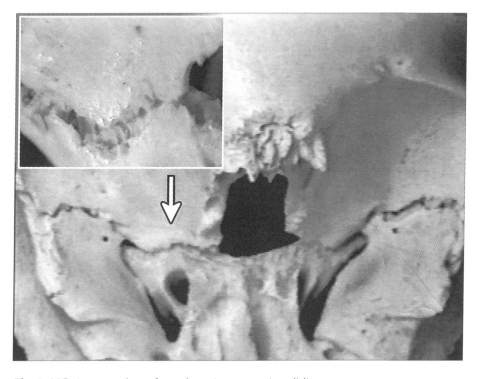

Fig. 7-82B Lesser sphenofrontal motion: posterior gliding

Articular Disengagement

CONTACTS

The optimal contact points for releasing the lesser sphenofrontal suture are located bilaterally on the frontal bone's inferolateral surface, anterior to the coronal suture and superior to the sphenofrontal suture. The other contacts are located on the lateral external surfaces of the sphenoid's greater wings (Fig. 7-83).

MANIPULATION

W-level compression is used to grasp the frontal bone's contacts, and W⅓R-level force is used to draw the frontal bone in an anterorostral direction. This maneuver elevates the frontal bone and separates the posterior orbital plate's articular margin from the overlapping edge of the sphenoid's lesser wings. Synchronously, W⅓R-level compression to the sphenoid's greater wings draws the contacts posteriorly. This locks the sphenoid to the remaining vault structures and secures its position against the maneuver on the frontal bone (Fig. 7-83).

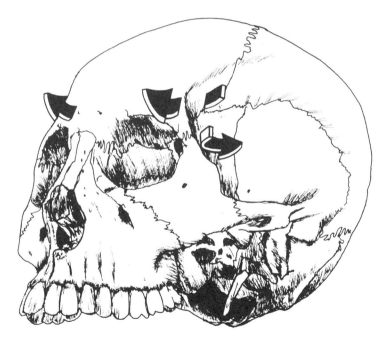

Fig. 7-83 Contact points and direction of manipulation (arrows) for releasing the articular surface of the lesser sphenofrontal suture

Articular Reengagement

CONTACTS

The optimal contact points for reengaging the lesser sphenofrontal suture are located on the frontal bone across the superior aspect of the superciliary arches and bilaterally on the external surface of the sphenoid's greater wings (Fig. 7-84).

MANIPULATION

W-level pressure is used to grasp the frontal bone's contact points, and W⅓R-level force is used to draw the frontal bone in a posterior direction against the sphenoid's anterior articular surface. W⅓R-level force on the sphenoid's contacts counters the frontal bone's motion, drawing the sphenoid in an anteroinferior direction. This compresses the sphenoid's overlapping anterior lesser wing articular surfaces against the invading frontal bone's surface, and secures the reengagement of the lesser sphenofrontal articular union (Fig. 7-84).

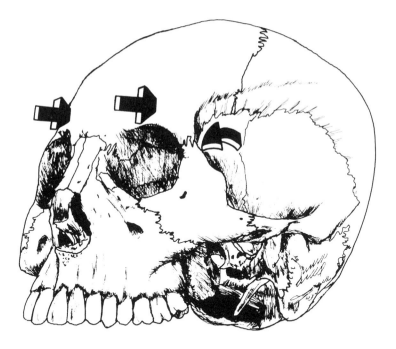

Fig. 7-84 Contact points and direction of manipulation (arrows) for reengaging the articular surface of the lesser sphenofrontal suture

Superior Sphenoethmoid Suture (Singular)

MORPHOLOGY

Located along the anterosuperior articular surface of the sphenoid's body, the superior sphenoethmoid suture is situated inferior to the lesser sphenofrontal suture and actually inserts under the protruding inferior ledge of the lesser sphenoid wings (Fig. 7-85). Although attempts to view this suture from inside the vault are hindered by the overlapping orbital plates of the frontal bone, a sagittal dissection reveals the sphenoid's anterosuperior margin as it extends under the lesser sphenofrontal articulation to overlap the ethmoid's posterior superior articular border (Fig. 7-86A).

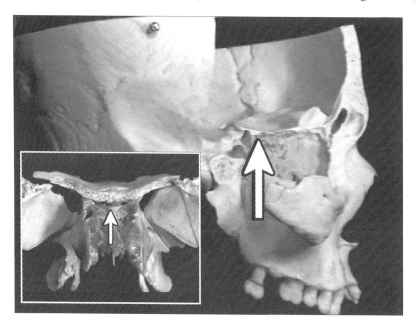

Fig. 7-85 Anterior and lateral exposures of the topographic location of the superior sphenoethmoid suture

Upon disarticulation, the suture exhibits three distinct pseudocondylar surfaces; consequently, the articulation can be subdivided into thirds (Figs. 7-86B and C). The ethmoid's condylar surfaces are slightly convex and extend rostrally to articulate with adjacent overlapping sockets implanted beneath the lesser wing's anteroinferior articular ledge (Figs. 7-86B and D). Slightly gouged to fit the ethmoid's medial condylar surface, the sphenoid's medial socket extends to the posterior margin of the ethmoid's cribriform plate. The sphenoid's lateral articular surfaces are positioned posteriorly, deeper into the suture's articular seam; they repeatedly display scooped-out condylar pockets that appear to function as rocking surfaces for the adjacent pseudocondylar projections of the ethmoid (Fig. 7-86C and D).

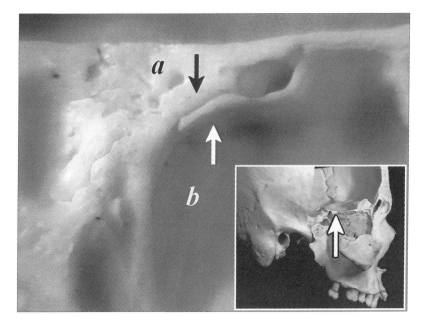

Fig. 7-86A Sagittal slice through the superior sphenoethmoid suture exposing the suture's articular junction between its medial and lateral condylar surfaces

a. Sphenoid's beveled overlapping articular surface
b. Ethmoid's underlying planed articular surface

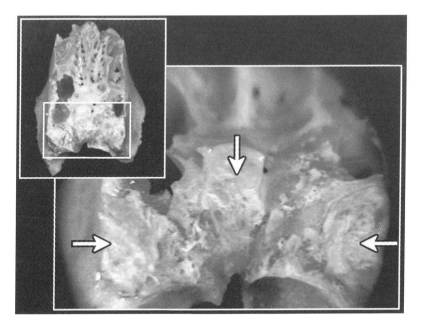

Fig. 7-86B Posterosuperior view of the ethmoid's superior sphenoid articulating surface. Arrows depict the ethmoid's three pseudocondylar formations.

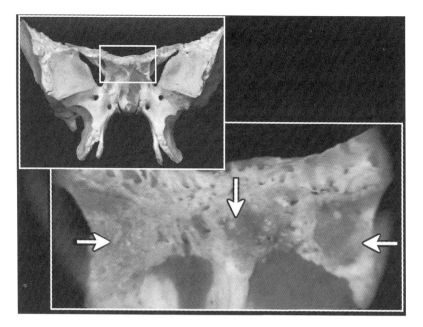

Fig. 7-86C Anterior view exposing the sphenoid's superior articulating surface to the ethmoid. Arrows delineate the sphenoid's three socket formations for the ethmoid's pseudocondylar projections.

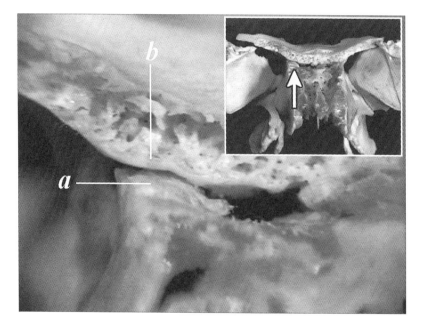

Fig. 7-86D Anterior exposure of the superior sphenoethmoid's right lateral articular seam. Note the condylar convexity of the ethmoid's articular surface.

a. Ethmoid's condylar surface
b. Sphenoid's concave articular border along the inferior surface of the sphenoid's lesser wing

MOTION

Because of its condylar configurations, anteroposterior rocking is the primary mode of motion. However, the pliability of the ethmoid's membranous osseous nature also appears to sanction transverse or multidirectional oblique gliding (Fig. 7-87).

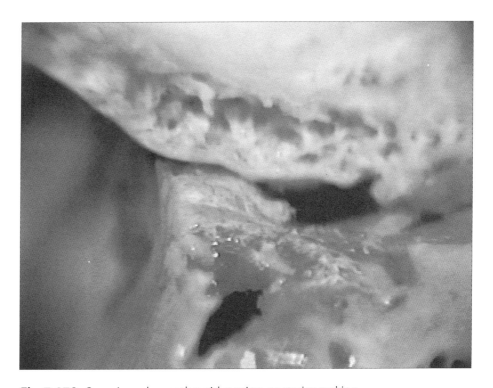

Fig. 7-87A Superior sphenoethmoid motion: posterior rocking

Compare with next photo →

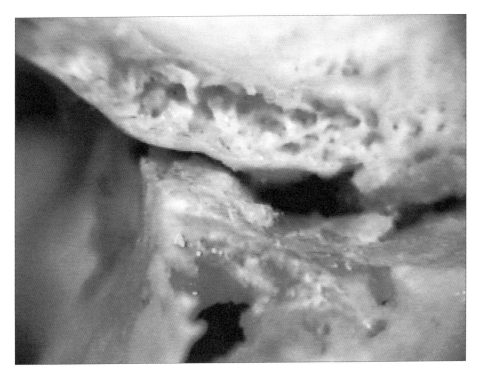

Fig. 7-87B Superior sphenoethmoid motion: anterior rocking

Articular Disengagement

CONTACTS

The optimal contact points for releasing the superior sphenoethmoid suture are located medial to the supraorbital notches along the right and left supraorbital margins of the frontal bone. The frontal bone's counter-contacts are bilaterally positioned on the zygomatic's frontal processes, inferior to the marginal tubercle (Fig. 7-88).

MANIPULATION

W⅓R-level force is used to compress the frontal bone's contacts and draw that bone in an anterorostral direction. This maneuver internally rotates the frontal bone's lateral ethmoid borders and secures the ethmoid within the frontal bone's ethmoid notch. The anterorostral force elevates the frontal bone's anterior nasal region and draws the ethmoid's posterior articular margin in an anteroinferior direction, unlocking the ethmoid's condylar formation from the sphenoid's articular sockets. A W⅓R-level steady compressive force toward the sagittal midline of the posterior ethmoid notch is applied on the zygomatic contacts. With this in place, the contacts are then drawn posteriorly with a W/R-level force. This maneuver compresses the zygomatic-sphenoid sutures and secures the zygomatic bones to the sphenoid's greater wings. The posterior force then secures the lesser wing's position as the ethmoid's articular surface is drawn away by the frontal bone's contacts (Fig. 7-88).

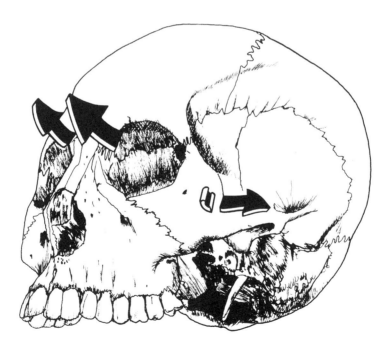

Fig. 7-88 Contact points and direction of manipulation (arrows) for releasing the articular surface of the superior sphenoethmoid suture

Articular Reengagement

CONTACTS

The optimal contacts for reengaging the superior sphenoethmoid suture are located inside the mouth on the medial tips of the right and left pterygoid processes, and on the glabella between the frontal bone's superciliary arches (Fig. 7-89).

MANIPULATION

W-level force is used to guide the pterygoid contacts posterosuperiorly toward the anterior lateral borders of the sphenobasilar junction. This maneuver rocks the sphenoid's body anteriorly and secures the lesser wing's articular surface against the ethmoid's posterior force. W/R-level force on the frontal bone's contact simultaneously compresses the glabella posteriorly toward the internal occipital protuberance. This drives the ethmoid posteriorly into the inferior articular socket of the sphenoid's lesser wing (Fig. 7-89).

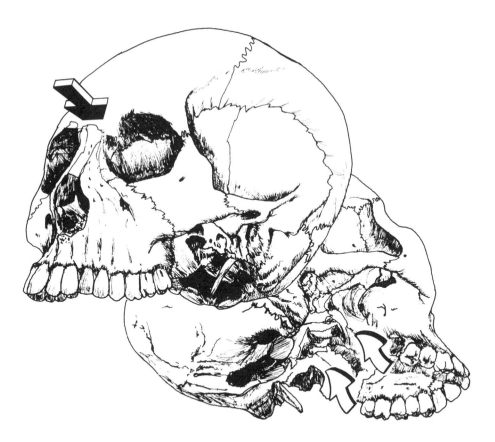

Fig. 7-89 Contact points and direction of manipulation (arrows) for reengaging the articular surface of the superior sphenoethmoid suture

Sphenopetrosal Fissure (Paired)

MORPHOLOGY

The sphenopetrosal fissure is located between the posterior floor of the sphenoid's greater wing and the anteromedial one-third of the petrous process (Fig. 7-90). Located in a caudal-anterior direction relative to its adjacent petrosal border, the sphenoid's articular surface is plane-like and is beveled to caudally overlap its adjacent petrosal surface. The petrous articular surface (also plane-like) is beveled to form an articular ridge that posterosuperiorly parallels the sphenoid's juxtaposed articular ridge (Fig. 7-91).

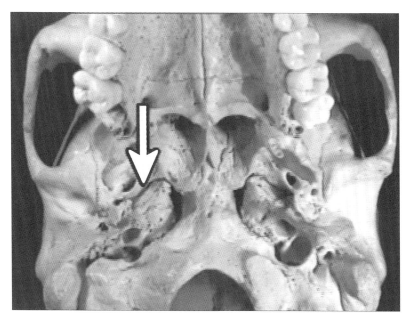

Fig. 7-90 Caudal topographic exposure depicting the sphenopetrosal fissure's location

Note: The petrous anteromedial apical tip is often found to articulate as a schindylesis with a small projecting tubercle extending from the postero-superior-lateral corner of the sphenoid's body. Characteristically, the enveloping apical articular surface is convex along its superior and caudal margins, and anteriorly wraps around the tubercle to secure it from anterior slippage. Two noteworthy characteristics of the sphenoid's tubercle are:

1. It consistently projects posterolaterally on a path that parallels the longitudinal axis of the temporal's petrous process.
2. The superior and inferior articular surfaces are gouged, allowing for rostral-caudal rocking (Fig. 7-92).

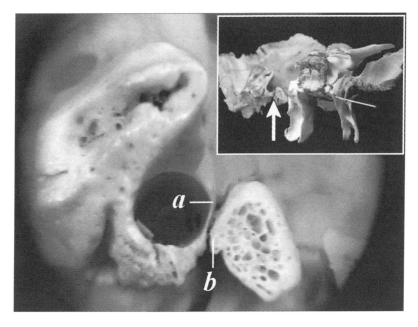

Fig. 7-91 Articular ridged surfaces of the petrous process and sphenoid

a. Petrous articular surface
b. Sphenoid's articular surface

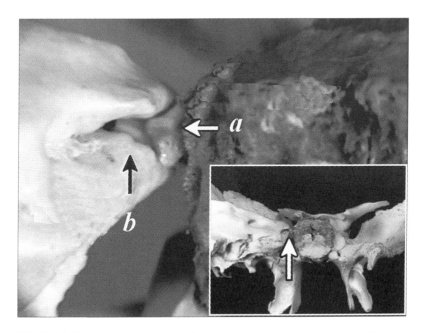

Fig. 7-92 Temporal's petrous apical groove and its encasement of the sphenoid tubercle

a. Sphenoid tubercle
b. Temporal's apical groove

MOTION

Although this is not a tight fitting articulation, the characteristic appearance of the ridged articular surfaces appears to encourage independent anteromedial (internal) to posterolateral (external) gliding. The tubercle's gouged contour and its enveloped articular association with the petrous apex suggests structural allowance for medial-caudal to lateral-rostral apical rocking (Fig. 7-93).

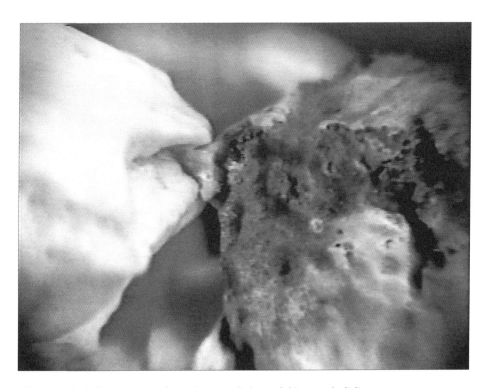

Fig. 7-93A Sphenopetrosal motion: medial-caudal internal gliding

Compare with next photo ➡

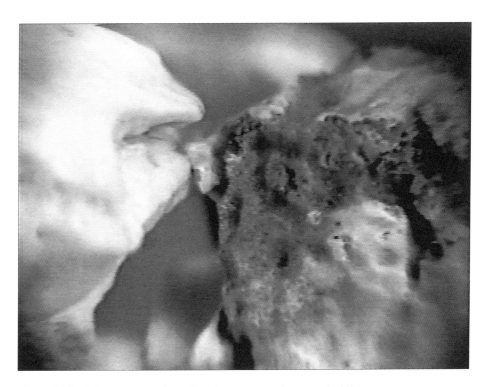

Fig. 7-93B Sphenopetrosal motion: lateral-rostral external gliding

Articular Disengagement

CONTACTS

The optimal contact points for releasing the sphenopetrosal fissure are located inside the mouth on the posterior surface of the medial pterygoid tip and along the anterior surface of the mastoid process posterior to the ear. *Note:* Both contacts are applied on the side of fissure fixation (Fig. 7-94).

MANIPULATION

W-level pressure is directed anteriorly on the pterygoid contact. The maneuver stabilizes the sphenoid's petrosal articular surface in an anteroinferior direction. Synchronously, W⅓R-level posterior force on the mastoid contact is used to glide the petrosal articular surface posterolaterally and separate its petrosal housing from the sphenoid's tubercle (Fig. 7-94).

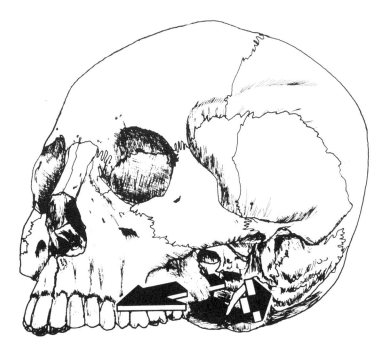

Fig. 7-94 Contact points and direction of manipulation (arrows) for releasing the left sphenopetrosal fissure

Articular Reengagement

CONTACTS

The optimal contacts for reengaging the sphenopetrosal fissure are located inside the mouth on the anterior surface of the medial pterygoid tip and along the posterior surface of the mastoid process. *Note:* Both contacts are applied on the side of fissure separation (Fig. 7-95).

MANIPULATION

Using W⅓R-level pressure, the pterygoid is directed posteriorly toward the occipital condyle of the same side. This guides the sphenoid's articular surface posteriorly toward its articular margin on the temporal's petrous process. Concurrently, W⅓R-level anteromedial compression toward the sphenobasilar junction is applied to the mastoid contact. This counterforce secures the articular surface of the petrous apex to the sphenoid's adjacent tubercle (Fig. 7-95).

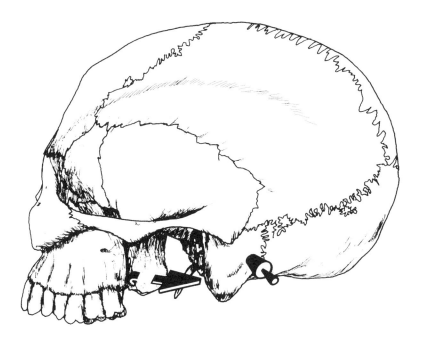

Fig. 7-95 Contact points and direction of manipulation (arrows) for reengaging the left sphenopetrosal fissure

Occipitopetrosal Fissure (Paired)

MORPHOLOGY

Located between the occiput and the petrous process of the temporal bone on the floor of the vault, the occipitopetrosal fissure runs from the antero-medial surface of the jugular foramen to the sphenobasilar junction (Fig. 7-96). The occiput's articular edge is often coarse and exhibits a ridge that extends along its superior longitudinal plane. The adjacent articular surface of the petrous process houses a longitudinal groove that envelops the occiput's articular ridge and extends medially under the ridge to form a supportive shelf for the occiput's inferior articular margin (Fig. 7-97).

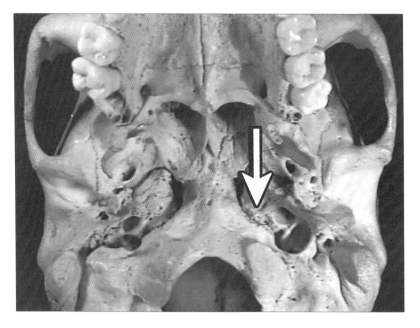

Fig. 7-96 Arrow depicts the occipitopetrosal fissure's topographic location

Fig. 7-97A Anterolateral exposure of the occiput's left petrous articular surface

a. Superior longitudinal ridge
b. Inferior medially shaved surface

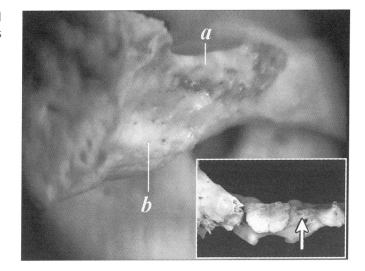

Fig. 7-97B Anteroinferior exposure of the left temporal's adjacent articular surface

Note: Arrow delineates the temporal's inferior articular ledge that appears to caudally support the occiput from below its superior ridge.

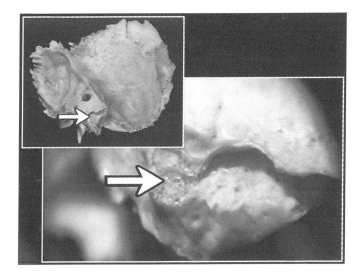

Fig. 7-97C Viewed from the anterior, the right occipitopetrosal fissure is coronally sliced to expose its articular junction.

a. Temporal's superior articular ledge
b. Temporal's inferior articular ledge
c. Occiput's superior longitudinal ridge formation

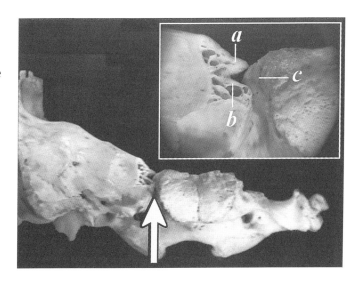

MOTION

Because of this fissure's articular configuration, it appears that independent superior or caudal motion is discouraged. However, the ridge-to-groove margin does create a track that encourages anteromedial to posterolateral gliding as well as superior to inferior pivotal rotation (Figs. 7-98 and 7-99).

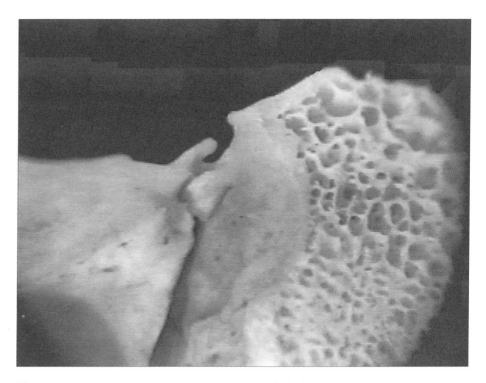

Fig. 7-98A Occipitopetrosal motion: anteromedial gliding

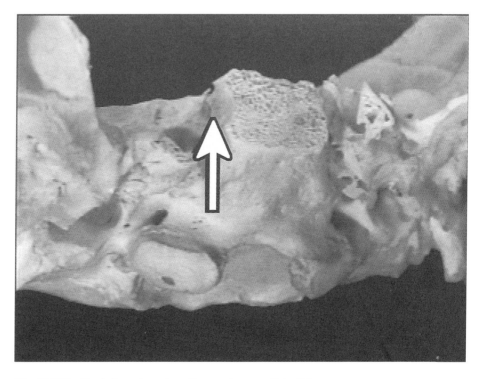

Fig. 7-99A Occipitopetrosal motion: anteromedial gliding

Compare with next photos ➡

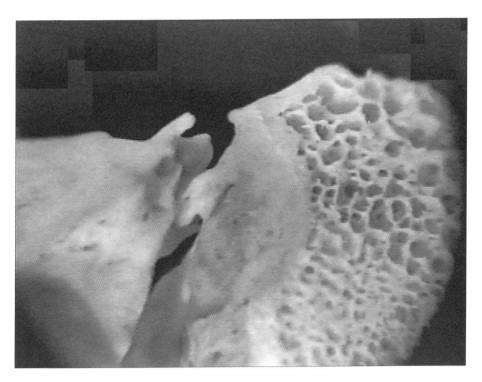

Fig. 7-98B Occipitopetrosal motion: posterolateral gliding

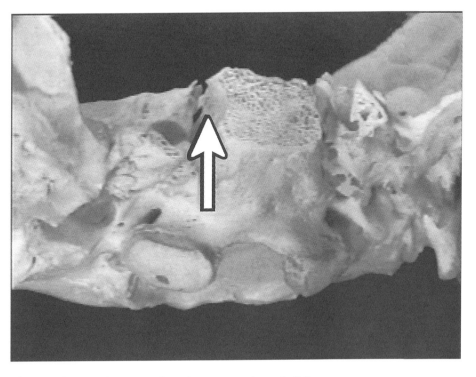

Fig. 7-99B Occipitopetrosal motion: posterolateral gliding

Articular Disengagement

CONTACTS

The optimal contact points for releasing the occipitopetrosal fissure are located posterior to the mastoid tip of the involved fixed side and anterior to the mastoid tip on the opposite healthy side (Fig. 7-100).

MANIPULATION

W/R-level force on the posterior mastoid contact directs the mastoid anterolaterally while simultaneous W¼R-level pressure is applied to the opposite mastoid contact to draw the healthy mastoid in a posterolateral direction. This maneuver allows the petrous process on the fixed fissure side to release from the occiput's articular surface as the force on the opposing healthy side secures the occiput into its occipitomastoid suture. This draws the occiput away from the fixed side (Fig. 7-100).

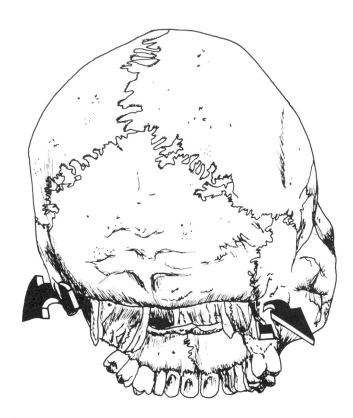

Fig. 7-100 Inferior view depicting the contact points and direction of manipulation (arrows) for releasing the left occipitopetrosal fissure

Articular Reengagement

CONTACTS

The optimal contact points for reengaging the occipitopetrosal fissure are located on the anterior mastoid tip of the involved unstable side and posterior to the mastoid tip on the healthy fissure side (Fig. 7-101).

MANIPULATION

W/R-level force on the anterior mastoid contact directs the mastoid posterolaterally while simultaneous W¼R-level pressure on the healthy mastoid contact draws that mastoid anterolaterally. This procedure allows the healthy mastoid side to draw away from its articular surface, causing the occiput's basilar region to laterally shift toward the unstable side. As the mastoid contact on the unstable side draws the mastoid posterolateral, its occipitomastoid suture locks and draws the occipitopetrosal articular surface together (Fig. 7-101).

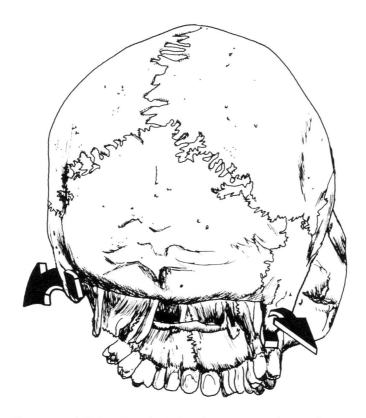

Fig. 7-101 Inferior view depicting the contact points and direction of manipulation (arrows) for reengaging the right occipitopetrosal fissure

Sphenobasilar Symphysis (Singular)

The morphology and motion of the sphenobasilar symphysis are described to complete the articular overview of the cranial base and vault. However, this articulation is not actually a sutural junction but a synchondrosis-based symphysis. With this structure, the approach used in this text of disengagement and reengagement is not applicable. Rather, treatment of the sphenobasilar symphysis is based on its realignment. This, therefore, falls outside the realm of the sutural techniques used in this text. For this reason, the manipulative techniques for the sphenobasilar junction will not be addressed here but will be discussed in a more appropriate future text on cranial meningeal technique.

MORPHOLOGY

Located in the center of the base of the cranial vault between the posterior body of the sphenoid and the anterior basilar surface of the occiput, this articulation is primarily a synchondrosis-based symphysis until the middle of the second decade of life (Figs. 7-102). After the twenty-fifth year, cancellous bone infiltration obliterates the symphysis junction and fuses the occiput with the sphenoid. Consequently, the practitioner is concerned with the articulation's realignment prior to its obliteration. After its ossification, the practitioner's focus shifts toward addressing the release of tension in the trabeculae of the symphysis.

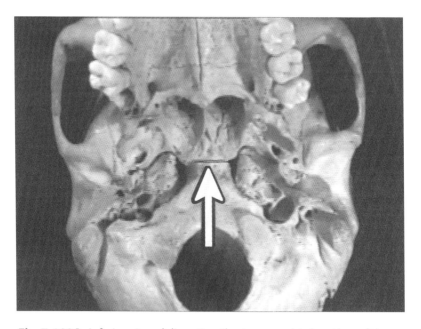

Fig. 7-102A Inferior view delineating the topographic location of the sphenobasilar symphysis

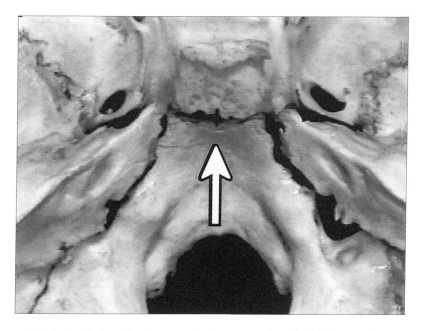

Fig. 7-102B Sphenobasilar symphysis as seen from inside the vault

During its cartilaginous phase, the occiput's basilar articular surface is bisected by a central vertical groove that appears to divide the basilar surface into two distinct condylar formations. Measuring approximately 1.2cm along its vertical convex axis and approximately 2.1cm across its concave horizontal axis, the basilar's bicondylar articular configuration is generally smooth and appears to support multidirectional gliding (Fig. 7-103A). Similar to the occiput's basilar surface, the sphenoid's adjacent articular surface is also bisected by a thin shallow vertical groove. Although the majority of the sphenoid's surface is flatter than its basilar counterpart, the vertical axis takes on a concave configuration by projecting a ledge from its rostral and caudal margins (Fig. 7-103B).

Fig. 7-103A Right anterior-oblique exposure of the occiput's basilar surface

a. Superior intercranial border
b. Inferior external articular border
c. Bisecting central vertical groove

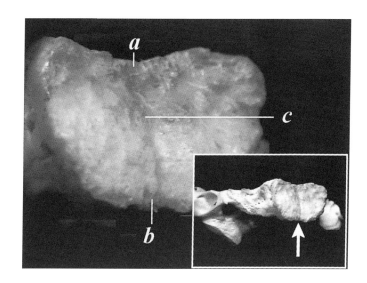

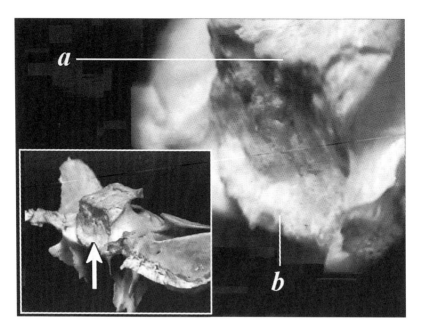

Fig. 7-103B Superior-posterolateral-oblique exposure of the sphenoid's basilar articular surface

a. Superior articular ledge
b. Inferior projecting articular ledge

MOTION

In its earlier stages the symphysis is truly the pivotal articulation of the skull. Its architectural configurations of convexities, concavities, condylar formations, and marginal ledges appear to support a multidirectional movement, including cephalad flexion, caudal extension, lateral flexion, vertical torsion, and anteroposterior expansion (Figs. 7-104 through 7-107).

Note: To address each of these distortions the practitioner must keep in mind that this structure is not a suture, and that it becomes ossified after the twentyfifth year of life. However, the anterior two-thirds of the sphenoid's body is a sinus cavity while the posterior third as well as the occiput's basilar portion is composed of spongy bone. This means that the junction has a certain degree of pliability and is capable of reacting to outside forces through its sinustrabecular association.

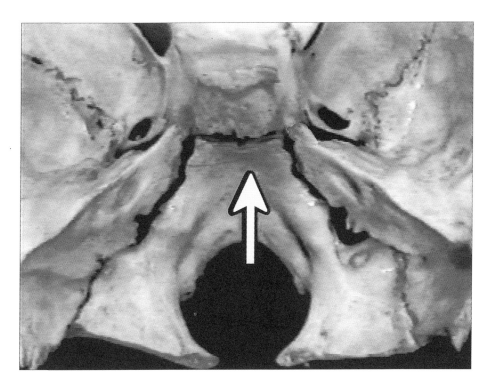

Fig. 7-104A Sphenobasilar motion: flexion

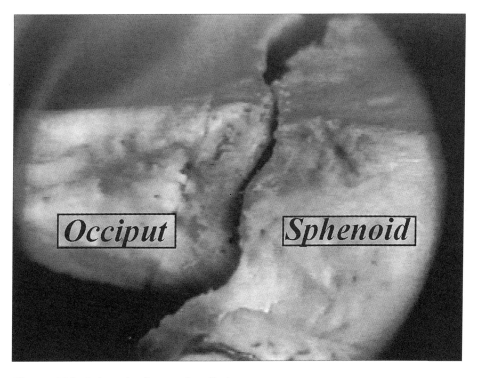

Fig. 7-105A Sphenobasilar motion: flexion

Compare with next photos →

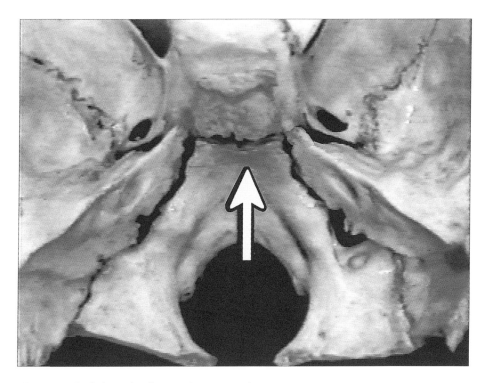

Fig. 7-104B Sphenobasilar motion: extension

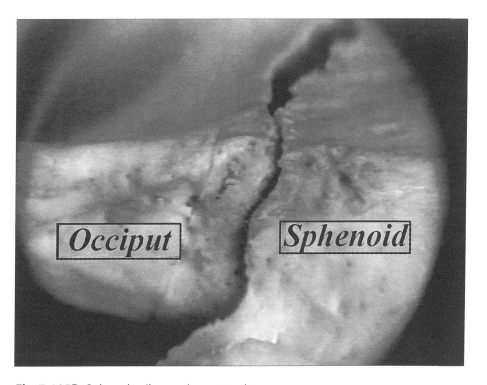

Fig. 7-105B Sphenobasilar motion: extension

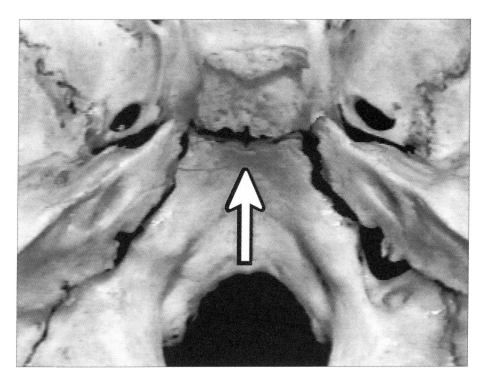

Fig. 7-106A Sphenobasilar motion: lateral flexion

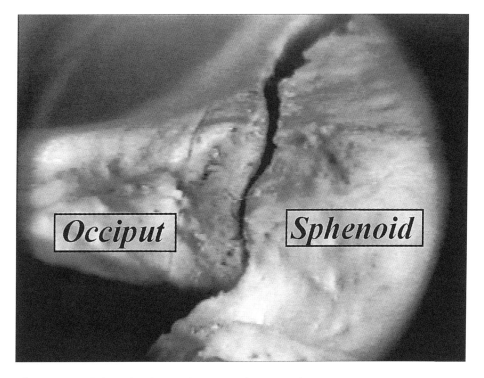

Fig. 7-107A Sphenobasilar motion: posterior expansion

Compare with next photos ➡

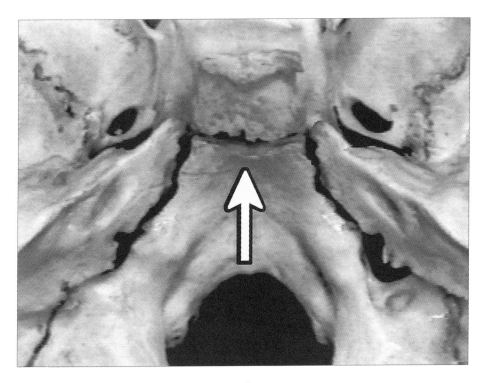

Fig. 7-106B Sphenobasilar motion: neutral

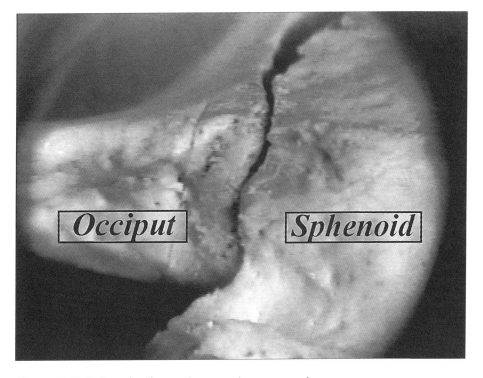

Fig. 7-107B Sphenobasilar motion: anterior compression

PART THREE

Manipulative Strategies For Tissue Aberrations

Aberrations are frequently found in distorted or displaced sutures. As a rule, these abnormalities usually evolve to compensate or support the articular surface, but they may also be the result of pathology. Etiologically, they may be generated by trauma, stress, infection, or chemical toxicity, or may be programmed by the individual's genes.

When addressing the sutural system, the presence of aberrations often obstruct the practitioner's attempts to reestablish sutural articular harmony. This can best be seen in a case where a fibrous adhesive bridge crosses a suture which is jammed along its articular junction. In this example, the practitioner may wish to disengage the suture's articular seam, but is prevented by the constant tension of the fibrous bridge. To address this condition, the fibrous bridge must first be "dissolved" or broken. Once this has been accomplished, the practitioner will find the jammed condition more amenable to attempts at sutural disengagement. Another example can be found in sutures that are constantly separated; in such distortions, edematous build-up may serve to discourage all attempts at sutural reengagement.

The following chapter outlines a series of manipulative strategies developed and refined by the Chinese over more than a thousand years.* The strategies are collectively called *tuina,* literally "push-pinch," or hand techniques, and are to be used by the practitioner when addressing the various pathological abnormalities often found within the suture's articular structures. The manipulative techniques are presented individually, and each maneuver is accompanied by its functional action. Using these additional alternative techniques, the practitioner is no longer restricted to selecting a singular articular approach. Rather, the practitioner can orchestrate a variety of alternative techniques to use before and after manipulation to best serve the patient's needs.

Although this text is primarily based in Western therapy, traditional Chinese therapeutic terms are periodically used for their elaborate depictions of aberrant conditions. Terms such as *stagnation, dampness, heat, cold, excess,* and *deficiency* are often used singularly or in combination to delineate a

---

* This information is based on the course in Traditional Chinese Medicine Orthopedics given by Dr. Hua Gu through the American Acupuncture Academy in 1993.

region's aberration while terms such as *tonify,* *drain,* or *disperse* are frequently used to describe therapeutic objectives. The following table contains a definition of these terms to help the reader's comprehension (Table 8-1).

Table 8-1 Descriptive Oriental medical terms used

Aberrant Qualities

Stagnation	Refers to fluid or respiratory rhythmic congestion.
Dampness	Refers to an accumulation or increase in regional fluid volume often related to blood, lymph, or cerebrospinal fluid.
Heat or cold	Signifies temperature variances that are often associated with increased or decreased metabolic activities.
Excess or deficient	Describes an increase or decrease in action or status.
Damp-heat	Describes areas of increased fluid accumulation and metabolic activity as found in the presence of infectious or traumatic conditions.
Deficiency heat	Describes conditions of dryness that may be associated with dehydration.
Excessive cold	Depicts areas that feel very cold due to diminished blood access.

Treatment Goals

Tonify	Procedures that result in strengthening qualities. They frequently involve enhancement of fuel delivery or increased metabolic activity.
Drain	Procedures designed to diminish vascular pressure or metabolic activity as in cases of sympathetic hypertonia or muscle spasticity.
Disperse	Procedures aimed at dissolving and diffusing areas of congestion as in cases of an edema or lactic acid accumulation.

CHAPTER EIGHT

Hand Techniques *(Tuina)*

Tui (Pushing)

TECHNIQUE

Applying pressure in one direction, usually with the palm, thumb, or thenar pad. W-level pressure is usually applied. The contact is slid along the surface of the involved structure.

ACTION

Pushing from distal to proximal is considered tonifying. Pushing from proximal to distal is considered draining.

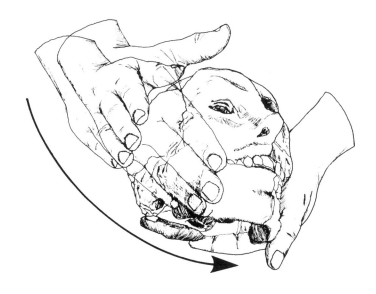

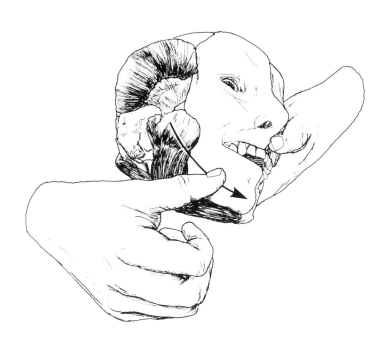

Na (Pinching)

TECHNIQUE

Repetitive lifting of muscles using the fingers and thumb.

ACTION

The purpose is to relax the muscles.

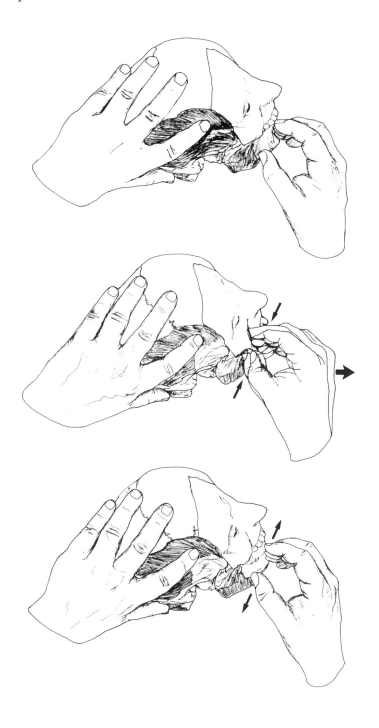

An (Pressing)

TECHNIQUE

Applying continuous pressure into an area using the thumb, finger, or palm. W- to R-level pressure is customarily used.

ACTION

The purpose is to drain and disperse stagnant cranial rhythmic impulses and blood.

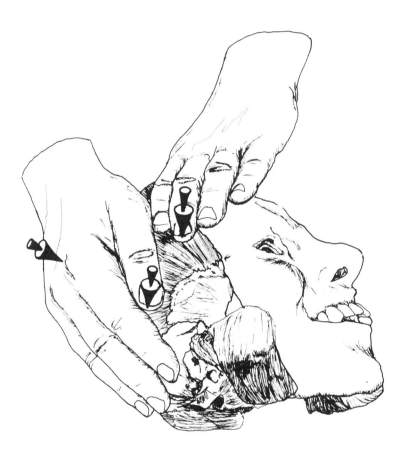

Mo (Circular Kneading)

TECHNIQUE

Gentle circular kneading of the skin using the palm or fingers. S- to W-level pressure is frequently used.

ACTION

The purpose is to increase blood circulation and draw the blood from inside the cranial musculature to the outer dermal layer.

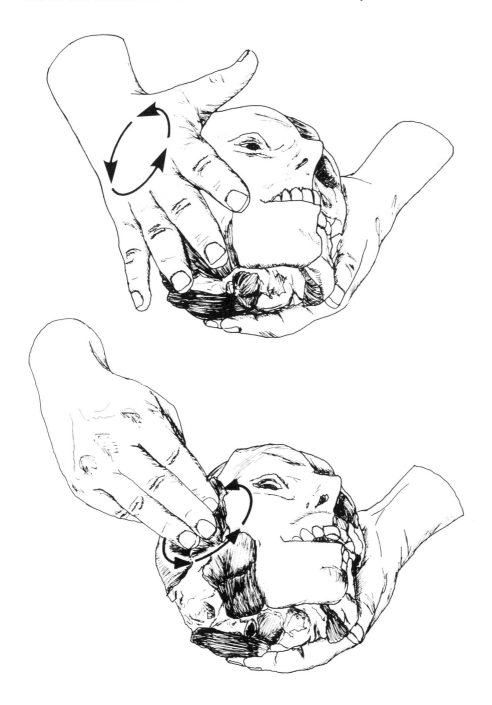

Yi Zhi Chan (Thumb Waving Pressing)

TECHNIQUE

Stabilizing the thumb on its tip and flipping back and forth.

ACTION

The purpose is to break through tissue fixations and improve blood flow.

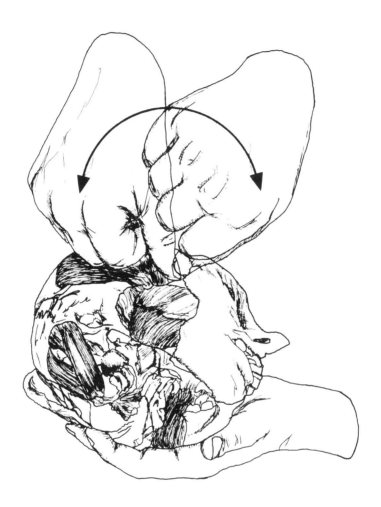

Gun (Rolling)

TECHNIQUE

Rolling pressure over a large area using the back of the hand. Start at the hypothenar surface.

ACTION

The purpose is to smooth out muscle spasms, drain pain, and disperse blood.

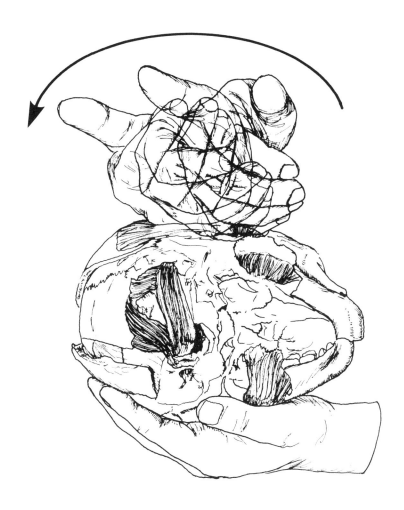

Rou (Stationary Circular Pressing)

TECHNIQUE

Rotating at 120 to 160 times per minute. This technique may be used anywhere on the body. Among the techniques that can be done separately or together are the following:

A. Rolling motion over the hypothenar of the hand
B. Circular motion with the tip of the thumb
C. Three-finger circular motion. Usually the index, middle, and ring fingers are used.
D. Palm circulation

ACTION

The purpose is to reduce or disperse muscle spasms, activate the blood, regulate the primary respiratory impulses (i.e., Qi), stop pain, reduce swelling, and remove fixations within tissues.

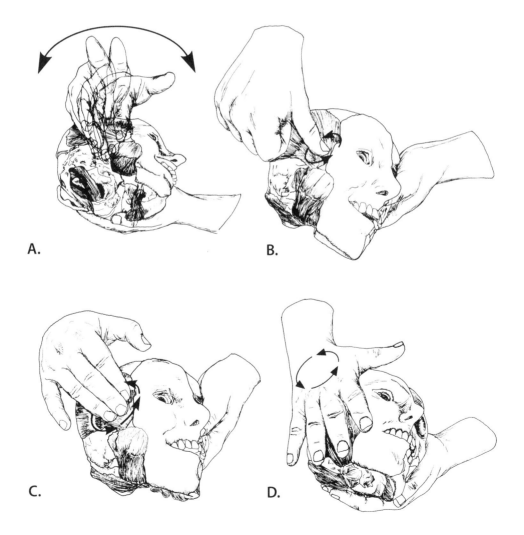

A.   B.

C.   D.

Ca (Rubbing)

TECHNIQUE

Back-and-forth rubbing over long distances in close contact with the skin surface. The technique is applied by a full hand contact or rubbing with the radial side of the index finger. W-level pressure is generally used.

ACTION

The purpose is to relieve pain, increase blood flow, and increase and regulate body temperature.

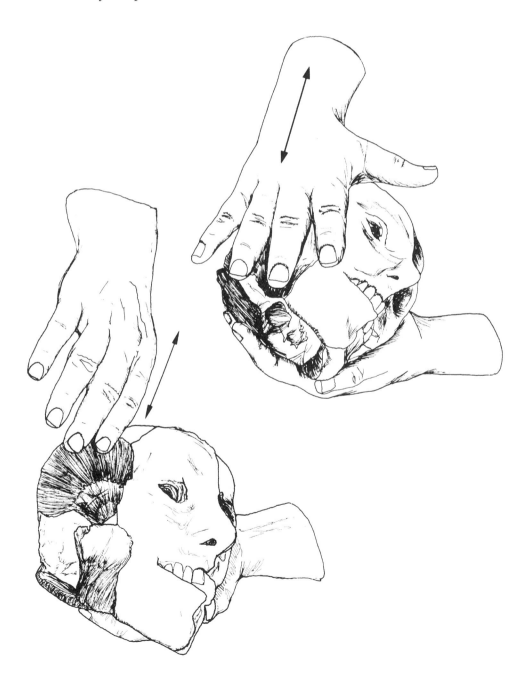

Ma (Wiping)

TECHNIQUE

Thumbs spreading away from each other, wiping along the skin. S½W-level pressure is usually used.

ACTION

The purpose is to dilate the blood vessels.

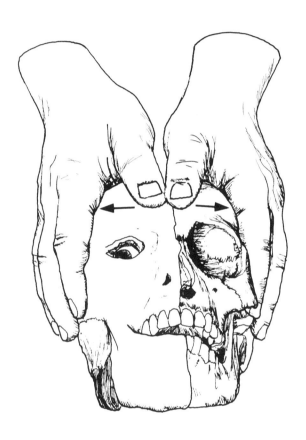

Cuo (Palm Twisting)

TECHNIQUE

An alternating rubbing of the scalp between the practitioner's palms. The technique is most often applied to the upper extremities but may be used on the cranial vault.

ACTION

The purpose is to relax the tissue and increase blood circulation.

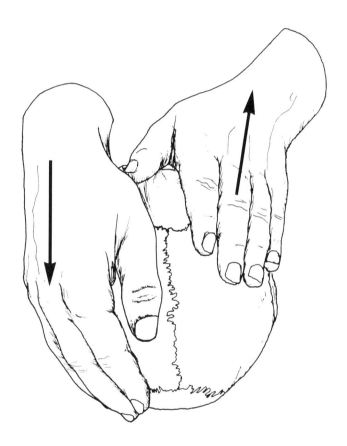

Tan Jin (Plucking)

TECHNIQUE

Grabbing the musculature between the fingers and thumb; pulling and holding the tissue for three or four seconds before releasing it quickly.

ACTION

The purpose is to smooth the muscle, separate adhesions, stimulate blood flow, and disperse primary respiratory energy.

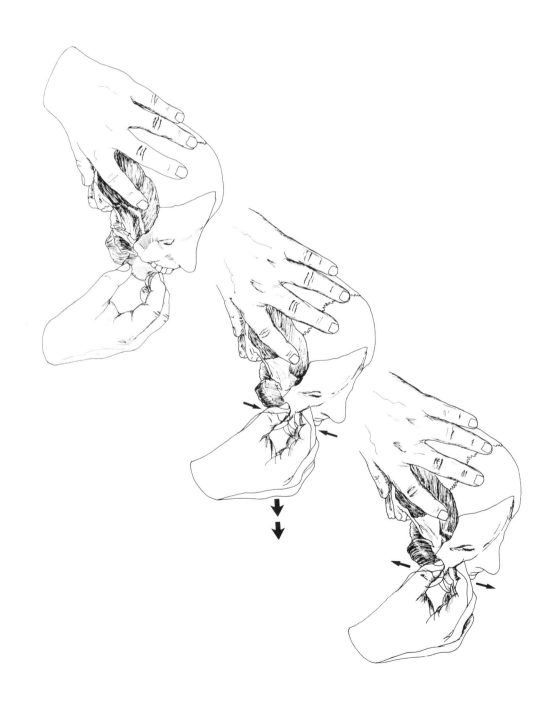

Fen Jin (Snapping)

TECHNIQUE

Stretching the tissue and snapping in opposing directions. Both thumbs are used.

ACTION

The purpose is to soften and break down adhesions and stimulate proper function within the articulation.

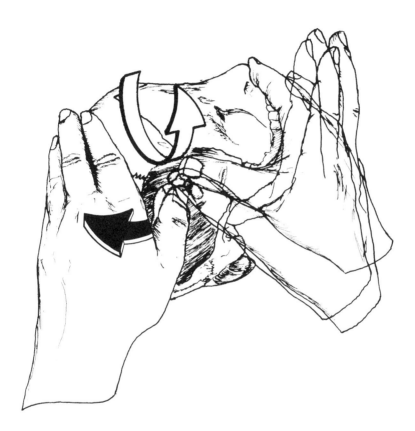

Pai (Patting)

TECHNIQUE

Cupped hand beating.

ACTION

The purpose is to smooth out muscles and stimulate blood flow.

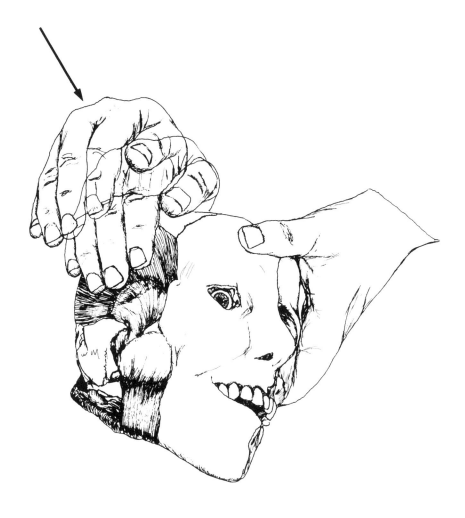

Ji (Beating)

TECHNIQUE

Continuous beating with the hypothenar aspect of the hand. The fingers are relaxed and separated.

ACTION

The purpose is to break up lymphatic congestion, activate blood flow, and relax muscle tissue.

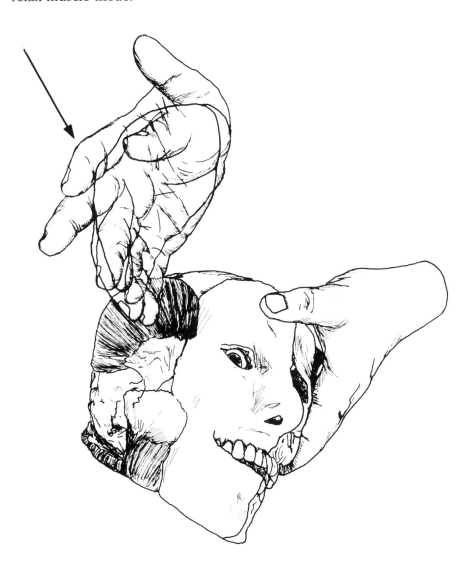

Zhen (Vibrating)

TECHNIQUE

Vibrating method. *Note:* This procedure is contraindicated in patient's with hypotension.

One of the following techniques is used:

A. A flat hand performs quick, short back-and-forth rubbing.
B. One hand encircles the index finger of the other. The encircling hand is placed on the vault so that contact is made by the hypothenar surface. The encircled index finger quickly wiggles back and forth, creating a vibratory motion into the patient's skull.
C. A hand vibrator may be worn over the dorsal surface of the applicator's hand while contact is made with the hand's finger tips or palmer surface.

ACTION

The purpose is to relieve pain, stimulate blood flow, and increase nerve transmission.

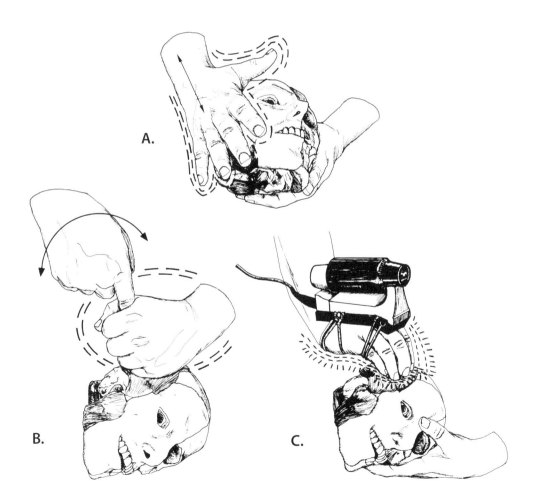

Ba (Traction)

TECHNIQUE

Pulling on various aspects of the skull from a proximal point to a more distal one.

ACTION

The idea is to open articular surfaces, decompress joints, or reverse osmotic pressure within the suture for the purpose of articular rehydration.

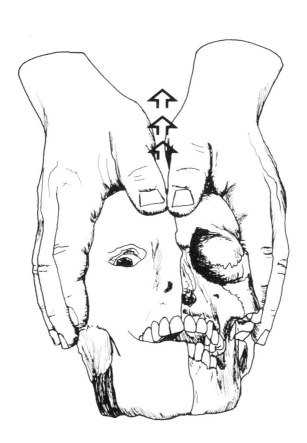

Yao (Rotating)

TECHNIQUE

Taking a joint through rotational movement.

ACTION

The purpose is to break and dissolve adhesions such as those often found in the temporal mandibular joint.

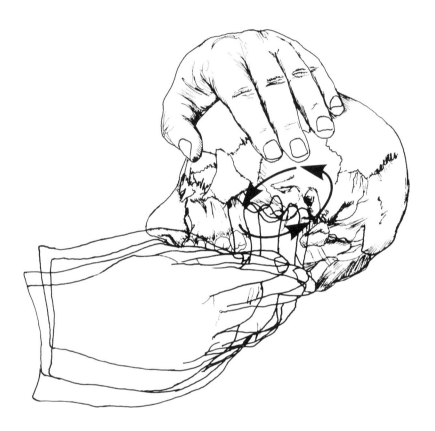

Ji (Squeezing)

TECHNIQUE

Compressing with the hands cupped together and fingers interlocked.

ACTION

The purpose is to compress sutures, disperse excess edema, or work injured suture tissue back into the articulation.

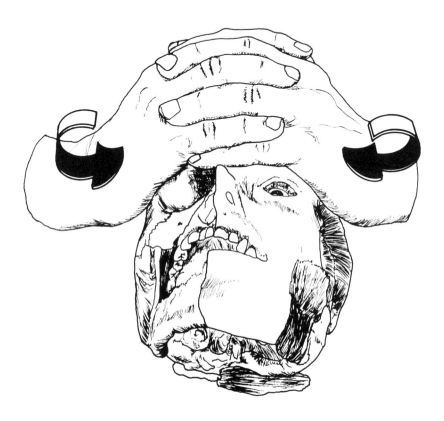

INDEX

A

J

L

T